SAMUEL READ

S0-BEP-111

Biologic Effects of Atmospheric Pollutants

LEAD

AIRBORNE LEAD IN PERSPECTIVE

*Committee on
Biologic Effects of
Atmospheric Pollutants*

DIVISION OF MEDICAL SCIENCES
NATIONAL RESEARCH COUNCIL

NATIONAL ACADEMY
OF SCIENCES

WASHINGTON, D.C.   1972

614.71
N213ℓ

NOTICE: The study reported herein was undertaken under the aegis of the National Research Council with the express approval of the Governing Board of the NRC. Such approval indicated that the Board considered that the problem is of national significance, that elucidation of the problem required scientific or technical competence, and that the resources of NRC were particularly suitable to the conduct of the project. The institutional responsibilities of NRC were then discharged in the following manner:

The members of the study committee were selected for their individual scholarly competence and judgment with due consideration for the balance and breadth of disciplines. Responsibility for all aspects of this report rests with the study committee, to whom sincere appreciation is expressed.

Although the reports of our study committees are not submitted for approval to the Academy membership nor to the Council, each report is reviewed by a second group of scientists according to procedures established and monitored by the Academy's Report Review Committee. Such reviews are intended to determine, inter alia, whether the major questions and relevant points of view have been addressed and whether the reported findings, conclusions, and recommendations arose from the available data and information. Distribution of the report is permitted only after satisfactory completion of this review process.

The work on which this publication is based was performed pursuant to Contract No. CPA 70–42 with the Environmental Protection Agency.

ISBN 0–309–01941–9

Library of Congress Catalog Card Number 71-186214

Available from
Printing and Publishing Office
National Academy of Sciences
2101 Constitution Avenue, N.W.
Washington, D.C. 20418

Printed in the United States of America

PANEL ON LEAD

PAUL B. HAMMOND, University of Minnesota College of Veterinary Medicine, St. Paul, *Chairman*

ARTHUR L. ARONSON, New York State Veterinary College, Cornell University, Ithaca

J. JULIAN CHISOLM, Jr., Baltimore City Hospitals and Johns Hopkins University Medical School, Baltimore, Maryland

JOHN L. FALK, Rutgers—The State University, New Brunswick, New Jersey

ROBERT G. KEENAN, George D. Clayton & Associates, Inc., Southfield, Michigan

HAROLD H. SANDSTEAD, Vanderbilt University School of Medicine, Nashville, Tennessee

BERTRAM D. DINMAN, School of Public Health, University of Michigan, Ann Arbor, *Associate Editor*

LOUISE H. MARSHALL, Division of Medical Sciences, National Research Council, Washington, D.C., *Staff Officer*

CONSULTANTS AND CONTRIBUTORS

ROY E. ALBERT, Institute of Environmental Medicine, New York University Medical Center, New York

FREDERICK M. BLODGETT, Marquette School of Medicine, Milwaukee, Wisconsin

THOMAS BROWN, Food and Drug Administration, Washington, D.C.

REID A. BRYSON, University of Wisconsin, Madison

T. J. CHOW, Scripps Institution of Oceanography, University of California, La Jolla

NORMAN COHEN, Institute of Environmental Medicine, New York University Medical Center, New York

ROBERT H. DAINES, College of Agriculture and Environmental Science, Rutgers—The State University, New Brunswick, New Jersey

PETER B. DEWS, Harvard Medical School, Boston, Massachusetts

BRUCE R. DOE, U.S. Department of the Interior, Branch of Isotope Geology, Geological Survey, Denver, Colorado

MERRIL EISENBUD, Institute of Environmental Medicine, New York University Medical Center, New York

ROBERT A. GOYER, University of North Carolina School of Medicine, Chapel Hill

KAMRAN HABIBI, Petroleum Laboratory, E. I. du Pont de Nemours and Company, Wilmington, Delaware

HARRIET L. HARDY, Occupational Medical Clinic, Massachusetts General Hospital, Boston

ROBERT A. KEHOE, Kettering Laboratory, University of Cincinnati College of Medicine, Cincinnati, Ohio

CHESTER C. LANGWAY, Jr., U.S. Army Cold Regions Research and Engineering Laboratory, Hanover, New Hampshire

JANE LIN-FU, Maternal and Child Health Services, Health Services and Mental Health Administration, Rockville, Maryland

L. N. LOCKE, Fish and Wildlife Service, Patuxent Wildlife Research Center, Laurel, Maryland

JAMES P. LODGE, Laboratory of Atmospheric Sciences, National Center for Atmospheric Research, Boulder, Colorado

LESTER MACHTA, Air Resources Laboratory, National Oceanic and Atmospheric Administration, Silver Spring, Maryland

CHARLES R. MALONE, National Research Council, Washington, D.C.

JAMES R. McNESBY, National Bureau of Standards, Washington, D.C.

DONALD F. MILLER, Food and Drug Administration, Washington, D.C.

JOHN M. MONTGOMERY, National Paint, Varnish and Lacquer Association, Inc., Washington, D.C.

JEAN M. MORGAN, Veterans' Administration Hospital, Birmingham, Alabama

BONNIE J. PEACOCK, Children's Hospital of the District of Columbia, Washington, D.C.

JOHN M. PIERRARD, E. I. du Pont de Nemours and Company, Newark, Delaware

FRANK J. RIZZO, Textile Research and Engineering Division, U.S. Army Natick Laboratories, Natick, Massachusetts

VINCENT J. SCHAEFER, Atmospheric Sciences Research Center, State University of New York, Albany

DAVID SHEMIN, Northwestern University, Evanston, Illinois

KATHRYN M. SIX, University of North Carolina School of Medicine, Chapel Hill

RALPH STREBEL, New York Medical College, New York

LLOYD B. TEPPER, Kettering Laboratory, University of Cincinnati College of Medicine, Cincinnati, Ohio

GARY L. TER HAAR, Ethyl Corporation Research Laboratories, Ferndale, Michigan

DONALD P. TSCHUDY, National Cancer Institute, Bethesda, Maryland

GERMUND TYLER, Department of Plant Ecology, University of Lund, Sweden

DAVID D. ULMER, Biophysics Research Laboratory, Peter Bent Brigham Hospital, Boston, Massachusetts

DENNIS J. VIECHNICKI, Ceramics Division, Army Materials and Mechanics Research Center, Watertown, Massachusetts

JOHN M. WOOD, School of Chemical Sciences, University of Illinois, Urbana

BERNARD C. ZOOK, George Washington University School of Medicine and Smithsonian Institution, Washington, D.C.

COMMITTEE ON BIOLOGIC EFFECTS OF ATMOSPHERIC POLLUTANTS

ARTHUR B. DuBOIS, School of Medicine, University of Pennsylvania, Philadelphia, *Chairman*

VINTON W. BACON, College of Applied Science and Engineering, University of Wisconsin, Milwaukee

ANNA M. BAETJER, School of Hygiene and Public Health, Johns Hopkins University, Baltimore, Maryland

W. CLARK COOPER, School of Public Health, University of California, Berkeley

MORTON CORN, Graduate School of Public Health, University of Pittsburgh, Pittsburgh, Pennsylvania

BERTRAM D. DINMAN, School of Public Health, University of Michigan, Ann Arbor

LEON GOLBERG, Institute of Experimental Pathology and Toxicology, Albany Medical College, Albany, New York

PAUL B. HAMMOND, Department of Physiology and Pharmacology, College of Veterinary Medicine, University of Minnesota, St. Paul

SAMUEL P. HICKS, University of Michigan Medical Center, Ann Arbor

VICTOR G. LATIES, University of Rochester Medical Center, Rochester, New York

ABRAHAM M. LILIENFELD, School of Hygiene and Public Health, Johns Hopkins University, Baltimore, Maryland

PAUL MEIER, Biomedical Computation Facilities, University of Chicago, Chicago, Illinois

JAMES N. PITTS, Jr., Statewide Air Pollution Control Center, University of California, Riverside

GORDON J. STOPPS, Haskell Laboratory, E. I. du Pont de Nemours and Company, Newark, Delaware

O. CLIFTON TAYLOR, Statewide Air Pollution Control Center, University of California, Riverside

JAROSLAV J. VOSTAL, University of Rochester Medical Center, Rochester, New York

T. D. BOAZ, Jr., Division of Medical Sciences, National Research Council, Washington, D.C., *Executive Director*

Preface

The United States Congress passed the Clean Air Act in 1963 and has since strengthened it through amendments. Responsibility for issuing air quality criteria guidelines to assist the states and cities in developing standards for air quality was assigned to the Environmental Protection Agency (EPA). The scope of the guidelines, as stated in the Clean Air Amendments of 1970, includes "effects on soils, water, crops, vegetation, man-made materials, animals, wildlife, weather, visibility, and climate, damage to and deterioration of property, and hazards to transportation, as well as effects on economic values and on personal comfort and well-being."

The National Academy of Sciences (NAS) was asked to prepare evaluative reports of current knowledge of selected atmospheric pollutants to serve as background for preparation of criteria documents and EPA decisions and to make recommendations for research where sound information is lacking. In the Division of Medical Sciences of the National Research Council (NRC), the Committee on Biologic Effects of Atmospheric Pollutants was formed to coordinate and supervise the activities of *ad hoc* panels of experts brought together to pool their knowledge of specific pollutants. Because most of the members of both the Committee and the Panel on Lead were biologists, this report treats the strictly biologic aspects thoroughly, whereas the material on nonbiologic effects of lead, which came from consultants, is brief.

The report reviews the scientific knowledge of the effects of lead on human health and welfare, enumerates the factors that alter these effects, and points out areas where data are lacking; it is an attempt to place in perspective the role of airborne lead in the biosphere. In its early planning, the Panel decided to consider biologic effects of lead not necessarily attributable directly to atmospheric sources and not necessarily at levels of exposure as low or as prolonged as those related to general ambient air. Such consideration was necessary because lead attributable to emission and dispersion into general ambient air has no known harmful effects. It was only by considering the circumstances in which lead is manifestly harmful that some perspective could be gained as to the significance of contributions from general atmospheric sources. The Panel was not asked to comment on air pollution standards and has not done so.

At the Panel's first meeting, in July 1970, a tentative timetable and outline were developed that seemed reasonable within the constraints of EPA's needs. Sections were then assigned to panelists and consultants, who prepared drafts that were revised by the full Panel and circulated to reviewers from the Committee, to outside specialists, to appropriate NRC divisions, and to the NAS Report Review Committee.

The bibliography is not intended to be exhaustive, but it contains the most important references to the primary literature sources on lead up to early 1971. Translations of most of the foreign-language reports are available from the National Translation Center.

Throughout the report, the units of measurement are consistent with common usage of workers in the area of the discussion. The term "lead particles" will be recognized as meaning "lead-containing particles."

Only by the cooperation of many persons was writing of the report within 9 months made possible. They responded generously, enthusiastically, and competently. Persons who prepared significant amounts of material for the Panel's review are A. L. Aronson (domestic animals, wildlife), J. J. Chisolm, Jr. (lead poisoning in man, disturbances of heme synthesis), T. J. Chow (geochemistry), R. H. Daines (plants), B. D. Dinman (occupational exposure), J. L. Falk (behavioral effects), K. Habibi (particle size determination), P. B. Hammond (input and disposition in man), R. A. Goyer and K. M. Six (cytoplasmic effects), R. G. Keenan (sources and uses, physical and chemical characteristics, analysis), H. H. Sandstead (metabolic effects, illicitly distilled whiskey), G. J. Stopps (epidemiology, organic forms), and G. L. Ter Haar (biosphere). The roster lists the names of contributors and consultants, to all of whom the Panel expresses great appreciation. In addition to the generous involvement of panelists, the response of EPA staff to requests for help was indispensable. The Panel's needs for information services were met in part by the NRC Advisory Center on Toxicology, the NAS Library, the National Library of Medicine, the Environmental Mutagen Information Center, and the Air Pollution Technical Information Center. Members of the Committee who had specific responsibilities to the Panel were Paul B. Hammond (Chairman, Panel on Lead), Bertram D. Dinman, Victor G. Laties, and Gordon J. Stopps.

The manuscript was edited by Norman Grossblatt, Editor of the Division of Medical Sciences. Much credit is due the staff officer for the Panel, Louise H. Marshall, for the successful completion of the document.

CHARLES L. DUNHAM
Chairman, Division of Medical Sciences

Contents

APPENDIXES

xi

Introduction

In the midst of currently intensified concern over the quality of the environment, it is both logical and proper to select lead for in-depth scrutiny, particularly from the standpoint of the consequences of atmospheric emissions. The amount of lead vented into the atmosphere over the United States as a result of combustion of lead-containing automobile fuel additives and from miscellaneous other sources is measured in hundreds of tons per day and is increasing in proportion to the ever-expanding use of the automobile. Because the uses of lead for purposes other than as a fuel additive are many and varied, it is important to develop a sense of perspective wherein the consequences of lead input into the environment from all major sources are evaluated.

Although this document is concerned with the hazards associated with the dispersion of lead into the environment, the consequences of dispersion should also be viewed from the standpoint of depletion of a natural resource. The earth's lead resources are being mined at the rate of 2.2×10^9 kg/year to meet worldwide needs.[59] The net loss relative to the earth's total lead resources, as with other minerals consumed by man, should be a factor in any decisions that will increase the rate of consumption of lead. "Only by supplementing our

1

fairly definite knowledge of measured and indicated reserves—or working inventory—with crude guesses and analogies tending toward the optimistic, can we at this time see sufficient reserves to equal lead demand during the balance of this century."[326]

The extensive mining and processing of lead dates back to pre-Christian times. Its low melting point (327 C), malleability, and ductility favored its early use for the manufacture of metal products. It also tarnishes in air and forms a film of oxide, which accounts for its not being readily corroded. This property also made it highly desirable for many applications.

In addition to numerous uses by civilized man, lead has contributed greatly to knowledge of geologic time. "Studies of lead isotopes in meteorites have been very fundamental to all of earth science,"[156] and have led to determination of the accepted age of the earth.[438] Lead has four radioactive isotopes (lead-210, -211, -212, and -214); lead-210, a natural β- and γ-emitter with a half-life of about 22 years, has been useful as an atmospheric tracer and in precipitation dating.[20,73]

Most of the salts of lead are highly insoluble, and, in nature, lead exists mainly as the least soluble of the common salts, lead sulfide (galena). Lead carbonate (cerussite), lead sulfate (anglesite), and lead chlorophosphate (pyromorphite) also are common naturally occurring forms. The interaction of lead with organic matter also results in the formation of stable complexes. Sulfhydryl, carboxyl, and amine coordination sites are all involved in the complexing of lead with organic matter. The low solubility of lead in the aqueous phase of natural systems is manifested in many ways directly relevant to the understanding of the behavior of lead in the environment. Some consequences of this fundamental characteristic are that lead is poorly transferred from soil to plants and that the concentration of lead in natural bodies of water is extremely low in proportion to the concentration in the beds of lakes and streams. In animal systems, the consequences are poor uptake and slow excretion. The net effect of these sluggish dynamics, however, is a high degree of accumulation with prolonged exposure. Animal tissues have excellent lead-binding characteristics. The persistence of lead added to segments of the environment to which man is exposed thus results in legitimate concerns over adverse cumulative effects.

The concern today is mainly over the possible hazards to living organisms that might result from the widespread dissemination of lead by man into the general environment, and particularly over the insidious effects of long-term exposure.

Because the mining, smelting, and commercial uses of lead have been so extensive for such a long time, a considerable body of knowledge already exists regarding the harmful effects of excessive exposure in man, animals, and plants. These effects generally have been observed only at levels of exposure higher than apply to the general populations of people, animals, and plants not near primary sources of man-made lead products. The primary goal of this report was to assess the likelihood that man, animals, and plants would be brought into the range of harmful levels of exposure now or in the near future and the circumstances that might make that possible. This goal required that the Panel address itself to questions pertaining to the magnitude and distribution of lead in the environment, both in the context of present conditions and in the context of likely future conditions, assuming the continuation of current technologic trends. It was also necessary to attempt to estimate minimal toxic exposure levels, drawing from the vast literature pertaining to the toxic effects of lead. The frustrations engendered by the attempt to do that found expression in the form of recommendations for future research.

1

Lead in the Ecosystem

NATURAL OCCURRENCE OF LEAD

"Pollution" implies the introduction of an undesirable substance. Any amount of a purely man-made substance in the environment is present obviously because man put it there. Other substances considered to be pollutants may occur naturally as well; that is the case with lead. Description of the source, magnitude, and distribution of man-generated lead pollution can hardly be undertaken without some knowledge of the natural background levels. Considering that man has mined and used lead for many centuries, accurate estimation of contemporary natural background of lead is difficult. Calculations of natural contributions have been made on the basis of geochemical information.

Natural sources apparently contribute only insignificantly to present-day concentrations of lead in the atmosphere. Natural concentrations have been estimated to be about 0.0005 $\mu g/m^3$ of air,[437] and result from airborne dust containing on the average 10–15 ppm of lead[121] and from gases diffusing from the earth's crust.[47] The latter source results in the presence of lead-210 in the atmosphere ranging from 7.1 $\times 10^{-3}$ dpm/kg of air at ground level to about 70 $\times 10^{-3}$ dpm/kg of air in the lower stratosphere.[73] Detectable quantities of lead-210 reach the earth's surface in precipitation and on dust particles.[186,254,322]

Perhaps the most useful records on natural concentrations of lead are to be found in chronologic layers of snow strata, available in quiescent ice sheets in perpetually frozen polar regions.* Annual layers of snow from Greenland and the Antarctic have been analyzed.[411] Annual ice layers from the interior of northern Greenland show that lead concentrations increase from less than 0.0005 μg/kg of ice at 800 BC to more than 0.2 μg/kg in AD 1965 (Figure 1–1). The ice layer corresponding to 1750 represents the beginning of the Industrial Revolution, and the lead concentration at that date is 25 times greater than natural levels. During the second half of the eighteenth century, lead concentrations tripled, and from 1935 to 1965, they abruptly tripled again. The sharpest rise occurred after 1940. Today, lead concentrations in Greenland snows are about 400 times the natural levels.

These data dramatically document the rise of lead in some components of the environment, but they must not be taken as representative of worldwide circumstances. For example, levels of lead in Antarctic continental ice sheets fail to show similar rises. Concentrations of lead in ice before 1940 were below 0.001 μg/kg and rose to only 0.02 μg/kg after 1940. The difference between lead concentrations in northern and southern polar snows is ascribed to barriers to north–south tropospheric mixing, which hinder the migration of aerosol pollutants from the northern hemisphere, where most industrial emissions occur, to the Antarctic.

Few chronologic records of lead concentrations are as complete as that described for polar regions, but there are data that reflect increasing lead concentrations in some other ecosystems. For example, it is estimated that the preindustrial lead content in marine water was about 0.02–0.04 μg/kg.[117] Today, surface waters in some areas of the Mediterranean and Pacific contain as much as 0.20 and 0.35 μg/kg, respectively, and only deep waters, below 1,000 m, appear uncontaminated (Figure 1–2). The lead content of fresh waters also has

---

*Reliable age data of annual layers have been obtained from radioactive (natural and artificial) and stable isotopic investigations of deep ice core samples—namely, total beta activity (primarily strontium-90 and potassium-40, useful for the last 10–20 years), lead-210 (for the last 100–150 years), silicon-32 (for the last 1,000 years), and oxygen-18 (combined with physical models, for the last 150,000 years).

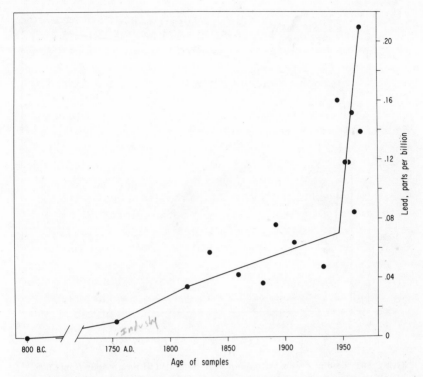

FIGURE 1-1 Increase of lead in snow at Camp Century, Greenland, since 800 BC. Reprinted with permission from Murozumi *et al.*[411]

increased in recent times. The available data suggest that the mean global natural lead content of lakes and rivers is 1–10 μg/liter.[359] The soil in rural areas of the United States has lead concentrations usually similar to the average content in the earth's crust, 10–15 μg/g.[121] But in many cities, the concentration of lead in soil is much higher, suggesting substantial but relatively localized pollution.

There are few examples of long-term trends in lead concentrations of biologic materials. Ruhling and Tyler[464] demonstrated chronologic increases in lead concentrations in Swedish mosses from 1860 to 1968 (Figure 1-3). The principal increases were believed to correspond to increased combustion of coal in 1875–1900 and of leaded gasoline in 1950–1968.

Other evidence of man's large contribution to total environmental lead is found in the geographic pattern of atmospheric lead concen-

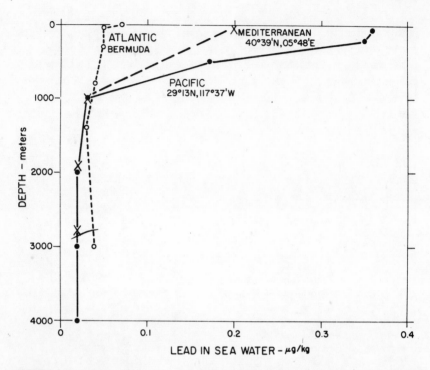

FIGURE 1-2   Lead profiles in the major oceans. Reprinted with permission from Chow.[117] (Atlantic waters were sampled at sites relatively free of continental influence.)

trations: high over major urban centers, lower by a factor of 10 or more over rural areas remote from human habitation, and lower than that by a factor of 100 over the mid-Pacific.[116,120]

A useful tool for distinguishing between industrially produced lead and lead that occurs naturally in contemporary soils and water has been analysis of its isotopic composition.[20,121] Many lead ores have a characteristic composition fixed during mineral genesis, and the isotopic composition of commercially important ores has been surveyed.[67] In addition, Chow and Earl[119] have determined the isotopic composition of several lead ores, gasolines, aerosols, waters, and marine sediments. The average isotopic composition of lead in sediments from the Pacific and Atlantic oceans is characteristic of lead from the Quaternary Period, deposited thousands of years ago. But lead in coastal surface seawater is characteristically from the Tertiary Period and is probably not the product solely of natural weathering. The isotopic compositions of lead in gasoline additives and in atmospheric aerosols from cities where the fuel was purchased are similar to each other and represent isotopically distinct lead ores of the Tertiary Period or earlier. Chow and Earl[119] infer that the aerosols could not be derived from weathering of natural surface material and that instead they come primarily from automotive exhausts. However, to ascribe this lead specifically to manufactured tetraethyl lead, one would have to know whether the isotopic composition of tetraethyl lead differs from that in all the other products of industry that contain lead and also enter the ecosystem by weathering, burning, and other routes.

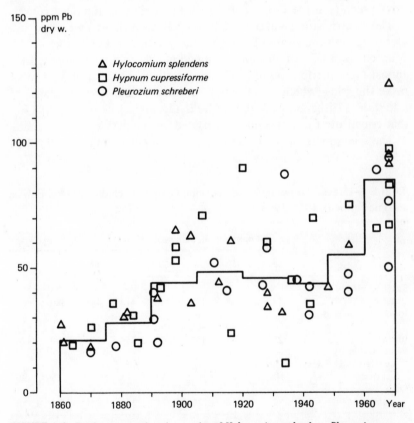

FIGURE 1-3 Lead concentrations in samples of *Hylocomium splendens*, *Pleurozium schreberi*, and *Hypnum cupressiforme* collected in Skane, Sweden, from 1860 to 1968. The line indicates 15-year averages. Reprinted with permission from Ruhling and Tyler.[464]

MAN-MADE SOURCES OF LEAD

Patterns of Lead Consumption

The consumption of lead in the United States has not increased substantially in the last 20 years (Table 1-1). More than one third of the lead consumed is recycled from previous consumption. This recycled fraction also has been fairly stable in recent years. There has been, however, a considerable shift in the pattern of lead consumption. Thus, while the use of lead for the manufacture of paint pigments has been decreasing, the use for manufacture of storage batteries and antiknock gasoline additives has risen dramatically (Table 1-2). As can be seen in Table 1-3, the uses of lead are diverse and numerous.

The electric-storage-battery industry has been the largest single user of lead in the United States for many years. In 1968, it accounted for 38.7% of all lead consumed in this country. There is an almost even distribution of lead between the metallic form used to make the grids (which contain 4-8% antimony) and lugs and the lead oxides (litharge, PbO; red lead, Pb_3O_4; and black oxide, Pb_2O) that constitute the active material pasted on the plates.

The second largest consumer of lead is the petroleum industry. In

TABLE 1-1   Lead Consumption in the United States (Excluding Alaska, Hawaii, and Puerto Rico), 1940-1968[a]

	Lead Consumption, Thousands of Tons							
	1940	1950	1955	1960	1965	1966	1967	1968[b]
Smelter, primary lead[c]	533	508	479	382	418	441	380	467
Recovery of secondary lead	260	482	502	470	576	573	574	551
Imports[d]	282	542	462	360	350	435	499	426
Stocks at primary smelters and refineries on Dec. 31	NA	NA	NA	250	83	NA	125	90
Consumption of metal, primary and secondary	782	1,238	1,213	1,021	1,241	1,324	1,261	1,318

[a]Adapted from U.S. Bureau of the Census.[549]
[b]Preliminary.
[c]From domestic and foreign ores and bullion.
[d]Includes lead imported for immediate consumption plus material entering country under bond; includes lead in pigs, bars, bullion, ores, and matte.

TABLE 1-2 Lead Consumption for Selected Uses in the United States[a]

	Lead Consumption, Thousands of Tons		
Year	As White Lead	In Gasoline Additives	In Storage Batteries
1935	80	37[b]	175
1940	66	50[b]	220
1945	36	76	60
1950	36	114	398
1955	18	165	380
1960	8	164	353
1965	8	225	555
1968	6	262	513

[a]Adapted from *Minerals Yearbooks*,[547] 1936–1968.
[b]Calculated from gasoline consumption × 2.04 g/gal.

TABLE 1-3 Lead Consumption in the United States, 1968, by Products[a]

Product	Lead Consumption, Tons	Product	Lead Consumption, Tons
Metal products	Subtotal 915,500	Chemicals	Subtotal 262,526
Ammunition	82,193	Gasoline antiknock	
Bearing metals	18,441	additives	261,897
Brass and bronze	21,021	Miscellaneous chemicals	629
Cable covering	53,456	Miscellaneous uses	Subtotal 23,106
Caulking lead	49,718	Annealing	4,194
Casting metals	8,693	Galvanizing	1,755
Collapsible tubes	9,310	Lead plating	389
Foil	6,114	Weights and ballast	16,768
Pipes, traps, and bends	21,098	Other, unclassified uses	17,924
Sheet lead	28,271		
Solder	74,074	Total[c]	1,328,790
Storage batteries:			
Battery grids, posts, etc.	250,129		
Battery oxides	263,574		
Terne metal	1,427		
Type metal	27,981		
Pigments	Subtotal 109,734		
White lead	5,857		
Red lead and litharge	86,480		
Pigment colors	14,163		
Other[b]	3,234		

[a]Adapted from *Minerals Yearbook*,[547] p. 647.
[b]Includes lead content of leaded zinc oxide and other pigments.
[c]Includes lead that went directly from scrap to fabricated products.

1968, this industry used almost 262,000 tons of primary forms of lead for gasoline additives (lead alkyls), or 19.7% of the total lead consumption. In addition, this industry uses lead in the form of pipe and sheets for the fabrication of corrosion-resistant equipment. Lead is used in heavy-duty greases—for example, in gear compounds for drilling machinery, and for use under water, where its lubricating properties are effective after exhaustion of the grease. About 1,000–2,000 tons/year are consumed in this use, which does not apply to automotive greases.

The paint industry uses white lead [basic lead carbonate, $2PbCO_3 \cdot Pb(OH)_2$] and red lead in paints intended only for outdoor use, for which their weathering characteristics make them valuable. About 50% of the white exterior house paints on today's market are oil-based and contain amounts of white lead that vary with the manufacturers' formulas. Lead chromates provided some 14,000 tons (as Pb) of yellow, green, and red pigment colors in 1968. These find many uses, for example, in traffic marking paints and printing inks.[596] The paint industry uses several other lead compounds, including white basic lead sulfate and blue basic lead sulfate. The lead associated with "lead pencils" is lead chromate in the yellow paint pigment.

Lead has found numerous applications in the ceramics industry. Glazes for china and structural clay products may contain lead oxides or lead silicates. Examples of the latter include glazed brick, lightweight aggregate, and porcelain enamels for aluminum and steel. During firing at high temperature, the interaction between lead and silica forms inert substances.

Miscellaneous uses of lead, on a tonnage basis, include the use of lead arsenate as an insecticide (decreasing since 1946) and the use of lead in electric cable insulation, hose, pipe, sheet, and floor coverings and as a stabilizer in vinyl plastics.

Emission of Lead to the Atmosphere

AMOUNTS

A national inventory of the sources of lead emission in the United States for 1968 by the Air Pollution Control Office has provided a data bank (summarized in Table 1–4) that shows that the inorganic emission from the combustion of leaded gasoline constitutes approximately 98% of the total emission of lead from the listed sources. It should be pointed out that this inventory does not include attrition

TABLE 1-4 Lead Emission in the United States, 1968[a]

Emission Source	Lead Emitted, Tons/Year
Gasoline combustion	181,000
Coal combustion	920
Fuel oil combustion	24
Lead alkyl manufacturing	810
Primary lead smelting	174
Secondary lead smelting	811
Brass manufacturing	521
Lead oxide manufacturing	20
Gasoline transfer	36
Total	184,316

[a]Data from National Inventory of Air Pollutant Emissions and Controls, a loose-leaf data bank on file at the Bureau of Air Pollution Sciences, Environmental Protection Agency, Research Triangle Park, North Carolina 27709.

of the innumerable lead-containing items that are subject to weathering and often are burned or otherwise disposed of after they have outlived their usefulness. The dispersion of lead compounds has many other sources: exhausting of workroom atmospheres; the abrasive action of automotive traffic on lead-painted lane dividers on streets and highways; resuspension of lead by high-speed cars; burning of lead-painted surfaces of houses, bridges, and other structures before repainting; welding of lead-painted structural or other steels; weathering of painted surfaces, with the resulting flaking and distribution into the atmosphere of a portion of the lead-bearing dust; incineration of leaded plastics and other materials whose usefulness has ended; recovery of lead from old battery cases, lead pipe, lead-sheathed cable, and sheet lead in secondary smelters; and, on a small scale, the welding and soldering operations conducted in plumbing and electrical repair shops. The magnitude of these additional sources of emission could be considerable and is unknown.*

In comparison with the burning of gasoline, the burning of coal has not been a serious source of atmospheric lead. In 1968, the production of coal in the United States amounted to 504 million tons. Analysis of 827 samples of domestic coal provided a weighted average of 7 parts of lead per million of coal.[1] This concentration would produce 3,528 tons of lead, of which 74% either remained in the

*Unpublished data (J. Wagman, personal communication) indicate that about 10% of the total particulate matter in municipal incinerator effluent may be lead.

clinker or was collected with the fly ash. (In modern furnaces burning pulverized coal, about 95–99% of the fly ash is removed by electrostatic precipitators, and only a small portion of the lead is emitted as aerosols.[180]) Probably no more than 920 tons escape to the atmosphere each year.

Significant amounts of lead used to be introduced into the atmosphere by smelting lead ores.[411] At the beginning of the Industrial Revolution, in 1750, smelting technology resulted in the loss of much lead fume. During the nineteenth century, smelting procedures were improved; and by the early twentieth century, it became economically feasible to recover lead smelter fume, which resulted in reducing the fraction of fume loss by a factor of 4. During the last four decades, the loss fraction has been further reduced by a factor of 8 (Table 1–5). Thus, the emission of lead into the atmosphere in the Northern Hemisphere from smelting currently is small, in comparison with the emission from burning gasoline. In 1968, for example (Table 1–4), the comparative values were 985 tons of lead emitted from smelting and 181,000 tons from burning leaded fuels.

PHYSICAL CHARACTERISTICS

Probably equal in importance to the absolute amounts of lead emitted to the atmosphere are its physical characteristics, in that they determine in large part its subsequent disposition. For example, the largest lead-bearing or pure lead particles will fall to the earth near the emission source and enter the ecosystem there, whereas the smallest particles will remain airborne and enter the ecologic cycle far from the emission source. The small particles

TABLE 1–5   Lead Aerosol Production in the Northern Hemisphere[a]

Year	Lead Smelted, Thousands of Tons	Lead Converted to Aerosols, %	Lead Aerosols from Smelters, Thousands of Tons	Lead Burned as Alkyl, Thousands of Tons	Lead Converted to Aerosols, %	Lead Aerosols from Alkyls, Thousands of Tons
1753	100	2	2	–	–	–
1815	200	2	4	–	–	–
1933	1,600	0.5	8	10	40	4
1966	3,100	0.06	<2	300	40	120

[a]Adapted from Murozumi et al.[411]

(less than 2 μm in mean equivalent diameter) become especially important when it is considered that they tend to be retained by the lungs and accessory airways when inhaled, to be absorbed or coughed up and swallowed later.

Aerosol lead may be emitted to the atmosphere in the form of dust, fume, mist, or vapor, depending on the source material and the method of generation.

Dusts are disperse systems of particles or aggregates of particles 1–150 μm in diameter that are thrown into the air by mechanical activities during blasting, crushing, drilling, grinding, and other industrial, constructional, or agricultural processes. Smaller particles tend to remain airborne longer, and particles less than about 10 μm in diameter can be inhaled into the respiratory tract.[83] Examples include the oxides and salts of lead that become airborne during handling or packaging.

Fumes are formed in chemical reactions, including combustion, and in such physical processes as distillation, sublimation, calcination, and condensation. Particle size is 0.2–1 μm. Examples are the fumes of metallic lead and lead oxide generated as vapors in smelters or foundries during melting operations and then condensed from the vapor state.

Mists are formed by the condensation of water vapor on submicroscopic particles of dust or gaseous ions or by the atomization of liquids.[272] Sprayed lead arsenate insecticide is probably the only example of a mist of a lead compound that is important in air pollution studies.

Vapors are formed from liquids by an increase in temperature. Like gases, they produce true solutions with the atmosphere. However, as soon as they regain their liquid state, from a decrease in temperature, they form mists and fumes. Evaporated lead alkyls are the best examples of vaporous forms of lead.

Particle size is the major determinant of the residence time of lead emitted into the atmosphere and of the degree of dispersion from the point of emission. Particle size also determines the degree to which lead is deposited and retained in the airways in man. Consideration of particle size distribution in ambient air therefore is of major importance. (A discussion of the measurement of particles appears in Appendix A.)

The particle size distribution of urban lead aerosols has been determined by a number of investigators. Robinson and Ludwig[454] report a mass median equivalent diameter (MMED) of 0.25 μm, with 25% of the particles smaller than 0.16 μm and 25% larger than 0.43 μm. Their data are from size-distribution analyses of samples collected from 59 urban sites with a modified Goetz Aerosol spectrometer in Los Angeles, San Francisco Bay area, Cincinnati, Chicago, and Philadelphia. There was little variation among these widely scattered places in MMED of the particles, and the results are representative of lead aerosols from a variety of urban sources, inasmuch as there was a fairly uniform division of samples between residential, commercial, and industrial areas in each of the five cities. In another study, the average MMED was 0.18 μm in Cincinnati and 0.42 μm in a nearby suburb.[340] In Cincinnati, 75% of the aerosol mass consisted of particles less than 1 μm in MMED, and in the suburb, 65% were smaller than 1 μm. Other studies, conducted in California,[407, 456] indicate that 50–90% of the lead particles in urban air are smaller than 1 μm.

A comparison of estimated emissions of lead from several sources in the Cincinnati area indicates that the principal contributor is the combustion of leaded gasoline,[380] each gallon of which contains about 2.4 g of lead as antiknock additive.

In 1962, Mueller and his associates at the California Department of Public Health determined the size of particles in the exhaust emissions of three popular makes of automobiles operated in cruise conditions.[80] They reported that 62–80% by weight of the particles were smaller than 2 μm in MMED, and of these, more than 68% were smaller than 0.3 μm. These results for cruising automobiles are in substantial agreement with those reported by Robinson and Ludwig[454] for general ambient air without specification as to source of lead.

In 1970, Habibi[223] used a new experimental system designed to study the wide range of particle sizes emitted in automobile exhaust in cyclic driving conditions.* He reported data obtained with an Andersen and a Monsanto impactor showing an MMED of 0.6 μm for lead particles during steady-state operation at 45 mph. This is in reasonably good agreement with the results of Mueller *et al.*[80] in cruise conditions with automobiles manufactured and tested in 1962.

---

*This consists of a programmed chassis dynamometer and a 40-ft tunnel in which the exhaust gases are diluted with filtered air in a known ratio, and proportional sampling is conducted under isokinetic conditions. In addition, a total exhaust filter was prepared by packing an 18-in.-diameter, 24-in.-long drum, with a high-efficiency fiber-glass medium. The filter was claimed to be capable of direct mounting on the tailpipe and could be used in direct road operation to determine exhaust emission rates as affected by road vibrations and thermal fluctuations associated with normal (start–stop) driving patterns.

However, of greater interest to researchers in the field of air pollution is Habibi's finding of heavy deposits of large "gritty" particles ranging from 300 to 3,000 μm in diameter. These deposits began to form along a 16- to 20-ft section on the floor of the dilution and sampling tunnel at the point where the exhaust gases expanded to the wall of the tunnel; the deposits appeared to be due to gravitational settling. More than 95% by weight of the lead so deposited was present as coarse particles, and the total quantity of this deposit amounted to 10% of the lead originally contained in the fuel consumed by the automobile.

CHEMICAL FORMS

Definitive data on the inorganic forms of lead in the atmosphere are lacking, except for the identification of several lead compounds emitted in the exhausts of automobiles using leaded gasoline as fuel. The chief lead emission products are (in particles of equivalent diameter between 2 and 10 μm) lead bromochloride ($PbCl \cdot Br$) and (in particles smaller than 1 μm) the alpha and beta forms of ammonium chloride and lead bromochloride ($NH_4Cl \cdot 2PbCl \cdot Br, 2NH_4Cl \cdot PbCl \cdot Br$), minor quantities of lead sulfate ($PbSO_4$), and the mixed oxide and halide ($PbO \cdot PbCl \cdot Br \cdot H_2O$). The chemical and physical characteristics of these unstable compounds are largely unknown and constitute a very difficult area of investigation that may be more important than is generally appreciated. It has been noted that little $2PbBrCl \cdot NH_4Cl$ was found in hot exhaust gas collected at the tailpipe. It was, however, found after cooling and mixing of the exhaust with the ambient air, and it has been suggested that this compound is less easily photolyzed than $PbCl \cdot Br$.[224] If phosphorus compounds have also been added to the fuel, up to 20% of the exhausted lead may be in the form of a phosphate–halide compound $[3Pb_3(PO_4)_2 \cdot PbCl \cdot Br]$. Data (J. M. Pierrard, personal communication) have been made available on samples collected near heavy traffic (at the Delaware Memorial Bridge tollgate) and in locales where the lead aerosols were assumed to have aged after emission. They apparently showed different surface compositions, which would be consistent with a conversion mechanism expected to release the less reactive hydrogen halide, rather than the more reactive molecular halogen, from the particles. A recent study[532] reported data on the effects of aging on automobile exhaust collected in a black bag. Using an electron probe, 75% of bromide and 30–40% of chloride compounds appear to have been lost 18 hr after the samples were collected, and the proportion of lead carbonates and lead oxides increased.

The literature contains only meager characterization of the inorganic forms of lead from other emission sources. Many of the oxides and salts of lead probably are dispersed into the atmosphere during their chemical preparation, use, and disposal and during the burning of lead-containing fuels, such as coal.

Very small amounts of tetraethyl lead (TEL) and tetramethyl lead (TML) in gasoline blends may escape to the atmosphere through vents on the carburetor and fuel system during evaporation of the fuel, as found in the three-city study,[554] described below. It was pointed out in that report, however, that, because these organic lead compounds are less volatile than gasoline, they tend to remain behind in the unevaporated portion. Furthermore, TEL and TML are light-sensitive and undergo photochemical decomposition when they reach the atmosphere.[554] The presence of TEL and TML in ambient air is discussed in greater detail in Chapter 6.

Nothing is known about the existence of organic forms of lead in the environment from biotransformation. The methylation of lead by bacteria has been studied in the laboratory using lead acetate (Pb^{2+}, the principal valence form of lead in exhaust emissions) as a substrate. No evidence was found of [^{14}C] tetramethyl lead formation from [^{14}C] methylcobalamin (J. M. Wood, personal communication).

The quantitative methods for determination of lead are discussed in Appendix B.

Lead in the Atmosphere

CONCENTRATION GRADIENTS

The concentration of lead in ambient air is closely correlated with the density of vehicular traffic, at least in the United States. It is highest in what might be termed "vehicular microclimates" in large cities, decreases with averaging of place-to-place variation within total city climates, then tapers off as one progresses into the suburbs or smaller towns and finally into rural areas. These gradients with reference to locale are also subjected to diurnal and seasonal cycles. The character of these patterns has been sampled only here and there, and the overall picture is still incomplete. Also, it is difficult to make reliable comparisons, because methods of sampling and techniques of analysis have not been standardized. Thus, it is impossible to compare lead concentrations of air taken close to traffic with that of air sampled from the roof of a tall building.

In the areas of highest concentration, the concentrations are considerably higher than would be encountered if values from various points in city air were averaged. Atkins, reporting the distribution of lead in the Palo Alto, California, environment[18] for very short sampling times (5 min), found up to 19 $\mu g/m^3$ a few feet from moving traffic. He also found close correlation between time of day and atmospheric lead concentrations; the concentrations were highest in the heavy-traffic hours around 8:00 a.m. and 4:00 to 5:00 p.m. In Los Angeles (Table 1-6), concentrations were highest in the morning

TABLE 1-6 Atmospheric Concentrations of Lead in Traffic—Los Angeles Area[a]

Route	Sampling Time	Days	Description	No. Samples	Lead Concentration, $\mu g/m^3$ Mean	Range
Parked along freeway[b]	0600–0900	Weekdays	Morning rush	7	38.0	26.9–54.3
Parked along freeway	0900–1600	Weekdays	Midday	7	24.1	16.6–31.1
Parked along freeway	1600–1800	Weekdays	Afternoon rush	7	18.4	8.7–25.4
Parked along freeway	–	Saturday	–	4	19.9	17.7–22.2
Freeway traffic	0600–0900	Weekdays	Morning rush	35	29.3	10.9–41.3
Freeway traffic	0900–1600	Weekdays	Midday	39	21.5	4.5–39.2
Freeway traffic	1600–1800	Weekdays	Afternoon rush	34	22.2	10.5–43.1
Freeway traffic	–	Saturday	–	32	25.3	10.0–71.3
Los Angeles downtown traffic	0600–0900	Weekdays	Morning rush	6	23.6	19.1–29.9
Los Angeles downtown traffic	0900–1600	Weekdays	Midday	4	10.5	8.4–12.2
Los Angeles downtown traffic	1600–1800	Weekdays	Afternoon rush	4	15.3	12.4–18.6
Los Angeles downtown traffic	–	Saturday	–	4	9.4	8.6–10.3
Pasadena downtown traffic	0600–0900	Weekdays	Morning rush	–	–	–
Pasadena downtown traffic	0900–1600	Weekdays	Midday	6	11.9	8.6–14.6
Pasadena downtown traffic	1600–1800	Weekdays	Afternoon rush	–	–	–
Pasadena downtown traffic	–	Saturday	–	2	12.4	12.3–12.4
Total				191		

[a]Adapted from Public Health Service Publication 999–AP-12.[554]
[b]Parked on shoulders of major freeway in downtown Los Angeles.

rush hour and for some reason never returned to the morning level during the afternoon rush hour. Regardless of the reasons, these microclimate concentrations in the vicinity of heavy traffic are of potential significance to the health of people who spend the working day in them. It should be noted that the mean concentrations of atmospheric lead did not fluctuate much during the day; at least this would appear to be the case in the Los Angeles samples cited.

The dilution of atmospheric lead from these points of high concentration is considerable. Even in Los Angeles, where vehicular traffic is unusually heavy, overall concentrations of lead are considerably lower in the ambient air than in the microclimates near vehicular traffic.

An extensive study to determine the variation in the annual, seasonal, monthly, and diurnal average distributions of lead and total particulate matter in the atmosphere of three U.S. cities was conducted by the Public Health Service in collaboration with the American Petroleum Institute, the Automobile Manufacturers Association, the California State Department of Public Health, E. I. du Pont de Nemours and Company, Ethyl Corporation, and the Kettering Laboratory, University of Cincinnati. Sampling sites were selected to represent four geographic and land-use classifications: rural, residential, commercial, and industrial. However, the samples were taken at various aboveground levels and therefore should not be compared. Atmospheric sampling was performed continuously from June 1961 through May 1962.[554] A summary of the results of the lead found during this period for Cincinnati, Los Angeles, and Philadelphia is presented in Table 1–7, which shows that the general urban concentrations ranged from about 1 to 3 $\mu g/m^3$, depending on the area sampled. The average concentration of lead for all samples collected during the year was 1.4 $\mu g/m^3$ in Cincinnati, 2.5 in Los Angeles, and 1.6 in Philadelphia. The highest average concentration for all samples collected during a single month at any single sampling site was 3.1 $\mu g/m^3$ in Cincinnati, 6.4 in Los Angeles, and 4.4 in Philadelphia. The highest individual concentrations were 6.4 $\mu g/m^3$ in Cincinnati, 11.4 in Los Angeles, and 7.6 in Philadelphia. A uniform sampling procedure was used in each of the cities, and the samples were analyzed by the same technique—those from Cincinnati by the Kettering Laboratory, those from Los Angeles by the California Department of Public Health, and those from Philadelphia by the U.S. Public Health Service Laboratory.

When monitored concentrations of airborne lead are averaged, it

TABLE 1-7 Concentration of Lead in Atmosphere[a]

	Atmospheric Lead Concentration, $\mu g/m^3$		
	Cincinnati	Los Angeles	Philadelphia
Annual average values			
Downtown	2	3	3
Outlying area	1	2	1
All stations	1.4	2.5	1.6
Seasonal distributions (all stations):			
Summer	1.3	1.9	1.4
Fall	1.7	2.8	1.9
Winter	1.3	3.1	1.9
Spring	1.3	2.1	1.4
Diurnal distributions (annual—all stations stated as a fraction of annual mean):			
2300–0300	1.3	1.0	0.9
0300–0700	1.1	1.1	0.8
0700–1100	1.4	1.2	1.4
1100–1500	0.8	0.7	0.8
1500–1900	0.9	0.8	1.1
1900–2300	1.0	1.1	1.1

[a]Adapted from Public Health Service Publication 999–AP–12.[554]

appears that higher mean concentrations of lead are correlated positively with size of city. This relation is illustrated in Figure 1–4, showing averages of composite samples collected quarterly and analyzed with a low-temperature ashing procedure and emission spectroscopy.

There is evidence of a decrease in lead concentrations as one moves outward from the core area of the larger cities. The National Air Surveillance Networks (NASN) of the Environmental Protection Agency is continually sampling the atmosphere for lead and other pollutants in many parts of the United States. In most cities, the average concentration of lead in the atmosphere in 1953–1966 ranged from 1 to 3 $\mu g/m^3$, but suburban and nonurban stations averaged 0.1–0.5 $\mu g/m^3$, and many concentrations at some of the very rural stations were less than 0.05 $\mu g/m^3$.[553,555-557,559,560] Data from the NASN for 217 urban stations during 1966 and 1967 showed an annual average lead concentration of 1.1 $\mu g/m^3$. Samples averaged quarterly at individual sites ranged from 0.02 to 19 $\mu g/m^3$. The nonurban stations showed an average of 0.21 $\mu g/m^3$ near the city, 0.096 at an intermediate distance from the city, and 0.022 in remote areas.[386]

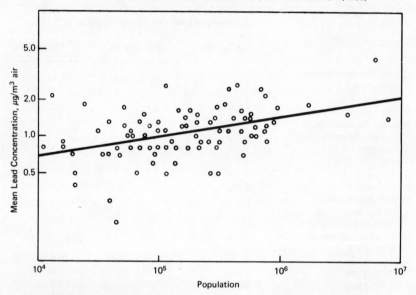

MEAN LEAD CONCENTRATION (1966-1967) VS. POPULATION (1960)

FIGURE 1-4 Mean lead concentration versus population for 87 urban stations having more than 30,000 persons in 1960, National Air Sampling Network, 1966 and 1967. The line is drawn through points determined by grouping the data geometrically by population intervals and finding the median concentration at the median population. (Data from R. I. Larsen, personal communication.)

YEARLY TRENDS

The consumption of lead alkyl fuel additives is increasing substantially every year. It cannot be assumed, however, that the concentration of lead in urban air is increasing in parallel. Indeed, the available data suggest that the concentration of lead in air, even over most of the large cities, is increasing only slowly. The most impressive data on this point come from analysis of the atmosphere in Cincinnati, Ohio, initiated by the Kettering Laboratory in 1938.[112] In 1941, a lead-monitoring program was inaugurated, and sampling was conducted intermittently and randomly at from 1 to 50 stations with electrostatic precipitators. In 1955, continuous sampling was begun at three representative sites with high-volume samplers fitted with tared glass-fiber filters; sampling took place over 24-hr periods, and particulate matter was collected from 2,000-m^3 air samples. During the 1961–1962 period, samplers with 3-μm membrane filters were used to collect samples continuously at four stations representative of industrial, commercial, central residential, and peripheral residential sites. These sampling periods ranged from 2 to 3 days. A mobile station was used intermittently to investigate special conditions. The 1961–1962 samples averaged 325 m³ and 480 m³ of air for the 2- and 3-day sampling periods, respectively.

The results of the study[112] with the same spectrographic and dithizone methods over the 20 years of the study showed a gradual, continual downward trend in the mean and median concentrations of lead in the atmosphere of Cincinnati. The mean and median concentrations were 5.1 and 3.4 μg/m³, respectively, in 1941 and 1.42 and 1.27 μg/m³ in 1962. It is important to mention that there is some bias in the results obtained during the earlier period of this 20-year study: a greater proportion of industrial and other specially selected sites were represented in the samples collected at that time. However, the investigator believed that there was little doubt about the downward trend when results obtained during the different periods and the sampling conditions were examined. Although the volume of traffic and the consumption of leaded gasoline increased greatly during the period of study, there was a simultaneous decrease in the quantity of coal consumed for heating purposes and in the mass of dustfall from all sources, resulting in less lead in the urban Cincinnati atmosphere. Furthermore, an increasingly effective enforcement of the smoke abatement ordinance, improved collection and disposal of particulate matter from industrial operations, and changes in traffic flow and land use in the metropolitan area of Greater Cincinnati each contributed to the decrease in atmospheric lead concentration during the 1946–1962 period.[554]

Landau et al.[325] of the Air Pollution Control Office discussed the average concentration of lead in air in 31 cities of the NASN sampling network for which data had been obtained in at least one year of each of three periods—1957–1961, 1962–1965, and 1966–1967. They reported that the average lead concentration had decreased slightly from the first to the second period. Lead concentrations for the third period were about double those of the second period. However, the data for the third period were obtained by an analytic procedure different from that used during the first two periods, and the authors assume that the increase in lead concentration between the second and third periods is due primarily to the change in analytic method. The NASN data cited earlier for 1953 through 1966 are from samples taken at many different sites, and exact information is not available as to when sites were changed. It is difficult, therefore,

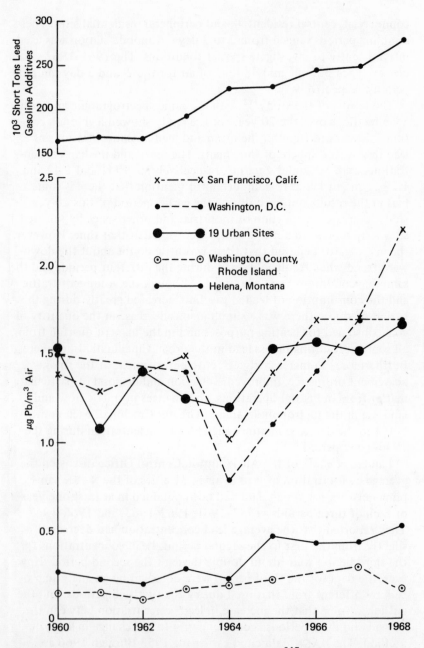

FIGURE 1-5 Amounts of lead consumed as gasoline additives[547] and mean lead concentration in air sampled at selected sites for 1960-1968, from analyses made with the new procedure; 14-18 sites averaged for each point. (Air data from R. I. Larsen, personal communication.)

to tell whether the atmospheric concentration of lead increased or decreased during that period, but the data seem to indicate that the concentrations remained fairly constant.

Nelson[419] reported concentrations of lead in air measured in suburban Salt Lake City during the period 1944–1965. Average lead concentrations for 5-year periods beginning in 1944 were 1.14, 0.75, 0.70, and 0.51 $\mu g/m^3$. For 1964 and 1965, the average was 0.30 $\mu g/m^3$. The reason for the decrease may be improvement in control of particulate matter emitted into the atmosphere from industrial sources.

The relation of some average airborne lead concentrations at selected urban and nonurban stations to lead consumed as gasoline additives is shown in Figure 1–5.

Chow and Earl[119] suggested that the lead concentration in San Diego is increasing at the rate of 5% per year. This estimate is based on weekly sampling at a single site and on yearly averages of NASN for 1959 and 1966 at this site of 1.12 and 1.84 $\mu g/m^3$, respectively. However, it is speculative to interpret citywide trends of lead in air from measurements taken at a single site, in that many investigations have shown that lead concentration decreases logarithmically with increasing distance from the source.

In view of the disparate results from different cities, it is not possible to make any generalization about trends. It should be added that still-unevaluated preliminary* data on samples taken in 1968–1969 for Los Angeles, Philadelphia, and Cincinnati indicate increases in average air lead concentrations of 56%, 19%, and 17%, respectively, since 1961–1962.[529] These studies involved 19 sampling sites; the average lead concentration increased at 17 and decreased at 2.

CYCLING OF LEAD IN THE BIOSPHERE

The fate of lead emitted into the atmosphere is poorly characterized. Figure 1–6 presents an ecologic flow chart that summarizes most of the major compartments and pathways taking part in the cycling of lead in the biosphere, a biogeochemical process. Because of the lack of significance attached to lead in natural systems in past years, there has been no comprehensive treatment of its movements within living

---

*The report from which these data are drawn notes that "all information presented at this time must be regarded as preliminary, since essential laboratory, statistical, and meteorological analyses, which might indicate the need for adjustments, have not been completed."[529]

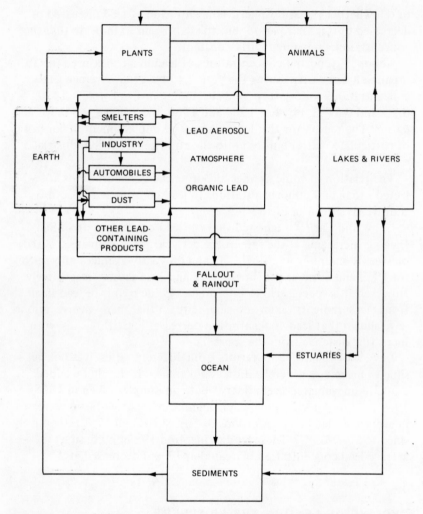

FIGURE 1-6 Ecologic flow chart for lead showing possible cycling pathways and compartments.

systems. There is insufficient information on the chemical forms, amounts, and rates of transfer of lead from one compartment of the environment to another to permit treatment of the subject in terms of systems analysis. However, fragmentary data afford some insight into the movement of lead in the biosphere. These data come primarily from studies of lead-210, a radionuclide important in tracing the pathways and determining flux rates of lead, as stressed by Burton

and Steward.[73] This section documents what is known about the
general movement of lead between compartments of the biosphere,
details of which are treated in subsequent chapters.

Lead in Precipitation

Lead is removed from the air by aggregation and by precipitation.
From analyses of lead-210 in rainwater, its residence time in the
atmosphere was calculated to be 7–30 days, depending on environmental conditions.[73, 186] Whether the residence times are valid for
atmospheric lead aerosols resulting from gasoline combustion is not
known, but Ter Haar et al.[533] found that stable lead and lead-210
were well mixed in air. If the residence time of atmospheric lead aerosols from automotive exhaust is 1–4 weeks, the turnover rate of these
materials may be such that a worldwide steady state of lead already
has been reached in the atmosphere.

Lazrus and co-workers[337] have sampled atmospheric precipitation
of lead at 32 U.S. stations and found a correlation between the number of gallons of gasoline used and the concentration of lead in rainfall in each area. The average lead concentration was 34 μg/liter in
precipitation, with the median somewhat lower, about 10 μg/liter;
the highest concentration found was about 300 μg/liter. The authors
pointed out that, on the average, at least twice as much lead is found
in atmospheric precipitation as in water supplies, from which they
infer the existence of a process by which lead is depleted after precipitation reaches the earth's surface. This conclusion is supported by
recent Russian studies[313] that indicate the tendency of lead to be
present in suspended matter, to be insoluble in surface waters, and to
be removed by natural sedimentation or filtration.

Ter Haar et al.[533] found, in a study carried out in a semirural area,
that an average of 1 μg of lead per square centimeter per year is precipitated out of the atmosphere. Although they had sparse data, there
seemed to be a correlation between the type of rainfall and its lead
concentration: showers had lower concentrations than slow, even
rainfall. Weather preceding the rainfall may affect the lead content,
in view of their finding of high concentrations after thermal inversions.

It seems likely that today the global mean natural lead content of
lakes and rivers lies between 1 and 10 μg/liter.[359] The average lead
content of 33 water samples of major rivers in North America was
6.6 μg/liter; and the average lead content of 440 lake and river water
samples in Maine was 2.3 μg/liter (range, 0.03–115 μg/liter).[310]

Goldberg[199] observed a rapid depletion of lead-210 in unfiltered samples along the paths from origins to outfalls of the Sacramento and Colorado rivers. Assuming that stable lead species and lead-210 have similar chemistry, he concluded that some inorganic or biochemical processes removed lead from solution.

In marine waters, Goldberg also found a rapid turnover and transfer of lead to deeper waters, which he credits to some process of biologic transfer.

Lead in Soils

The natural concentration of lead in soils is primarily a function of the geologic source of the parent material.[229] The usual range is about 2–200 ppm, exclusive of areas near deposits of lead ores.[265,406,590] Specific areas of increased concentration due to man-made sources (e.g., mining and fallout from industrial operations and motor vehicles) have been discussed earlier. In addition to these sources, soils receive on the average 1 $\mu g/cm^2$ per year from precipitation (discussed previously), and 0.2 $\mu g/cm^2$ per year may be deposited in dustfall. Using these averages, Ter Haar et al.[533] estimated the contribution of stable and radioactive atmospheric lead to soil at about 0.2% of the existing natural burdens of soil lead per year. This amounts to about 0.04–4 $\mu g/g$ per year and might explain the failure of most investigators to detect a significant accumulation of lead in soils remote from heavy traffic and industrial areas.

There appears to be a natural mechanism by which lead tends to be moved upward in the earth's crust. Many workers have shown that a sharp lead profile, higher at the surface than at underlying depths, is frequently found. Swaine and Mitchell,[523] in a study of lead profiles of eight soils in Scotland, found that the lead content was approximately halved in going from the surface to a depth of 50 in. Wright et al.[590] reported a similar result for virgin soils of four great soil groups of Canada. Soils in both studies were from uncultivated areas far from industrial contamination. Goldschmidt[200] and Hibbard[251] also reported higher concentrations of lead and other elements in the upper horizon.

Swaine and Mitchell,[523] in their study of Scottish soils, found a thirtyfold decrease in lead with depth in some cases. They stated:

The surface accumulation of Pb is the outstanding effect observed in the total trace-element contents of the profiles examined. . . . Ten-fold increase calculated on the basis of the air-dry material in the surface horizon, is not uncommon. The effect is greatest in organic-rich uncultivated surface horizons, and is even more pronounced when expressed on a mineral matter or ash basis. . . . These soils are generally remote from industrial areas and from high-density motor traffic; being uncultivated, contamination from tractors is excluded. The obvious explanation would appear to be an accumulation of Pb through plants, much more pronounced than for other elements. Presumably an insoluble complex which holds the Pb in the surface horizon—whether organic or inorganic is not yet established—is being formed on the decay of the plant material.

Numerous investigators have studied the concentration of lead in depth profiles of soils along highways. All reported decreasing lead content of these soils with distance from the highway and with depth beneath the surface. The data of Lagerwerff and Specht[323] (Table 1–8) typify these findings. There was a reduction of about 65–75% in the lead content of the top 5 cm of soil as the sampling site was moved from 8 m away to 32 m away from a highway with traffic densities ranging from 7,500 to 48,000 cars per day. Further exami-

TABLE 1-8   Lead Content in Roadside Soil and Grass as a Function of Distance from Traffic and Grass Depth in Profile[a]

		Lead Content, μg/g Dry Weight			
Site	Distance from Road, m	Grass	Soil Profile Layer, 0–5 cm	Soil Profile Layer, 5–10 cm	Soil Profile Layer, 10–15 cm
I	8	68.2	522	460	416
West of U.S. 1, near Plant	16	47.5	378	260	104
Industry Station, Beltsville, Md.	32	26.3	164	108	69
II	8	51.3	540	300	98
West of southbound lanes,	16	30.0	202	105	60
Washington-Baltimore Parkway, Bladensburg, Md.	32	18.5	140	60	38
III	8	21.3	242	112	95
West of Interstate 29,	16	12.5	140	104	66
Platte City, Mo.	32	7.5	61	55	60
IV	8	31.3	150	29	11
North of Seymour Road,	16	26.0	101	14	8.2
Cincinnati, Ohio	32	7.6	55	10	6.1

[a]Adapted from Lagerwerff and Specht.[323]

nation shows that, at a depth greater than 5 cm, four soil samples taken 16–32 m from a highway with a traffic density of 23,000 cars per day provided analytic values of lead that are lower than the frequently cited 16 ppm (16 μg/g of dry soil). Although comparable samplings gave higher values than these, it is apparent that the penetration of lead into the soil drops rather uniformly, as interpreted from the data in Table 1–8.

The concentration of lead in street dust and surface soil of large cities is extremely high. In a study of 77 midwestern cities ranging in population from 100,000 to 1,000,000,[266] the average concentrations of lead in dust collected from residential and commercial sites were 1,636 μg/g and 2,413 μg/g, respectively.[499] The concentration of lead in surface soils in city parks is also very high: Balboa Park, San Diego, 194 μg/g; Golden Gate Park, San Francisco, 560 μg/g; and MacArthur Park, Los Angeles, 3,357 μg/g.[116]

Lead in Biota

Studies of lead-210 also have provided knowledge of the movement of lead into plants. For example, Wilson and Cline[586] concluded that soil lead is largely unavailable for uptake by plants, only 0.003–0.005% of the total amount of lead in soil being available for such uptake. Several investigators have concluded that the primary source of the lead taken up by plants is rainfall, not soil.[185,253,377] However, Tso et al.[545] believe that a significant amount of soil lead is available to plants. In any event, soil lead is not absorbed by most plants.[389]

An interesting situation exists with regard to the concentrations of lead-210 in animals of the Arctic, where relatively high concentrations have been found in the biota. This occurs because the lead nuclei tend to accumulate on the sedges and lichen, which attain high concentrations because of their slow growth. This vegetation forms a large part of the diet of the caribou and reindeer, which in turn constitute a substantial fraction of the diet of predators in these regions. The concentrations of lead-210 found by Holtzman[258] in the reindeer and the caribou were 7 and 11 picocuries/g of bone ash, respectively. The flesh of the reindeer contained 0.05 picocurie/g wet, and that of the caribou, 0.08 picocurie/g. However, the wolf, which preys on these animals, was found to have only 1 picocurie/g of bone ash and 0.02 picocurie/g of flesh. The reason for the lower concentrations of lead-210 in the wolf than in the animals it eats is that lead-210 is a bone-seeker; thus, the concentrations tend to be higher in bone than in flesh. Because the predators are flesh-eaters, the lead concentration in the predator tends to decrease as one follows the food chain. Accumulation of lead in bones of vertebrates may be a general rule, inasmuch as this also was observed in fish, with lead-210 in bone exceeding that in muscle by a factor of over 50.

SUMMARY

The relative inertness and malleability of lead enhance its usefulness to man; it occurs in nature chiefly as a sulfide. Lead radionuclides are useful in geologic dating and in documenting the cycling of the metal in ecosystems. Current world production is about 2.5 million tons per year, about 40% in the United States. Yearly U.S. consumption of primary and secondary (recycled) lead is about 1.3 million tons and has almost doubled in the last 30 years. The largest consumer is the electric-storage-battery industry (39%), followed by the petroleum industry, which uses 20% of the total for gasoline additives. Lead consumption for these two uses has increased with the production of antiknock gasoline and batteries at the same time that the manufacture of lead-containing paints and insecticides has decreased, but the magnitudes of the absolute amounts differ widely.

Patterns of lead emission to the atmosphere have changed in modern times. The initial increase due to smelting and coal-burning that started with the Industrial Revolution has been checked by improved industrial controls, but the decrease in those emissions has been more than offset by emissions from automotive exhaust fumes. Today, about 98% of the airborne lead that can be traced to its source comes from combustion of gasoline. Geographically, there is a logarithmic increase in atmospheric lead concentration from mid-ocean, to remote high mountains, to seashore, to suburban and urban environments. In spite of the rapid increase in the consumption of lead alkyls used in automotive fuels, however, the concentration of lead in urban air is, in general, rising only slowly, presumably because of dispersion.

The disposition of lead emitted to the atmosphere (and indirectly to other ecologic compartments) depends on its physicochemical form and on meteorologic factors that help to dissipate it. About half the lead-containing particulate matter from automotive exhausts is removed from the air by gravity within a few hundred feet of roadways. The remaining lead consists of aerosols that are largely airborne until removed by precipitation. The mean residence time of lead in the atmosphere, calculated at 7–30 days, reflects the efficiency with which the aerosols are removed by precipitation. Much of the lead entering aquatic systems via precipitation and runoff is not water-soluble and apparently is removed from water by sedimentation. The low solubility of lead in water also is an important factor in terrestrial systems, because it affects the ability of plants to assimilate lead. Precipitation tends to increase the lead content of soils gradually, but little of this lead enters food chains because of its limited availability to primary producers. The role of microorganisms in the biotransfer of lead and almost all aspects of transfer rates between compartments of the ecosystem are two areas in which there is little or no information.

2

Lead and Plants

Lead in plants could arise from several sources, including (a) lead present in the soil, either naturally or added artificially (e.g., by spraying or as a result of industrial activity); (b) lead present in rain-water and groundwater; and (c) lead present in the air. Each of these sources may in turn affect the roots, stems, and leaves of plants in a different manner.

EFFECT OF LEAD IN SOIL

Lead is a natural, but minor, constituent of agricultural soils and plants. Swaine[522] gave a range of lead in agricultural soils of 2–200 μg/g. Most investigators report soil lead concentrations within these limits; however, a few have found a higher lead content in some soils. The average concentration of lead in soil is thought to be about 16 μg/g.[522] The lead content of the soil is not constant with depth. It is normal for the lead content of undisturbed soil to decrease with depth. This and the lead gradients in soils near busy highways are discussed in detail in Chapter 1.

The amounts of lead reported in plant material have varied widely.

33

The lead content of the leaves of different species growing in three wooded areas in New Jersey ranged from less than 0.3 to 30 μg/g.[194] In several crop plants, it averaged less than 10 μg/g.[570]

In discussing plant uptake of lead from soil, it is probably more appropriate to consider soluble lead than total lead. Brewer[65] gives a range of 0.05–5 μg/g of soluble lead in soils. Difficulty arises, however, when one tries to decide what should be used as the extracting agent that simulates the root of the plant. At best, a correlation can be made between the extractability of lead and the ease with which the soil releases its lead to the plant. The relation of extractability of lead chloride added to the soil, its organic matter content, and pH was demonstrated by MacLean et al.[369] using oats and alfalfa. This work showed that low humus content and high acidity favor lead uptake by plants from soil. It also showed that when large amounts of lead (1,000 μg/g) were added to the soil, the availability of the lead to the extracting agent, 1N ammonium acetate, could be correlated roughly with the availability of lead to the plant.

The typical effects of adding lead to soil are summarized in the work of Baumhardt.[36] He added lead to soils in field plots in amounts varying from about 20 to 1,000 μg/g of soil. Corn (Zea mays L.) was then grown on this soil for 2 years. He concluded that there was no reduction in germination on any plot treated with lead and that it had no effect on plant height, date of silking, or grain yield. The lead content of the leaves was significantly greater when the amount of lead added was about 250 μg/g, but there was no detectable increase in the lead content of the kernel at any lead concentration studied. The results showed that the length of time after the addition of lead has an influence on its biologic availability. Thus, the lead content of the plant portion without the grain grown in soils receiving more than 250 μg/g was about half as great in the second year of harvest as in the first year. Extraction with ammonium acetate confirmed that the lead was less available in the second year. Keaton[292] also noted the decrease in soluble lead with time. The importance of soluble lead versus total lead is further shown by a greenhouse experiment conducted by Marten and Hammond,[372] in which an eightfold increase in the total lead content of a soil did not result in a significant increase in the lead content of bromegrass grown in it.

The trace amounts of lead absorbed by plants from soils can be increased by increasing the lead content of the soil or by decreasing the binding capacity of the soil for lead. Motto et al.[406] reported on the absorption of lead by plants from solutions. In a greenhouse experiment, five crop plants—carrots (a root crop), potatoes (a tuber crop), tomatoes (a fruit), corn (a grain), and lettuce (a leafy vegetable)—were grown in acid-washed sand to which complete nutrient solutions were added daily until the plants were well established. When the plants were established in the sand culture, the sand was washed by leaching with distilled deionized water. Each culture was then treated with nutrient solutions that contained no phosphorus and either no lead or 1, 2, or 4 μg/g of lead as lead nitrate. These solutions were added to the growing plants daily for a week; then the sand was washed and complete nutrient solution was added daily for a week. This was repeated until the crops were ready for harvest. All harvested plant parts were washed in distilled deionized water to which detergent had been added. The results of this experiment are recorded in Table 2-1. The roots of each crop absorbed soluble lead and translocated some of it to aboveground parts, except the leaves of potatoes, fruits of tomatoes, and the grain of corn, which showed little or no increase in lead. In lettuce, potatoes, and tomatoes, the small feeder roots were analyzed, and their lead content was very high; in corn and carrots, larger roots were analyzed, and their lead content was much lower, indicating poor translocation even in the roots.

In these and other experiments using solution culture,[352] the concentrations of lead in the nutrient solution were very high, compared with the concentrations of lead that might be expected in solutions in soil, but the overall amount of lead in the plants was not extremely high. This further confirms the poor translocation of lead in plants. Studies by Motto et al.[406] in the field indicate similar results. They found that lead was absorbed through the root system with some translocation to other parts of the plant. The fruiting and flowering parts of the plant contain the smallest amount of lead and show little effect of changes in the amount of lead supplied.

Several studies have been made of the relative importance of air, water, and soil as sources of lead in plants. Dedolph et al.[147] studied the effects of lead in air, water, and soil on the concentration of lead in perennial rye grass and radishes. Filtered air was used for half the plots. Both grass and radishes were found to derive about 2–3 μg of lead per gram of dry matter from the soil when the concentration of lead in air and in water was zero. They concluded that there are substantial amounts of soil-derived lead within plants and that soil has long been and remains an important source of lead in plants.

Ter Haar,[531] in a similar study, investigated the effects of lead in

TABLE 2-1 Concentration of Lead in Plants Grown in Acid-Washed Sand in a Greenhouse in 1968, μg/g Dry Weight[a]

Plant	Treatment, ppm Pb			
	0	1	2	4
Carrot				
Tops	8.7	16	19	27
Roots	3.1	7.9	18	21
Corn				
Tassel	7.8	8.1	7.4	9.2
Leaves	11	19	39	88
Stalk	0.6	11	28	44
Husk				
Outer	2.9	7.9	15	23
Inner	3.9	7.3	13	16
Roots	3.7	12	22	35
Kernel	1.0	1.7	2.8	3.3
Cob	2.4	2.7	4.3	10
Lettuce				
Leaves	5.7	12	16	37
Roots	7.6	108	182	332
Potato				
Leaves	11	7.8	12	12
Stems	7.6	29	55	123
Roots	30	200	451	764
Tuber	1.0	0.6	2.6	1.2
Tomato				
Leaves	8.1	8.1	15	16
Stem	3.6	24	89	87
Root	17	418	690	739
Fruit	3.6	2.5	2.3	2.1

[a]Derived from Motto et al.[406]

air and soil on the lead concentration of the edible and inedible portions of several important types of food crops. These were studied by growing crops in greenhouses supplied with filtered and unfiltered ambient air and in plots planted in long rows perpendicular to a busy highway. The lead content of the soil varied from 65 μg/g near the road to 25 μg/g remote from the road. On the basis of these crops, the conclusion was that lead occurring naturally in the soil is the main source of lead in the edible portion but that, in the concentration range studied, the variation of lead content of the soil did not affect the lead content of the crops (Tables 2-2, 2-3, 2-4).

These studies further showed that fresh unprocessed foods grown in filtered air contained quantities of lead similar to those in foods in the marketplace. Thus, it seems that food as purchased probably is not significantly contaminated with lead unless processing is done in a careless manner.

Schuck and Locke[483] studied five crops—cauliflower, tomatoes, cabbage, strawberries, and oranges. In spite of their being grown near heavily traveled highways used by up to 50,000 cars per day, the amount of lead found in the five crops in an untreated state was never greater than 1 μg/g fresh weight, and the average lead concentration for the entire crop area studied was only one tenth or even one hundredth of that.

Although their conclusion that crops are not inclined to absorb lead through the root system disagrees with those of some of the authors cited earlier, it may be that the pH of their soil, or some other physical or chemical characteristic of the soil, led to this conclusion. Little systematic work has been done on the uptake of lead from soil of different types, in which the effects of pH and other physicochemical variables may account for the differences found.

EFFECT OF LEAD IN WATER

The effects of lead in soil discussed in the preceding paragraphs are undoubtedly actually the effects of trace amounts of lead in "soil

TABLE 2-2   Lead in Crops, Greenhouse Studies, μg/g Dry Weight[a]

	Unfiltered Air	Filtered Air	LSD[b]
Air	1.45 μg/m^3	0.09 μg/m^3	–
Soil	17.1	17.1	–
Leaf lettuce	6.6[c]	3.2	1.3
Cabbage head	1.0	1.1	0.35
Cabbage—unharvested leaves	4.5	5.8	1.6
Tomatoes	0.59	0.72	0.26
Beans	1.4	1.2	0.52
Bean leaves	20.9[c]	7.9	8.8
Sweet corn			
Kernel	0.22	0.27	0.22
Cob	0.43[c]	0.69	0.24
Husk	6.9[c]	1.8	1.5
Carrots	1.7	2.1	1.9
Potatoes	0.30	0.33	0.12
Wheat	0.18	0.16	0.06

[a]Modified from Ter Haar.[531]
[b]Least significant difference.
[c]Different from other values in row at 95% level of confidence.

TABLE 2-3   Lead in Crops, Highway Studies, μg/g Dry Weight[a]

	Feet from Road			
	30	120	520	LSD[b]
Air	2.3[c] μg/m^3	1.7[d] μg/m^3	1.1 μg/m^3	–
Soil	65[c]	40[d]	25	–
Leaf lettuce	6.5	5.0	4.8	3.1
Cabbage head	0.56	0.86	0.83	0.44
Cabbage–unharvested leaves	6.4[c]	8.9[d]	4.0	1.3
Tomatoes	1.3	1.2	1.6	1.3
Beans	1.9[c]	1.2	0.90	0.47
Potatoes	0.48	0.64	0.40	0.27
Sweet corn				
Kernel	0.39	0.21	0.83[c]	0.31
Cob	0.74	0.55	0.68	0.21
Husk	12.6[c]	6.6	5.7	3.6
Soybeans				
Beans	0.28[c]	0.12	0.10	0.10
Husk	15.9[c]	8.0[d]	5.3	0.22
Oats				
Kernel	0.47	–	0.53	0.37
Chaff	31.4[c]	15.5	12.8	15.5
Carrots	1.6	–	1.5	0.61
Wheat				
Kernel	0.62	0.42	0.48	0.17
Chaff	17.8[c]	9.8[d]	6.2	1.6

[a]Modified from Ter Haar.[531]
[b]Least significant difference.
[c]Single letter shows this value different from others in row at 95% level of confidence.
[d]Two letters in same row show these values different from others at 95% level of confidence.

TABLE 2-4   Lead in Rice, μg/g Dry Weight[a]

Road	Sample	Feet from Road		LSD[b]
		30	700	
U.S. 90	Grain	0.17	0.18	0.04
	Hulls	3.9[c]	1.9	0.98
	Straw	4.1	2.5	1.2
I-10	Grain	0.23	0.24	0.04
	Hulls	4.9[c]	2.9	1.6
	Straw	5.83[c]	2.13	0.35

[a]Modified from Ter Haar.[531]
[b]Least significant difference.
[c]Different from other values in row at 95% level of confidence.

solution." The factors of soil type and probably pH, which strongly affect the uptake of lead, influence the amount of lead in solution in the groundwater. In nearly all cases, this concentration will be very low because of the strong coordination of lead to soil.

The effect of lead in rainwater on lead concentration in plants was studied in work mentioned earlier[147] in which the lead-in-rainwater variable was separated from the lead-in-soil and lead-in-air variables. There was no detectable change in the lead concentrations in any part of grass and radishes sprayed with 40 μg/liter of lead chloride.

EFFECT OF LEAD IN AIR

Many authors substantiate the conclusion that lead in air increases the concentration of lead in the leafy parts of plants near highways but does not affect the compact portion of the plant. Kloke and Riebartsch[311] found higher concentrations of lead in grass grown near busy highways. Cannon and Bowles[83] found higher concentrations of lead in vegetation grown near a highway than in that grown some distance away. Warren and Delavault[570] correlated lead content in plants with highway traffic. They determined lead in tree stems collected from an area remote from highway traffic and in stems of the same species collected in an area of heavy traffic. The lead values for the remote area ranged from 0.4 to 2.0 μg/g dry weight, and for the heavy-traffic area from 2 to 52 μg/g dry weight. Everett et al.[173] measured the lead content of unwashed privet leaves collected from sites along main highways and remote from highways in England. They found an average of 86 μg/g dry weight in the leaves near the highway and 45 μg/g dry weight in the sites away from the highway.

Ruhling and Tyler[464] have studied the concentrations of lead in mosses. They observed that, because the mosses obtain their minerals chiefly from precipitation and settled dust, they could be used as an index for surveying deposition of airborne heavy metals. They found in southern Sweden that the concentration of lead in mosses has risen from about 25 μg/g in the nineteenth century to the present average of about 100 μg/g. The interpretation of these findings is discussed in Chapter 1.

The experiments of Dedolph et al.,[147] cited earlier, using filtered and unfiltered air, showed no effect of lead in air on radishes, but the concentration of lead in grass was about doubled when the lead concentration was raised from zero to about 1 μg/m^3. Studies near a busy highway confirmed these results. Grass grown at increasing distances from the road contained concentrations of lead that could be correlated with the concentration of lead in the air.

The study by Ter Haar,[531] cited earlier, concluded that airborne lead contributed about 0.5–1.5% of the lead content of the U.S. diet. Of the ten crops studied—wheat, potatoes, tomatoes, sweet corn, carrots, cabbage, oats, rice, leaf lettuce, and snap beans—eight were not affected by the concentration of lead in air. In both field and greenhouse tests, the inedible portions of the plants (bean leaves, cornhusks, soybean husks, and oat, wheat, and rice chaff) showed a 2- to 3-fold increase in lead concentration when grown near the road or in the greenhouse with unfiltered air (Tables 2-2, 2-3, 2-4).

Leh[343] compared rye and potato plants growing within 15 ft of traffic with similar plants growing more than 300 ft from the highway. The lead contents of chaff and green tops from near the highway were higher by a factor of about two, whereas those of kernels and tubers were unaffected.

Motto *et al.*[406] grew five commercial crops (lettuce, tomatoes, corn, potatoes, and carrots) along highways supporting 12,500, 47,100 and 49,000 cars every 24 hr. These crops were grown 30, 100, and 250 ft from each of the three highways. The soil in all locations was a sassafras loam. All the plants except the corn were grown to usable maturity; the corn was harvested after the kernels became hard. The data (Table 2-5) demonstrate the tendency for lead from air to accumulate on leaves and other exposed aboveground plant structures. These washed samples indicate that the lead from the air or the soil did not increase in the portions of plants consumed by man, except for lettuce leaves, which exhibited a highly significant increase in lead in the samples gathered near the highways supporting the most traffic.

All investigators reach the same conclusion. In a narrow band near the highway, the concentration of lead on the surface of foliage is proportional to the concentration of lead in the air. On the protected portions of the plants (e.g., seeds and roots), which in almost all cases are the edible portions, little or no effect is noted.

SEASONAL VARIATIONS

The importance of the growing state of the plant in the plant's lead content is noted by several investigators. Daines *et al.*[135] report an increase in atmospheric lead during the winter months, increasing the

TABLE 2-5   Concentration of Lead in Five Crops Grown at Three Field Sites in 1968[a]

	Traffic Volume								
	12,500 Cars per 24 hr			47,100 Cars per 24 hr			49,000 Cars per 24 hr		
Distance from highway, ft	30	100	250	30	100	250	30	100	250
Air lead, $\mu g/m^3$	1.4	1.1	1.0	4.5	2.7	2.4	5.2	3.3	2.5
Soil lead, ppm at 0–6 in.	54	38	33	134	138	300	229	130	89
Lead content, ppm, of:									
Carrot									
Tops	18	11	14	37	26	21	53	22	17
Roots	3.8	5.3	3.9	6.2	9.5	9.4	9.1	10	5.0
Corn									
Tassel	31	7.4	7.8	179	144	69	–	–	–
Leaves	19	17	14	86	47	36	88	51	40
Stalk	3.6	3.7	0.9	5.6	3.6	0.2	6.2	3.4	3.6
Husk									
Outer	11	5.0	6.8	} 3.0	5.0	2.6	–	–	–
Inner	5.0	5.2	2.4				–	–	–
Roots	6.0	3.9	5.4	19	14	19	54	19	–
Kernel	3.8	3.6	3.1	0.0	0.2	0.2	–	–	–
Cob	8.0	3.2	2.6	0.4	0.0	0.4	–	–	–
Lettuce									
Leaves	12	13	–	24	21	14	56	35	–
Roots	16	15	–	24	27	39	61	32	–
Potato									
Leaves	36	31	21	87	47	29	–	–	–
Stems	12	8.4	7.8	15	11	14	–	–	–
Roots	22	23	18	33	49	58	–	–	–
Tuber	0.5	1.5	1.0	2.6	3.0	3.0	–	–	–
Tomato									
Leaves	36	25	17	76	82	40	88	52	44
Stem	9.0	9.8	6.9	27	25	31	29	13	7.7
Root	11	15	14	27	35	50	37	12	9.6
Fruit	2.8	3.0	2.4	4.6	2.7	2.8	3.6	1.2	3.2

[a] Adapted from Motto et al.[406]

opportunity for lead to be deposited from the air. During the summer months, plants are normally growing, thus diluting the lead deposited on their leaves with new tissue. The lead deposit on leaves would be expected to increase with increasing exposure time. Chadwick and Chamberlain[95] also found that less lead remained if it was applied during the summer to grass than if it was applied the winter after the same weathering period. The lead content in privet foliage was greater during September through April than during May through August.[173]

Mitchell and Reith[393] found that there is an increase in lead in the aboveground portion of the plant when active growth stops. In autumn, the lead content of the aboveground portion of pasture herbage begins to rise from about 1 μg/g dry weight to 10 μg/g dry weight. It may reach 30–40 μg/g in the winter. The authors believe that the increase in lead content of the aboveground portion when the plant is dormant may indicate translocation of lead from roots to tops during the winter months or loss of organic matter through respiration, rather than uptake from the soil. They ruled out the possibility of surface contamination from lead in air and soil contamination. This study indicates that caution is necessary when comparing lead concentrations in plant materials. If they are harvested in different seasons, the results may not be comparable. More work is needed to learn the influence of seasonal variation and the effect of aging stress on lead uptake.

One further point should be made. Even in the absence of lead in air, the leafy portions of plants are often higher in lead than the rest of the plant. Ter Haar[531] observed this in his greenhouse study. Goldschmidt[200] observed it as early as 1933. He stated that the mineral solution enters the plants through the roots and concentrates at the point of greatest evaporation—namely, the leaves.

The concentration of lead in grass near a highway is of special interest, because animals may consume it. Chow[118] found up to 60 μg/g dry weight in grass cut within about 40 ft of U.S. Highway 1 in Maryland and the Baltimore–Washington Parkway. With an increase in traffic from 11,000 to 32,000 cars per 12 hr, Kloke and Riebartsch[311] found an increase in roadside grass from 16 to 60 μg/g dry weight. Leh[343] found 180 μg/g dry weight on the median strip, 120 μg/g dry weight 6 ft from the edge, and 35 μg/g dry weight about 20 ft from the edge of a road reported to carry 30,000 cars in 12 hr.

Dedolph et al.[147] found that, for a road carrying 30,000 cars per day, the concentration of lead in grass was correlated with the concentration of lead in air. Forty feet from the road, the lead in air was 2.3 μg/m^3, and the grass contained 15 μg/g dry weight. At 120 ft from the road, the lead in air was 1.7 μg/m^3, and the grass contained 8.4 μg/g dry weight.

Motto et al.[406] analyzed grass clippings gathered at seven distances

(0–225 ft) from highways supporting 12,800–54,700 cars daily
(Table 2–6). All samples were divided: One portion was washed in
four changes of distilled deionized water to which a small amount of
detergent was added for the first washing; the second portion was
analyzed without washing. The average lead content of unwashed
orchard grass clippings gathered at the highway edge (255 $\mu g/g$ dry
weight) was more than five times that of grass gathered 225 ft from
the highway. It was of interest that the decrement in lead content
was steepest in the first 75 ft from the highway. If the average lead
content of the grass samples reported by Motto et al. were charted
against distance from the highway, the curve would be very similar to
that of Daines et al.[135] for atmospheric lead versus distance from a
highway. Daines et al. reported a decrease in atmospheric particulate
lead of over 50% between 10 and 150 ft from the highway.

Motto et al.[406] further report that washing the grass removed lead
from all samples studied; however, those gathered in the first 75 ft
lost the greatest amount of lead (nearly 50%) in washing. The fact
that lead can be removed from leaves by washing and that lead in
grass is correlated with lead in air demonstrates that all or much of
the lead on leaves that comes from the air is, as stated by Schuck and
Locke,[483] present "as a topical dust coating."

RESPONSE OF PLANTS TO LEAD

Although a considerable volume of literature is devoted to studies of
lead in soils and plants, there seems to be no reliable evidence that
lead injures plants in nature. In fact, extensive investigations summarized by Bradshaw et al.[64] show that some species of plants have
adapted to habitats near mining operations that contain lead, zinc,
and copper in amounts that are toxic to nonadapted populations of
the same species. Jowett[283] showed that a high tolerance to lead had
developed in many populations of *Agrostis tenuis* (colonial bentgrass)
growing on disused lead mines in mid-Wales. The tolerance mechanism
is specific for the metals separately, and it is known that there is no
significant difference between tolerant and nontolerant plants in the
amount of toxic metal absorbed. However, tolerant plants can be
distinguished from nontolerant by both calcium and phosphate response.[284] Wilkins[582] reported that lead tolerance in *Festuca ovina*
(sheep fescue) seemed to depend on a single gene with large effect.
Toxic effects on plants of experimentally administered lead have

TABLE 2-6 Lead in Roadside Grass Samples[a]

Distance from Highway, ft	12,800 Vehicles per 24 hr	14,700 Vehicles per 24 hr	17,700 Vehicles per 24 hr	19,700 Vehicles per 24 hr	41,000 Vehicles per 24 hr	45,600 Vehicles per 24 hr	48,600 Vehicles per 24 hr	48,600 Vehicles per 24 hr	54,700 Vehicles per 24 hr	Average
					Lead Content, Not Washed, ppm					
0	—	—	—	133	141	118	—	664	219	255.0
25	63	—	—	84	66	192	154	454	139	164.6
75	76	—	—	65	103	—	66	198	83	98.5
125	—	—	31	41	—	66	45	139	78	66.7
175	—	—	—	41	60	46	66	—	61	54.8
225	—	35	—	34	56	41	48	68	59	46.3
Av.	—	—	—	66.3	85.2	92.6	75.8	304.6	106.5	112.0
					Lead Content, Washed, ppm					
0	40	40	91	133	136	71	128	492	98	136.6
25	37	23	64	58	85	80	62	262	83	83.8
75	64	34	46	59	80	—	50	77	60	58.8
125	58	43	26	58	55	46	36	59	45	47.3
175	47	35	—	18	46	31	45	—	62	40.6
225	50	31	—	36	58	32	31	44	43	40.6
Av.	49.3	34.3	56.8	60.3	76.7	52.0	58.7	186.8	65.2	69.8

[a]Modified from Motto et al.[406]

44

been manifested by a variety of signs.* There are reports of delay in germination of seeds of cress and mustard after treatment with concentrations of lead ion above 0.01% and of retardation of subsequent growth;[152] of delay in root growth and leaf and flower production in hyacinth bulbs exposed to lead ion;[46] and of contributory effects to frenching of tobacco.[140]

At the cellular level, toxic effects on plants have been found experimentally affecting cell walls, nuclei, and mitochondria. From studies using *Allium cepa* (onions), *Zea mays* (corn), and *Vicia faba* (broad bean), Hammett[231] reported the concentration of lead within the nuclei and cell walls of the growing portions of roots. He found that lead retarded cell proliferation while allowing cells to increase in size. In further studies, he noted that the mitotic (dividing) nuclei of the growing roots "have a special avidity for lead," and that a reaction between lead and an organic sulfhydryl occurred in the area of normal rapid elongation. Of interest is the comment that "the sulfhydryl group stimulates cell proliferation in mammals and in lower organisms."

Mitosis induced by lead nitrate has been found indistinguishable from that induced by colchicine, with spindle disturbances and chromatid formation in root tips of *Allium cepa.*[347] In a small number of experiments, barley seeds soaked for 7 hr in 0.2 *M* solutions of lead nitrate seemed to be more susceptible than controls to x radiation.[519]

Koeppe and Miller,[312] using corn mitochondria, found that lead chloride (50–62 μmoles/liter) in media containing either potassium chloride or sucrose stimulated oxidation of exogenous reduced nicotinamide adenine dinucleotide. This increased oxidation was not affected by the presence of phosphate. These studies further indicated that lead chloride (12.5 μmoles/liter) inhibited oxidation of succinate in the absence of phosphate. Inasmuch as phosphate is essential for plant growth, the effect on succinate oxidation would seldom be encountered in nature. The effects of high concentrations of lead on animal cell mitochondria are described in Chapter 4.

In all the experiments discussed here, the concentrations of lead bore no resemblance to the concentrations present in soil solutions. In all cases, effects were noted only at concentrations several orders of magnitude higher than would be present in the soil solution, even in a soil highly polluted with lead.

---

*During the period when lead arsenate was used as an insecticide on fruit trees, injury to apple and peach foliage was common. However, this phytotoxicity was produced by the arsenical and not the lead part of the compound.

SUMMARY

1. Plants can absorb soluble lead through their roots and translocate some of it to their aboveground portions. There is a natural concentration of lead in plants that comes from the natural lead content of the soil.

2. Widely varied concentrations of lead in soil have little effect on the lead content of the plant. The lead naturally occurring in soils is largely unavailable to plants, as is the airborne lead in soils along heavily traveled highways.

3. Lead in air does not measurably increase the lead content of the edible portions of most plants.

4. Leafy portions of plants within about 75 ft of busy highways contain higher concentrations of lead than do plants growing farther away. This is true for a narrow band on both sides of the highway. There is little or no evidence that this lead can be translocated downward to the underground portions of the plant.

5. Because about 50% of the lead on leaves of plants growing near busy highways can be removed by a water wash, it must be concluded that much of the lead is present as a surface deposit. Although the lead particles in the air are small enough to enter the open stomata of plants (unless prevented by electrostatic forces), there is no evidence that lead particles from air enter the leaf.

6. Even in the absence of lead in air, leafy portions of plants generally contain more lead than the other parts.

7. Rainwater does not appear to be a significant source of lead in crops.

8. Stresses on a plant, such as senescence, may increase the concentration of lead in it.

9. Evidence that lead, as it occurs in nature, is toxic to vegetation is lacking. However, in studies using roots of some plants and very high concentrations of lead, lead has been reported to concentrate in cell walls and nuclei in mitosis and to inhibit cell proliferation but to allow the continued increase of cell size. In addition, on the basis of corn mitochondria, it has been reported that lead chloride stimulated the oxidation of exogenous reduced nicotinamide adenine dinucleotide and decreased the oxidation of succinate in the absence of phosphate. Because phosphate is essential for plant life, the importance of the effect of lead chloride on the oxidation of succinate in plant cells is uncertain.

3

Input and Disposition of Lead in Man

Lead has been detected in all tissues of man and animals, even in environmental settings remote from man-made sources of lead. In assessing the potential hazards of environmental lead, the foremost consideration is the margin of safety between ordinary rates of input and rates that are demonstrably toxic. Subsidiary considerations are the relative contributions of air, food, water, and other sources and the relative importance of the several portals of entry into the body.

This chapter emphasizes the input and disposition of lead in man under ordinary conditions, in contrast with extraordinary exposure to lead, which is the subject of Chapter 4. Some animal data are cited, but mainly as evidence of what is thought to occur in man.

SOURCES AND ROUTES OF INPUT

Food, water, and other beverages are the major sources of lead input in man and probably in most animals. There have been numerous studies of the concentration of lead in various foods and beverages.

47

Diet

Exposure to lead from drinking water is influenced by the water's source, treatment, and distribution system. These facts have been known for many years, as evidenced in a letter by Benjamin Franklin[187] on the "bad effects of lead taken inwardly." One of the sources of lead that Franklin cited was rainwater collected from lead roofs overhung with trees that shed acid-producing leaves. Modern work has now documented Franklin's observations.

The lead content in public water supplies of the 100 largest cities in the United States in 1962 ranged from traces to 62 μg/liter;[163] the higher concentrations reflect sizable additions of lead from pollution in some localities. Continuous monitoring of the water supplies of the United States since 1962 has demonstrated that their lead content has in general not exceeded the U.S. Public Health Service's prescribed standard of 50 μg/liter.[552] Kehoe[298] found values of 3–40 μg/liter for water from 35 U.S. towns and cities and pointed out that the lead content of drinking water may be high if the piping or joint luting used contains lead or if the water stands undisturbed in lead pipes or luting of a new building for a weekend. In such conditions, concentrations as high as 920 μg/liter have been obtained. Aside from those special circumstances, lead concentrations in drinking water have been observed to be little different from those in the oceans, in rural ponds and streams, and in well water.

Ettinger[172] points out that samples from surface-water stations in heavily populated and industrialized areas where waste pollution is high contain only small amounts of lead in solution, probably because of rapid precipitation and coordination of insoluble lead from waters containing silt, which acts as excellent coordination sites for precipitating lead. Organic species in the water also coordinate lead and aid in removing it from water. A recent report[379] of 2,595 distribution samples found that 25% contained no measurable lead and about 73% contained less than the mandatory 50 μg/liter; 41 samples contained more than this limit.

From all these findings, it is evident that drinking water contributes, on the average, a small amount of lead to the body burden. On the basis of the data cited, it seems unlikely that many people drink water containing more than 50 μg/liter with any consistency. The average intake of lead from water and water-based beverages cannot be stated with any precision, but, assuming 20 μg/liter and a daily consumption of 1 liter, the lead consumed from water would be 20 μg/day. This estimate would apply to an adult; for an infant or young child, it would be proportionally greater (i.e., on the basis of body weight).

The amount of lead input in man from food depends on the natural lead content of foods, factors that may increase it, and the amount of food ingested. Of prime interest is the effect of exposure to automobile exhaust on the lead content of comestibles. Also to be considered are factors associated with the storage and preparation of foods.

Kehoe *et al.*[304] found lead in every item of food obtained from the field and from dwellings of the inhabitants of a primitive region far from industrial and mining activities. Patterson[437] estimated that the natural lead content of food should be 0.01 μg/g wet weight (0.01 ppm) and concluded that most of the lead present today in food is from industrial sources. The lead content of food today is considerably greater than 0.01 μg/g. Schroeder and co-workers[480] have made extensive examinations of lead in food. On a fresh-weight basis, they found about 1.2 (range, 0–1.5) μg/g in condiments, 0.5 (range, 0.2–2.5) μg/g in fish and seafood, 0.2 (range, 0–0.37) μg/g in meats and eggs, 0.4 (range, 0–1.39) μg/g in grains, 0.2 (range, 0–1.3) μg/g in vegetables, and no lead detectable by his analyses in fresh whole milk. Monier-Williams[398] and Warren and Delavault[570] estimated about 0.2 μg/g of food.

The contribution of atmospheric lead to the amount in vegetables and fruits is not clearly known. If significant, it is probably not due to direct uptake by plants from the air or water.[147,406,531] Two recent studies[406,483] have defined the extent of the contribution of lead dispersed into the atmosphere along highways to the lead content of vegetation. Both investigations (which are discussed in detail in Chapter 2) showed that the amount of lead found on soils and plants in such areas tends to decrease with distance from the highway and that one half to two thirds is removable by washing, except in the case of rough-surfaced foods, such as strawberries. In the case of unwashed animal feed, lead may find its way from aerially contaminated grasses and other vegetation to meats consumed by man. There is no evidence that this possible source of food contamination has measurably altered the concentrations of lead in animal food products, such as meat and milk, over the last 30 years. Because milk is a major source of nutrition for infants and young children, there is special concern for the contribution of this food to total dietary lead intake. The concentration of lead in milk was reported in connection with an outbreak of bovine lead poisoning.[232] The concentration of lead in milk was linearly related to the coexistent concentration of lead in the blood of nine cows having varying degrees of lead exposure. In this same study, concentrations of lead in the milk of eight cows not known to be exposed to an unusual amount of lead averaged 0.009 mg/liter. This average is slightly lower than the values reported by another group in 1940.[302]

The total dietary intake of lead is generally estimated to be about the same in recent years as it was in 1943, if the estimates of Cholak and Bambach[114] are compared with those of Kehoe,[298] Schroeder et al.,[480] Harley,[239] and Lewis.[350] Assuming that a person consumes about 2,000 g of food and drink per day, Schroeder and Tipton[482] estimated that lead intake averages 100–500 μg/day, depending on the foods eaten. Cholak and Bambach[114] estimated the intake of lead in food to be about 300 μg/day; Kehoe,[298] whose analytic work was performed by associates in the Kettering Laboratory, estimated a similar amount on the basis of a large number of duplicate daily samples of food and beverages.

Harley[239] conducted an especially useful study in New York City. He has determined the lead concentration in various foods and estimated the yearly intake of lead on the basis of the Department of Agriculture consumption statistics for food for an adult man at 103 mg or about 285 μg/day, a figure that is consistent with other investigations.

Lewis[350] points out that no food or group of foods is either a large or a constant contributor to lead in man, because man's diet is composed of a wide variety of individual items, and various foods contribute various amounts of lead. Lewis estimated the average daily dietary intake of lead at about 300 μg, with a range for most people of 100–2,000 μg. The range can vary markedly from person to person and from city to city, on the basis of choice, opportunity, and specific habits.

The daily dietary intake of lead of persons 1–3 years old without unusual nondietary exposure has been estimated at 130 μg,[34,110] on the basis of the daily fecal excretion of lead (with urinary losses not accounted for). The greater lead intake of infants, compared with adults, on a unit-body-weight basis, probably is related to infants' higher caloric and water requirements. It is not known whether the apparent greater intake is accompanied by a correspondingly greater total output; the critical balance studies have not been conducted, as they have in adults.

Respiration

Inhalation of air is a smaller potential source of input than ingestion of food and water. In view of the great variations of lead in air with season and locale, the potential intake by this route is as variable as the potential intake from food and water. For example, data cited in Chapter 1 indicate that the median concentration of lead in the air of Los Angeles in 1962 was 2.5 $\mu g/m^3$, although some stations in the city recorded concentrations as high as 16.9 $\mu g/m^3$. In most suburban areas, by contrast, the concentration probably seldom exceeds 0.5 $\mu g/cm^3$, and for rural areas, 0.1 $\mu g/m^3$. Thus, there is at least a five-fold variation in atmospheric lead exposure, depending on whether one is a resident of downtown Los Angeles or of a typical suburb (2.5 $\mu g/m^3$ versus 0.5 $\mu g/m^3$). The variability of potential lead intake by inhalation is further increased by the variability of total air inhaled, which depends, for example, on the degree of physical activity engaged in. A man doing light work for 8 hr a day would inhale more than twice (22.8 m^3 versus 10.8 m^3) as much air as a man at rest all day (Table 3-1). If one superimposes on this range a 25-fold difference in atmospheric lead concentration between rural and urban air, the potential daily intake of lead could vary from 1.1 μg for a rural man at rest all day to 57.0 μg for a man engaged in light work in downtown Los Angeles and residing there continually while not at work (Table 3-1). The comparable amount of lead potentially inhaled by a suburbanite who commutes to the city for light work is 30.6 μg.

As in the case of dietary intake, potential respiratory intake in infants is greater than that in adults on a unit-body-weight basis for

TABLE 3-1 Potential Daily Intake of Lead by Inhalation

Activity Level[a]	Air Inhaled, m^3	Potential Lead Intake, μg		
		@ 0.1 $\mu g/m^3$	@ 0.5 $\mu g/m^3$	@ 2.5 $\mu g/m^3$
8 hr working ("light activity")	9.6	0.96	4.8	24.0
8 hr nonoccupational activity	9.6	0.96	4.8	24.0
8 hr resting	3.6	0.36	1.8	9.0
Total	22.8	2.28	11.4	57.0

[a]Of a "standard man" weighing 70 kg, 20–30 years old, 175 cm tall, and having a surface area of 1.8 m^2.

exposure to comparable concentrations of airborne lead. A 1-year-old child inhales 6 m³ of air per day, compared with the 23 m³ per day inhaled by an adult.[515] Again, the significance of this proportionally greater inhalation of lead per day is obscure because of lack of studies of the metabolism of lead in infants. The proportionally greater intake might be accompanied by a correspondingly greater rate of excretion.

ABSORPTION AND EXCRETION

Although food and water are generally a greater potential source of lead in man than is the air, there are still many uncertainties as to their relative contributions, mainly because of the imperfect state of knowledge concerning the fate of the lead that is inhaled. The contributions of food and water to the total daily assimilation of lead have been studied extensively. Much was learned from detailed, prolonged balance studies conducted in man at the Kettering Laboratory, University of Cincinnati, under the leadership of R. A. Kehoe. By analysis of samples of all the food, water, and incidental beverages ingested and of the total urine and feces excreted, the net balance of intake versus output in a number of men was determined over a period of many months. This was done in conditions of both normal and abnormally high intake. The results of these studies have been reported over a span of many years and were summarized in 1961.[298] They show that at normal intake the amount of lead excreted generally exceeds slightly the amount ingested in food, water, and incidental beverages. The failure of lead intake to match lead excretion was thought to be due to the unmeasured contribution to the intake made by lead inhaled in air. A typical set of data is presented in Table 3–2. It is apparent from these data for the first seven periods of 8 weeks each that any one period may yield either a slight increase or a slight decrease in the total lead content of the body without any apparent relation to the small fluctuations in the level of intake. In the case of this particular subject, a change in residence and in diet at the end of the seventh period resulted in approximately a doubling of the rate of lead intake, with a pronounced accumulation of lead. In conditions approximating a steady state, in which oral input roughly parallels urinary and fecal output, the urinary excretion of lead is about 10% of the oral input. In this respect, the data in Table 3–2 are typical of Kehoe's findings in human subjects, and it is inferred that net absorp-

TABLE 3-2 Lead Ingestion and Excretion of a Normal Human Subject[a]

8-Week Periods	Lead Ingested, mg	Lead excreted, mg			Net Change in Body Lead, mg
		Total	In Feces	In Urine	
1st	13.59	11.95	10.45	1.50	+1.64
2nd	13.31	15.13	13.63	1.50	−1.82
3rd	13.16	13.82	12.45	1.37	−0.66
4th	11.51	11.59	10.41	1.18	−0.08
5th	9.30	8.93	7.88	1.05	+0.37
6th	9.24	9.05	8.16	0.89	+0.19
7th	12.75	13.74	12.86	0.88	−0.99
Subtotal	82.86	84.21	75.84	8.37	−1.35
8th	22.21	17.61	15.85	1.76	+4.60
9th	18.17	15.05	13.76	1.29	+3.12
Subtotal	40.38	32.66	29.61	3.05	+7.72
Total	123.24	116.87	105.45	11.42	+6.37

[a]Adapted from Kehoe.[298]

tion of lead from the gastrointestinal tract is approximately 10%. The contribution to total excretion of lead assimilated through the airways was not determined. Inclusion of this additional factor would have resulted in a reduction of the estimated proportion of gastrointestinal absorption. More complete studies involving normal ambient air lead and normal dietary lead have not been reported.

In additional studies by the same author, a change from slight decrease to increase in body lead (i.e., lead accumulation) was demonstrated with addition of small daily doses of a lead salt to the diet[298] continually for as long as 4 years (see Figure 3-1). Although the urinary excretion of lead increased roughly in proportion to the daily intake of lead, new levels of equilibrium were not reached within the period wherein urinary and fecal excretion consistently equaled or exceeded oral intake. Inasmuch as increasing the level of oral intake of lead resulted in an increase in urinary excretion, it can be concluded that a small fraction of the lead ingested is indeed absorbed. The time required for approximate balance between input and outgo to be achieved when lead is added to the diet is unknown, but it is more than 2 years.

It is not known how long it takes to achieve a new steady state when intake is substantially increased, or whether indeed a steady state ever is achieved. For that matter, the rate at which approximate equilibration of intake and outgo is achieved under usual dietary con-

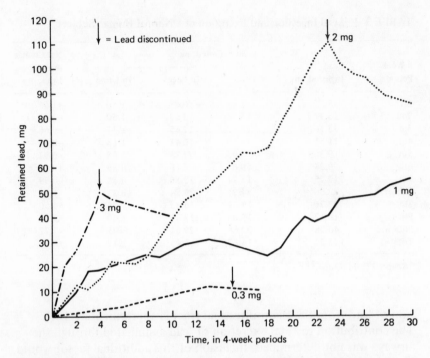

FIGURE 3-1   Retention of lead in four human subjects at daily doses of 0.3, 1, 2, and 3 mg of lead. Modified from Kehoe.[298]

ditions is not known. Virtual equilibration certainly does not occur during fetal life. The concentration of lead increases rather rapidly throughout fetal life in the bones, whole body, and, to a lesser degree, liver.[261]

Some confirmation of Kehoe's work is provided in two Japanese studies as to the approximate balance of dietary intake with outgo and the persistence of accumulation of lead in the body during long periods of abnormally high oral intake.[260,270] Further consideration is given to the long-term accumulation of lead in man in a later section.

The influence of dietary factors on the absorption of lead in man has been studied to some degree by Kehoe.[298] Increases and decreases in dietary calcium and phosphorus, alone and in combination, had no significant influence on the retention by the body of small daily doses of lead (1 mg). Studies in rats indicate that high dietary levels of both calcium and phosphorus decrease the amount of dietary lead retained,[512] whereas vitamin D has the opposite effect.[511]

The relative contributions of the gastrointestinal and urinary routes to total excretion of lead under a variety of conditions are not clearly known. The data presented in Table 3–2 indicate that about 90% of the dietary lead is eliminated in the feces. Some of this lead has probably been absorbed and re-excreted into the gastrointestinal tract by biliary secretion and by secretion and epithelial exfoliation elsewhere in the gastrointestinal tract. After the intravenous administration of lead-212 to four men, the average urinary excretion in the first 24 hr was 4.6% of the dose and practically ended in that period.[268] During the first 48 hr after administration, only 0.18% of the dose appeared in the feces. Owing to the slow appearance in the feces of substances excreted in the upper bowel, it is not certain that these results reflect the true relative contributions of urine and feces. Booker *et al.*[58] conducted similar studies in two human subjects. They found no lead-212 in the feces during the first 24 hr after injection and 4.42% in the urine. During the second 24 hr, however, they found 1.42% in the urine and 1.5% in the feces. This suggests that the fecal route of excretion may well contribute as much as the urinary route to total excretion. Long-term studies of lead excretion in the baboon indicate that the ratio of urinary to fecal excretion of lead is approximately 2 : 1.[166] Similar studies in rats[92] and in sheep[50] indicate that in these species the fecal excretion of lead is even greater than that in urine; in these two studies, biliary excretion was found to be much greater than excretion elsewhere in the gastrointestinal tract.

Knowledge concerning the contribution of respired air to the total amount of lead entering the body is insufficient to allow anything better than general approximations. A reasonably sound estimate can be provided for the fraction of the inhaled lead that is deposited in the airways, but very little is known concerning its fate once deposited. Lead particles deposited in the nasopharyngeal region may be swallowed or ejected by nose-blowing or expectoration. Particles deposited in the trachea and bronchi may migrate up to the pharynx by ciliary-mucus transport to be swallowed or expectorated later, or they may enter the systemic circulation. Even particles deposited in the alveolar bed may be phagocytized by migratory macrophages and conveyed back up the airways to be swallowed and passed through the gastrointestinal tract largely unabsorbed.

The degree to which inhaled lead is initially deposited in the respiratory system has been studied by a number of investigators. Mehani[387] reported an average deposition of 37% for nonindustrially exposed men and 39% and 47% for two groups of industrially exposed men.

Unfortunately, he did not report the particle size distribution for the inhaled lead.

In recognition of the fact that particle size is an important determinant of the deposition and retention of inhaled particles, some investigators have characterized the particles under study in this regard. The information available concerning the size distribution of lead particles in the environment (see Chapter 1) seems to indicate that the major concern in respiration should be the fate of respired lead particles with mass median equivalent diameters (MMED's) in the range of 0.1–1.0 μm and that the average MMED in the general atmospheric environment is about 0.25 μm.

There are only two reported studies in which the deposition of lead in the lungs was measured and particle size was recorded. The first of these studies was by Kehoe.[298] The lead was in the form of lead sesquioxide generated by burning tetraethyl lead. Particles of two size groups were used: an average diameter of 0.05 μm with 90% from 0.02 to 0.09 μm; and a median diameter of 0.9 μm with 90% less than 2 μm. Diameters were determined by electron microscopy. A diameter of 0.05 μm for lead sesquioxide as seen in the electron microscope represents an MMED of approximately 0.25 μm, which is identical with the MMED for lead reported for the general atmospheric environment by Robinson and Ludwig.[454] Particles of lead sesquioxide having a diameter of 0.9 μm as viewed in the electron microscope would, by contrast, have an MMED of 2.9 μm, which is considerably higher than is encountered in the general environment. (See Appendix A for particle-size conversion.) In both cases, the concentration of lead in the air was 150 μg/m³, which is much higher than is encountered in the general environment. The deposition in the respiratory tract associated with exposure to the smaller particles was 36%, a value almost identical with the 37% reported by Mehani for nonindustrially exposed men.[387] Deposition of the larger particles was 46%.

The other major study of lead deposition was reported by Nozaki.[425] Many particle sizes were compared, and an effort was made to distinguish between pulmonary and tracheobronchial deposition. The concentration of lead was 10 mg/m³, which is extremely high, even for an industrial situation. The source of lead was fumes generated in a high-frequency induction furnace. Particle size, which was closely controlled,[259] varied from 0.05 to 1 μm and, as in Kehoe's studies, was determined visually with an electron microscope. Deposition was observed in conditions of both rapid shallow respiration and slow deep respiration. For particles having a diameter of 0.05 μm (by electron microscopy), the total deposition in the respiratory tract for slow deep respiration was similar to that reported by Kehoe, but was appreciably lower for rapid shallow respiration (Table 3-3).

The observations by Mehani,[387] Kehoe,[298] and Nozaki[425] suggest that the deposition in the respiratory tract of lead from the ambient air is approximately 37%. All these studies were deficient in one respect or another, and more extensive studies are needed in which particle size and respiration rate and depth are controlled and varied in a systematic fashion, preferably using lead concentrations in the general range to which the public is currently being exposed.

Very little is known about the clearance of lead from the respiratory tract. Only one investigator has provided any useful information on the retention characteristics of lead in a form similar to that in general ambient air, but it was at a concentration much higher than would be ordinarily encountered. In the respiratory experiments cited earlier, Kehoe determined the excretion of lead in urine and feces before, during, and after termination of inhalation of small and larger particles of lead oxide (average MMED, 0.25 μm; median MMED, 2.9 μm). During the long periods of inhalation, the excretion of lead of both size groups in urine increased. Only during inhalation of the larger particles, however, was the excretion of lead in feces increased. The increase was attributed to passage of inhaled lead into the gastrointestinal tract by swallowing. It was estimated that 40% of the lead deposited in the airways was transferred to the gastrointestinal tract. In this case, 50% of the lead particles were greater than 2.9 μm in MMED. It was probably the particles in this range of diameter that were transferred to the gastrointestinal tract. Even assuming total retention, the usual amount of input of lead via the airways is prob-

TABLE 3-3 Deposition of Lead Inhaled by Man[a]

10 Respirations/min; 1,350 cc Tidal Air		30 Respirations/min; 450 cc Tidal Air	
Particle Diameter, μm	Particle Deposition, %	Particle Diameter, μm	Particle Deposition, %
1.0	63.2	1.0	35.5
0.6	59.0	0.6	33.5
0.4	50.9	0.4	33.0
0.2	48.1	0.2	29.9
0.1	39.3	0.1	27.9
0.08	40.0	0.08	26.5
0.05	42.5	0.05	21.0

[a]Adapted from Nozaki.[425]

ably less than that via food and water. Given 37% deposition and even total retention, a lead concentration of 2.5 $\mu g/m^3$ of air, and inhalation of 23 m^3 of air per day, a person would absorb 21 μg of lead per day originating in the air, compared with roughly 30 μg/day originating in food and water. In the specific case of the data cited in Table 3–2, the estimated concentration of atmospheric lead at that time and place was 2.0 $\mu g/m^3$. Adding the amount of lead absorbed from inhaled air would convert a net decrease of 1.35 mg observed during the first seven 8-week periods to an increase of 5.3 mg.

Work is in progress on a study that is mentioned because it may have important implications regarding the retention of lead inhaled by man at low concentrations. These studies should be viewed with the caution due preliminary findings (T. B. Griffin, J. C. Russell, L. Golberg, F. Coulston, and J. Bradley, personal communication). Rats and rhesus monkeys (*Macaca mulatta*) have been exposed to continuous inhalation of lead sesquioxide particles at an atmospheric concentration of lead of 21.5 $\mu g/m^3$ for 1 year. Also, more than 20 human volunteers have been exposed 23 hr daily to inhalation of 10.9±3.1 $\mu g/m^3$ for up to 4 months. These studies may provide much needed information concerning the retention of lead inhaled by man at relatively low concentrations for a prolonged period.

In evaluating the relative contributions of various environmental sources of lead to total input in the general population, dermal contact cannot be totally ignored. Some finite amount of lead is continuously coming into contact with the skin from air, water, and clothing (see Chapter 7). These contacts are not considered significant,[84, 530] although critical experiments of the type conducted to evaluate the significance of normal dietary intake have not been reported. Because the output of lead in urine and feces is so nearly accounted for by oral and respiratory input, dermal absorption is surely insignificant in usual conditions of lead exposure. Fat-soluble lead alkyl compounds, however, are readily absorbed from the skin and constitute an occupational hazard (see Chapter 6).

Lead is lost in sweat, falling hair, and discarded and desquamated skin to some variable, imprecisely known degree. The concentration of lead in sweat approaches that in urine.[298,496] It has been observed that, during long-term constant intake of lead added to the diet, accumulation of lead in the body decreased in the summer months, but this was accounted for by increased losses in urine and, perhaps, feces.[300, 301] Thus, at least in the temperate zone, the role of sweat in total lead balance seems insignificant.

The influence of ambient temperature on lead metabolism has been studied to some degree because of the known seasonal variation in the incidence of lead poisoning in infants, the incidence being appreciably higher in the summer months than during the rest of the year (see Chapter 4 and Figure 4-9). The mechanism has been investigated in rats and mice.[24,25,75] The enhancement of toxicity by high ambient temperature was accompanied by considerable reductions in both fecal and urinary lead excretion and was favored by dehydration. The effect was most pronounced when exposure to high temperature was delayed until after the administration of lead. The finding in experimental animals that lead excretion decreased when ambient temperature was high does not agree with the observations in man mentioned earlier. The apparent difference between man and animals in this respect is not understood.

DISTRIBUTION IN THE BODY

In ordinary conditions (steady state or nearly steady state of lead retained by the general population), over 90% of the total amount of lead in the body is in the skeleton.[482] The concentration found in the tissues is variable, being highest in bone, intermediate in liver, kidney, and aorta, and low in muscle and brain. The concentration in most other tissues lies between those in kidney and muscle.

The data reported by Schroeder and Tipton[482] indicate that the concentration of lead is greater in the tissues of North Americans than in those of some foreign populations, particularly Africans and Swiss (Table 3-4).

Distribution of lead in the body is discussed further in the summary of Chapter 4.

LEAD IN THE BLOOD

What is known about the relation of the concentration of lead in the body to its toxicity has been learned mainly by study of the relation of symptomatology and exposure to the concentration in biologic fluids, principally the blood, especially under the conditions of occupational exposure at known levels. Lead in human (and animal) blood is associated predominantly with the erythrocytes. In one recent analysis of the distribution of lead in blood, the concentration in

TABLE 3–4 Lead in Adult Human Tissues According to Geographic Area[a]

Tissue	Median Lead Concentration, ppm Ash					
	Nine U.S. Cities (150 Cases)	San Francisco (27 Cases)	Switzerland (9 Cases)	Africa (54 Cases)	Middle East (37 Cases)	Far East (74 Cases)
Aorta	140	220	*32*[b]	71	140	*91* (95%)[c]
Liver	130	160	59	*64*	70	*97* (99%)
Kidney	98	54	45	*36* (96%)	62	62
Pancreas	49	65	42	24	34	39
Lungs	47	38	32	*28* (98%)	42	*43* (99%)
Testes	12 (95%)	20	23	29	*32*	*35*
Heart	5 (57%)	10	14	5 (65%)	*24* (95%)	*19*
Brain	5 (69%)	5 (96%)	5	5 (71%)	*14* (88%)	10 (81%)
Spleen	27 (96%)	44	20	21 (80%)	40	33 (95%)
Bone	43	–	–	–	*26* (95%)	*30* (94%)
Total body, mg[d]	121.6	137.2	61.9	63.2	78.4	93.7

[a]Adapted from Schroeder and Tipton.[482]
[b]Numbers in italics indicate significant difference ($p < 0.001$) from "nine U.S. cities."
[c]Percent of samples in which lead was found; if no figure is given, lead was found in all samples. Data calculated from Tipton.[538]
[d]Estimated by comparison of values.

erythrocytes was approximately 16 times greater than the concentration in serum.[75] Analytic data are usually reported as micrograms per 100 ml of whole blood or micrograms per 100 g of whole blood.* Obviously, some serious errors of interpretation can result from comparing whole-blood concentrations in people with low hematocrit values with those in people with normal hematocrit values (see Chapter 4).

The manner in which lead is associated with erythrocytes is not well understood. There have been numerous studies involving the addition of lead *in vitro*. The validity of such studies is questionable, because lead added *in vitro* can be removed by dialysis with EDTA (ethylenediaminetetraacetic acid) for 24 hr, whereas lead originally in the cells is not affected.[124] This study and others indicate that lead normally associated with erythrocytes is only slowly exchangeable with lead in plasma. It is reasonable to suppose that the concentration of lead reflects the contemporaneous exchangeable material in the tissues perfused by blood. A similar rationale applies to the lead concentration in urine. Indeed, during periods of change in the rate of dietary lead intake, the changes in concentration of lead in blood and urine occur more or less proportionally, with blood exhibiting a somewhat lesser fluctuation than urine.[298]

The concentration of lead in blood is considered more useful than that in urine, because blood is not subject to large fluctuations in water content, as is urine, or to the influence of changes in renal excretory capacity. However, it should be pointed out that no data exist concerning the correlation between the concentration of lead in blood and that in other tissues of the same persons. The difficulties of making such a study are compounded by the distribution of the body burden of lead in exchangeable and nonexchangeable pools.

The concentration of lead in the blood of the general population has been studied extensively and found fairly stable. When the analyses are performed competently, the 90% range found in various population groups, such as post office employees and city health department employees, roughly doubles.[554] The constancy of blood lead content is further evident in that it does not change significantly with age, either among North Americans[554] or among some foreigners.[262] Similarly, there is no increase in the concentration of lead in serum with age in U.S. citizens.[75]

---

*Throughout this document, blood lead content is expressed as amount per 100 g of whole blood, because it is a more accurate measure than volume, which would be about 5% higher.

Although it is valuable (in terms of degrees of exposure) to know how much lower lead concentrations are in the blood of the general population than in the blood of persons who experience overt signs of lead toxicity, what one really wishes to know is the difference in lead intake between healthy and lead-poisoned people. That is what makes the relation between lead concentration in blood and lead exposure important.

The relation between lead concentration in the blood of the general population and total lead input into the body per unit time is not known and cannot be known in the individual case because of the great variety of opportunities for exposure to lead in the modern environment. Although a few studies have been reported in individual experimental subjects in which the balance between dietary lead intake and excretion was determined, in no case was a determination also made of the actual concentration of lead being inhaled throughout the entire 24 hr of every day of the experimental period. Ideally, one would wish to know the amount of lead absorbed per unit time by persons whose blood lead concentrations are also known. Even a knowledge of the amount of lead inhaled and ingested and the contemporaneous concentration of lead in the blood would be useful as an index of lead absorption.

Taking what information is currently available, an analysis has been reported by Goldsmith and Hexter[80] of the relation between blood lead and estimated exposure to atmospheric lead. In the analysis, air sampling data and blood lead determinations that were not necessarily taken at the same time and place had to be used. A dose-response relation was suggested by a plot of lead concentration in blood against concentration in air. This relation was elaborated by the inclusion of data from experimental subjects exposed to high, known concentrations of lead sesquioxide.[202] The regression line for the data was calculated solely on the basis of the epidemiologic data, and the point was made that the experimental data only reinforce the validity of the relation (Figure 3-2). The blood data used were those from men only, because the concentration of lead is known to be lower in women than in men living in similar environmental circumstances.[554] The validity of calculating a regression line from these data has been challenged on the basis of the variability of the absorption of lead from larger sources (e.g., food), but not the general proposition that the atmosphere is a source of lead that can be absorbed.[520] A significant regression, in any case, could not be said to exist for the data below the value of approximately 2 $\mu g/m^3$.[201] Thus, the regres-

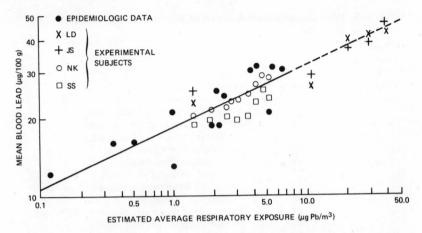

FIGURE 3-2 Mean blood lead concentration for epidemiologic and experimental respiratory exposures with regression from epidemiologic data only. Redrawn from Goldsmith and Hexter.[202]

sion line cannot be applied with confidence to the exposure conditions affecting the general population; this is so even for the general population of most large urban centers, inasmuch as average ambient air concentrations even in these centers do not generally exceed 2 $\mu g/m^3$.

The most extensive study of the relation between exposure to atmospheric lead and lead concentration in blood was conducted under the auspices of the U.S. Public Health Service from 1961 through 1963.[80] Several thousand atmospheric samples were collected and analyzed for lead, as well as samples of blood and urine from over 500 persons. The study was conducted in the metropolitan areas of Los Angeles, Philadelphia, and Cincinnati, which were selected because their atmospheric lead concentrations were known from prior investigations. A general trend was noted toward an increase in the concentration of lead in the blood of the different groups as they varied from rural or suburban areas to the central cities in their place of residence or work (Table 3-5). It was inferred that atmospheric lead contributes to total blood lead, although differences in dietary lead intake among the groups might have contributed to the differences in blood concentrations. In a preliminary examination of data from a more recent study involving 1,441 women, no relation could be detected between exposure to lead in the ambient air (0.17–3.39 $\mu g/m^3$) and blood lead (L. B. Tepper, personal communication).

TABLE 3-5   Lead Concentration in Blood of Selected Groups of Males[a]

Mean Lead Concentration in Blood, mg/100 g[b]	No. Subjects	Group
0.011	9	Suburban nonsmokers, Philadelphia
0.012	16	Residents of rural California county
0.013	10	Commuter nonsmokers, Philadelphia
0.015	14	Suburban smokers, Philadelphia
0.019	88	City employees, Pasadena
0.021	33	Commuter smokers, Philadelphia
0.021	36	City health department employees, Cincinnati
0.021	155	Policemen, Los Angeles
0.022	11	Live and work downtown, nonsmokers, Philadelphia
0.023	140	Post-office employees, Cincinnati
0.024	30	Policemen, nonsmokers, Philadelphia
0.025	191	Firemen, Cincinnati
0.025	123	Policemen, Cincinnati
0.025	55	Live and work downtown, smokers, Philadelphia
0.026	83	Policemen, smokers, Philadelphia
0.027	86	Refinery handlers of gasoline, Cincinnati (1956)
0.028	130	Service-station attendants, Cincinnati (1956)
0.030	40	Traffic policemen, Cincinnati
0.030	60	Tunnel employees, Boston
0.031	17	Traffic policemen, Cincinnati (1956)
0.031	14	Drivers of cars, Cincinnati
0.033	45	Drivers of cars, Cincinnati (1956)
0.034	48	Parking-lot attendants, Cincinnati (1956)
	1,434	Total

[a]Adapted from Three Cities Study.[554]
[b]Values are those determined for the 1965 study, except where otherwise indicated.

In the studies cited above, cigarette smokers have slightly higher blood lead concentrations than nonsmokers of similar residence and place of work. This can be attributed to the inhalation of additional lead from cigarettes, because each cigarette generates about 1–2 μg of airborne lead when burned.[128] However, although the majority of workers have found consistently increased blood lead content among cigarette smokers,[345] others have failed to confirm this finding (M. McLaughlin and G. J. Stopps, personal communication).

The purpose of the Goldsmith-Hexter regression line (Figure 3-2) was to adduce evidence concerning the contribution of atmospheric lead to the body burden of lead in the general population. The same approach has been used by Danielson in an effort to describe a dose-response relation between total daily lead assimilation and lead concentration in blood.[138] The author used the epidemiologic data of Goldsmith and Hexter for blood lead and for presumed atmospheric lead. He then assumed that all these groups were receiving the same amount of lead, 350 μg/day, in their diets, and were inhaling 15 m³ of air per day. To get from potential input to actual input, he assumed 10% retention of dietary lead. Data for two experimental subjects receiving 1 and 2 mg of lead per day added to their diet were included. A regression line was then plotted, giving a dose-response relation. Although this approach seems sound, the assumptions are somewhat at variance with available information. The retention of lead in the lungs probably is considerably lower than the 50% assumed in this particular report. Even if one assumes total retention of lead deposited in the respiratory tract, the data available suggest that lung deposition should be about 37% for particles of the size usually encountered in ambient air, and not 50%. Another assumption that seems to have been in error was that an average man inhales 15 m³ of air per day. Current information suggests that 23 m³ would be a better estimate for "reference man" engaged in light working activity (Table 3-1).

Using epidemiologic data for lead concentrations in the blood of various groups of men whose exposure to atmospheric lead differed[80] and data for two experimental subjects whose dietary intake of lead was known and who were exposed to atmospheric lead estimated at 2 μg/m³ (subjects E. B. and M. R.[298]), the relation between blood lead and daily lead intake can be estimated (Figure 3-3). This is a revision of the dose-response relation discussed above,[138] using the same sources of data on lead in inhaled air and blood and assuming complete retention of the 30% or 37% deposited from inhalation of 23 m³ of air per day and oral intake of 300 μg of lead per day with 10% absorption.

Some may find it difficult to accept the assumption that all the lead deposited in the airways is retained and absorbed. The only evidence available on this point was provided by Kehoe.[298] His study of the inhalation of lead sesquioxide suggested that all the particles deposited in the airways are retained if the particles are small (0.25 μm MMED). On inhalation of such an aerosol for 22 weeks, 8 hr/day, the urinary excretion of lead doubled within 2 weeks and persisted at that level for the duration of the period of exposure. Essentially total freedom from the swallowing of lead moved upward from the lungs and their passages, and total retention of the lead deposited in the respiratory tract is inferred from the absence of a corresponding in-

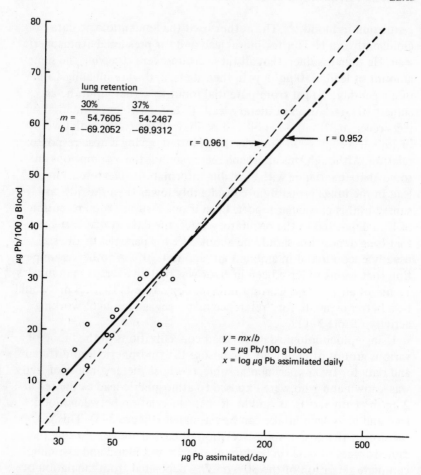

FIGURE 3-3 Relation between total absorption of lead and concentration of lead in blood. Calculations based on assumptions of 23 m³ of air inhaled per day, absorption of 10% of 300 µg of lead per day oral intake, and retention of 37% (solid line) or 30% (broken line) of inhaled lead. See Appendix C for original data (solid line) and calculations.

crease in fecal excretion of lead. Retrograde movement of lead from the airways back into the nasopharynx therefore seems not to have occurred. By contrast, Kehoe's experiments with the larger lead particles (50% larger than 2.9 µm MMED) suggest that only particles exceeding 2.9 µm in MMED are subject to such retrograde movement. This is inferred from the estimate that approximately 40% of the total lead, by weight, in this experiment was swallowed after lung deposition. The rest was probably retained in the airways and eventually absorbed into the body. The tendency for particles to be deposited in the nasopharynx, as opposed to the lower airways, increases with particle size. Thus, if 50% of the particles exceeded 2.9 μm in MMED and only 40% of the lead, by weight, was transferred to the gastrointestinal tract, almost all the particles below 2.9 μm in MMED were probably retained in the lungs. Inasmuch as 90% of the lead particles in ambient air are smaller than 1.6 μm in MMED,[456] it would seem from Kehoe's data that retention of deposited lead particles of the size found in ambient air is essentially complete. Even if one were to assume only 30% retention of the inhaled lead, the calculated total intake of lead over the range of 20–80 μg/100 g of blood would differ by less than 10% from the amount calculated on the assumption of 37% retention (Figure 3–3).

It is not the purpose of this chapter to discuss the biologic effects of lead. However, it will be established in Chapter 4 that biologic effects, including clinical lead poisoning, can be related to blood lead concentrations, if only in a general way.

ACCUMULATION

The extensive balance studies performed by Kehoe led him to conclude that in normal environmental circumstances man achieves a steady state with regard to lead fairly early in life and maintains this steady state, wherein the rate of output approximately equals the rate of input.[296,299,302] In support of this conclusion, he cited a limited study of the concentration of lead in the bones of people of various ages in which no age-related increase was apparent. More extensive studies have been conducted regarding the concentration of lead in human tissues. Some investigators report no marked variation with age;[426,538] others report substantial increases.[261,482] In these studies, the concentration of lead in bone (expressed in terms of ash) increased up to the age of 40 and perhaps beyond. A similar age-related increase was noted in the wall of the aorta;[482] the possibility that the increase might be due to disease (e.g., calcification) was not ruled out. The rising concentrations of lead in bone and aorta were found in both U.S. and foreign populations. Age-related increases were also found in some other organs of North Americans, but not of some foreign populations.

There are two possible explanations for these increases. The first is that the older people were formerly exposed to higher concentrations of lead than they are today and have retained this lead in their dense bone. This is probably not true with regard to oral intake of lead in food, but it may be true of lead in drinking water. One can only speculate as to changes in respiratory exposure, because air sampling programs are too new to allow comparison of today's air with the air of 30 years ago.

The other possibility is that lead is sufficiently accumulative to result in increasing concentrations through middle life, even at a constant rate of intake. Studies of the rate of loss from the body of single doses of radioactive lead in rats,[55, 366] rabbits,[525] and dogs[39] have been reported. In all cases, the rate of loss conformed to power-function kinetics. That is, the fraction of the dose remaining in the body was less and less readily excreted with the passage of time, perhaps as the lead slowly moved into the dense bone and became metabolically inaccessible. These observations were made on animals and were of relatively short duration, compared with the life-span of man, but they are nonetheless compatible with the data that suggest some accumulation over man's life-span.

Accumulation of lead in the body is not necessarily paralleled by an increase in hazard. The concept of biologic availability must be considered. Elements whose accumulation is accentuated by progressively decreasing availability for excretion are bone-seekers. They are poorly excreted because they become relatively isolated from the blood as they move into dense bone matrix, which is a compartment having a very low turnover rate. In the case of radioactive bone-seekers, such as strontium-90, burial in the matrix of bone does not result in biologic inactivation, because the emitted radiations influence biologic processes that occur well beyond the immediate atomic environment. In the case of stable elements, such as the species of lead (lead-207) that is the major source of environmental contamination, isolation in dense bone is equated with biologic inactivation. The accumulation of lead in the body with age may also involve some soft tissues, such as the wall of the aorta. The biologic availability of lead in soft tissues may similarly decrease with age. The lack of age-related increase in the concentration of lead in the blood or blood serum of adults (see above) suggests an absence of increase in the readily exchangeable or biologically available lead with age.

SUMMARY

The diet is the major source of lead in man and probably in most animals. The lead content of most water supplies in the United States

does not exceed 50 μg/liter, and general distribution samples have
the same content. The daily intake of lead from this source for an
adult is probably about 20 μg.

The natural lead content of food has been estimated at 0.01 ppm,
but some analyses show higher levels—up to 2.5 ppm, depending on
the type of food. On the basis of the accepted average of 0.2 ppm,
the daily adult intake, depending on factors determining the food
eaten, is 100–500 μg. The daily average oral intake of lead in this
country is thus about 300 μg, and limited data indicate that this figure
has not changed significantly during the last 30 years. Infants on a
mixed diet are estimated to take in 130 μg/day, proportionally more
than adults on a body-weight basis but not on the basis of metabolic
rate or caloric requirement.

The atmospheric contribution to the lead content of foods is probably not significant; near heavy sources, such as highways, lead contained in particulate matter is largely washed from plant parts consumed by man. Fallout probably contributes significantly to the
intake of animals only under very unusual circumstances.

The net absorption of lead from the gastrointestinal tract is 5–10%
if the intake is not substantially increased. Under usual dietary conditions, therefore, about 30 μg of lead are absorbed daily by man
from food and beverages. Calcium and phosphorus intake seem not
to alter absorption substantially; nothing is known of other dietary
influences in man. Data on normal fecal and urinary excretion and
on excretion after administration of lead-212 in man and experimental animals suggest that the fecal route is at least as important in lead
loss as the urinary route.

The contribution of inhaled lead to the total daily assimilation of
lead in man is not clearly known. Speculation as to its contribution
is based on limited studies of lung deposition and on data concerning
atmospheric lead concentrations in the general environment, rather
than in the specific environment determined continuously for periods
of weeks or even days. Lung deposition is estimated to be approximately 37% in man. The lung clearance of inhaled lead is largely unknown. What little information there is suggests that, in the particle
size range found in ambient air, lead deposited in the respiratory tract
undergoes very little, if any, oral transfer to the gastrointestinal tract.
For all practical purposes, all the lead deposited in the lung seems to
be retained. On the basis of all the above considerations, it is to be
expected that the atmospheric contribution of lead to the total daily
assimilation by a standard man engaged in light activity would be

extremely variable, depending on where he lives and works. Epidemiologic data gathered to date have not provided convincing evidence that inhaled lead contributes to the concentration of lead in the blood at atmospheric concentrations below $2–3$ $\mu g/m^3$. There is some evidence of a contribution when the atmospheric concentration of lead is higher.

The exposure of people in the general population to lead results in some accumulation in the body up to and perhaps beyond the age of 40, as determined by analysis of tissues. There is no apparent concurrent increase in lead circulating in the blood. The biologic significance of and reason for the increase are not known.

4

Biologic Effects of Lead in Man

Knowledge of the biologic effects of lead in man is based largely on the study of persons with overt clinical lead poisoning and on experience in the medical supervision of workers industrially exposed to lead. Exposure to lead in these groups is considerably greater than exposure likely to be encountered by the general population, whose intake of lead is derived from normal food sources and the ambient air. Similarly, most of the available experimental data on intact animals are based on studies in which high doses of lead have been administered. Although the effects of high doses of lead in man and experimental animals do not necessarily permit precise estimates of possible biologic effects of lower doses, they do point to areas of metabolism and function in man in which further study of the dose-response relations at the subclinical level is appropriate. Types of exposure associated with clinical lead poisoning are also important, because they represent clear and present risks to some segments of the population. Because the total amount of lead absorbed by a person may be derived from several sources, airborne lead must be considered in relation to other sources to which various population groups may be exposed.

ETIOLOGY OF LEAD POISONING IN MAN

Uncontrolled industrial exposure to airborne lead, the eating of lead-pigment residential paints by children with pica, and the drinking of illicitly distilled lead-contaminated whiskey are responsible for most of the cases of overt clinical illness due to lead poisoning today. What information is available concerning dose-response relations in man is derived largely from the study of groups poisoned in those ways. The burning of discarded battery casings in the home and contamination of food and drink by improperly lead-glazed earthenware vessels have also been responsible for severe illness from time to time.

Industrial Exposure to Lead and Its Compounds

A brief perusal of Table 1–3 should indicate which population in the United States stands at greatest risk of suffering untoward effects engendered by lead and its compounds. Review of those data indicates that metal products and miscellaneous and unclassified uses account for 72% of the lead consumed in the United States. Consideration of each of the products in these groups in terms of the biologic availability of the lead therein makes it apparent that as finished products they do not, in normal use, pose threats to human health. However, because fabrication may include heating, grinding, dissolution and volatilization, spraying, or other manipulations productive of biologically available forms of lead, workers engaged in each type of manufacture shown in Table 1–3 represent industrial populations that are at risk of lead absorption. By contrast, normal use of the products poses essentially no risk to the general population of users.

The ubiquity of lead—in contrast with other nonferrous metals—in industry is indicated by a U.S. Public Health Service list of 113 potential occupational exposures[192] attended by a risk of lead poisoning. A reliable definition of the extent of the risk of occupational lead exposure is unavailable. In contrast with numerous other technologically advanced nations, the United States has no data on the prevalence of occupational lead poisoning. Except for a few of the states—whose reporting systems are of questionable adequacy—no data of this nature are available. It is hoped that the Occupational Safety and Health Act of 1970 will lead to the accumulation of such data.

Estimates of the magnitude of the industrial health problem posed by lead exposure are fragmentary. H. E. Stokinger (personal communication), in a canvass of the persons in public agencies largely responsible for control of industrial lead exposure, attempted to collate their estimates of the trends in reported cases. In this survey, evidence based on lead measurements in air and urine indicated that "lead exposures had decreased by a factor of several magnitudes in ... 7 or 8 major categories representing the major uses of lead since 1934." On the basis of hitherto unassembled data, it seems that this decrease had "continued but at a slower rate since 1945."

Such impressions require some amplification. These reports represented mostly workers employed in relatively large corporations; large employers are more accessible to regulatory agencies than small shops. Furthermore, large corporations often provide lead-exposure control and medical surveillance programs, because they are economically better able to afford such environmental and medical controls. The potential magnitude of the problem of occupational lead poisoning is not clarified if one considers that approximately two thirds of all workers in the United States work for employers of 100 persons or fewer. There are also large groups of peripatetic workers—for example, in construction—for whom few data are available.

Stokinger, in 86 surveys of 26 different operations over a 4-year period, found indications of excessive exposure to lead, as judged by blood analysis, in 10–35% of exposed workers (Table 4–1). It should be emphasized that these data do not represent systematic sampling; often, they represent only the blood samples of persons thought to be suffering from lead poisoning, and many workers possibly suffering from lead absorption were not sampled. The manpower resources

TABLE 4-1 Percentage of Workers Tested Having Blood Lead Concentrations above Allowable Limits[a]

Year	No. Blood Specimens	Blood Samples Indicating Lead Poisoning		Estimated No. Exposed[b]
		No.	%	
1966	214	74	35	430
1967	114	17	15	215
1968	136	13	10	483
1969	104	14	13	276
Total	568	118		1,404

[a]From H. E. Stokinger, personal communication. Allowable limit = 100 μg/100 g of whole blood.
[b]Estimates might be incorrect by a factor of 2 or 3.

of the few effective official agencies are insufficient to permit representative sampling, and blood samples were sought from employers (usually large corporations) who were aware of the risks of lead exposure.

To place occupational exposures in their proper perspective as regards the general population risk, it is appropriate to consider the atmospheric concentrations associated with clinical occupationally induced lead poisoning. Data generated over many years indicate that cases of overt lead poisoning usually are associated with air concentrations of over 0.5 mg/m^3. A blood concentration of 80 μg/100 g of blood may produce symptoms and signs of lead poisoning in an exposed worker, and a concentration of 100 μg/100 g of blood will usually produce clinical manifestations. However, some investigators[196,491] have found 50–80 μg/100 g of whole blood associated with mild lead poisoning symptoms.

The magnitude of the differences between workers' exposure to atmospheric lead (and their blood lead concentrations) and community exposures (and the general population's blood lead concentrations) should place in proper perspective the risks of the occupationally exposed. These differences, coupled with a large potential working population at risk, should indicate the relative gravity of the occupational lead problem, compared with the lead problem of any other population group. It is reasonable to assume that any ill-defined potential health risks associated with long-term lead exposure that the general population may carry are also present among the large group occupationally exposed to lead. Thus, the occupationally exposed carry both the risk of overexposure, usually minimal in the general population, and a relatively higher risk of whatever lead-related harm may befall the general population as a result of community exposure.

Lead-Based Paints on Housing Surfaces

The clear association between lead poisoning in children with pica and old deteriorating and dilapidated urban housing in the United States, England, and Australia is well-documented.[188,221,271,273,358,397,514,583] The source of the lead is lead-pigment paints in one or more of the layers of paint applied to the woodwork and plastered and papered walls of dwellings before World War II, when lead pigments were common constituents of both interior and exterior house paint. In such paint, lead may constitute 5–40% of the final dried solids. These layers persist in flaking multilayer paint chips, crumbling plaster, and cracking wall paper in old substandard housing that is still in use. Within the dwellings, windowsills and frames are apparently most often nibbled by young children.[30,110] According to the 1960 U.S. Housing Census, 30.6 million dwelling units occupied in 1960 were built before 1940.[357] Of these, 5.6 million were classified in 1960 as deteriorating and 1.8 million as dilapidated. (Comparable data from the 1970 U.S. Census will not be available until after January 1972.) In Baltimore, 90% of the reported cases of lead poisoning are in children who live in multiple-dwelling, rented housing units.

Chisolm and Harrison[110] reported that old paint containing more than 1% lead (by weight) could be found on at least one of the surfaces of the home accessible to a young child in almost every case of poisoning. In 102 of 105 cases, at least one source containing more than 5% lead was found at the child's residence. In a survey of 100 randomly selected blocks of dwellings in Baltimore, lead in excess of 1% in paint was found on interior surfaces in 70% of 667 dwelling units.[484] Similar surveys of old housing in Philadelphia[271] and London[33] have likewise revealed that 70–80% of interior painted surfaces contained more than 1% lead. In these three surveys, only a few samples from each dwelling unit were analyzed. Extrapolation of a limited survey in Baltimore[484] indicated a 98% probability of houses with positive findings for lead if a greater number of samples per dwelling unit had been analyzed. In the investigation of actual cases, the analysis of 20–25 different samples is usually required to identify all the interior surfaces that are both positive for lead (more than 1% lead) and accessible to young children. Geographic spot maps have been kept by the Baltimore City Health Department during the last 30 years. They indicate that, as old inner-city dwellings are replaced by urban renewal and other modern construction, the location of reported cases moves outward from the center of the city and that cases are now found in older housing in nearly all parts of the city (E. W. Dahle, Jr., personal communication). In 1955, the American Standards Association developed a standard specifying that paints for toys, furniture, and the interior of dwellings should not contain "harmful quantities" of lead. The standard, now known as ANSI Standard Z66.1, limits the lead content to less than 1% lead in the final dried solids of fresh paint. This excludes lead pigments (usually white lead or lead carbonate and lead sulfate in oil-based paints), but it does not necessarily eliminate other lead additives in the total paint formulation. ANSI Standard Z66.1 also limits the concentrations of antimony, arsenic, cadmium, mercury, selenium, and barium in paints conforming to the standard. This standard was developed on the basis of a number of factors, including the observation that clinical cases of poisoning were associated with sources containing more than 1% lead in paint and the use of semiquantitative gravimetric methods of analysis at the time for testing paint samples.[288] Newer methods of detection based on the principle of x-ray fluorescence may call for revision of this 1% w/w standard, inasmuch as the result obtained by x-ray fluorescence analysis is expressed as weight of lead per unit of exposed wall surface (mg/cm^2).[334] Several prototype portable nondestructive detectors for *in situ* detection of lead in housing surfaces are now available. Their use can simplify and greatly speed detection. Because the detectors measure the amount of lead in 10 or more layers of paint, they provide a more useful value in terms of the dose of lead contained in multilayered flakes of paint of various thicknesses. For example, 10 layers of paint containing 1% lead would contain 10 times as much lead per unit area as one layer containing 1% lead, although both the 10-layer and the one-layer paint flakes would give a concentration of 1% by traditional gravimetric analysis. One report[110] showed four paint fragments with a surface of approximately 5 cm^2 weighing 2.68 g and containing 9.5% lead, or 254 mg of lead; had these fragments contained 0.95% lead, their removal would not have been required under the 1% gravimetric standard, although they would have contained 25 mg of lead. (The 1% gravimetric standard is the basis of all currently applicable municipal ordinances.) The amounts of lead found in the feces of children with lead poisoning[110] (range, 0.37–225 mg/24 hr) correspond to the amounts of lead found in multilayer paint chips with an exposed surface area of 1–5 cm^2.

Before 1940, lead pigments were widely used in both interior and exterior paints. Beginning about 1940, titanium dioxide, a less expensive white pigment, began to replace lead pigments, especially white lead, in interior paints. Even so, in Baltimore, for example, lead-pigment paints could still be bought for interior use until 1958, when a municipal ordinance designed to prohibit their sale was passed.[484] As of 1970, approximately 50% of exterior oil-based paints contain some lead in their pigments; the other 50% are latex paints and do not contain lead, except for small amounts that might be used for tinting purposes, according to information supplied by the National Paint, Varnish and Lacquer Association.* The laws and ordinances pertain-

*R. A. Roland, letter dated October 16, 1970.

ing to the labeling, use, and removal of lead-based paints in effect in October 1970 are summarized in Table 4–2. At that time, four states had laws pertaining to one or two of these aspects of the problem, and 10 municipalities had ordinances prohibiting the use of paints containing more than 1% lead in interior paints and requiring the removal by scraping or other means or covering of interior surfaces painted with high-lead paints accessible to children in dwelling units occupied by children with blood lead concentrations greater than 60 μg/100 g of whole blood. In some cities, enforcement has been difficult and far from satisfactory, especially where enforcement has been under criminal codes.[357] In Baltimore and Philadelphia, enforcement is carried out as a civil proceeding under the Hygiene of Hous-

TABLE 4–2 State and Local Laws and Ordinances Pertaining to Use of Lead in Interior House Paints (October 1970)[a]

	Labeling[b]	Use Prohibited	Removal Required[c]
State			
Connecticut	1967	1967[d]	–
Illinois	1958	–	–
Kansas	1958	–	–
New York	–	1970[e]	–
Municipality			
Baltimore, Md.	1958	1958	1951
Cincinnati, Ohio	1960	1960	1960
Cleveland, Ohio	1970	1970	1970
Jersey City, N.J.	1962	1962	1962
New Haven, Conn.	–	1968[f]	1968[f]
New York, N.Y.	1959	1970	1970
Philadelphia, Pa.	1966	1966	1966
St. Louis, Mo.	1970	1970[g]	1970[g]
Washington, D.C.	–	1970	1970
Wilmington, Del.	1963	1963	1963

[a]According to information supplied by National Paint, Varnish and Lacquer Association, Inc., Washington, D.C. (legislation thought to be pending in Minneapolis-St. Paul, Minn., and Newark, N.J., as of October 1970).
[b]Label on paint can conforms to ANSI Standard Z66.1, which identifies paints containing <1% lead as safe for interior use. Label must state whether paint conforms to this standard.
[c]Ordinances invoked in dwelling units of children found to have blood lead concentrations >60 μg/100 g of whole blood in most cities listed.
[d]Prohibits use of paints not conforming to ANSI Standard Z66.1 on interior of dwellings owned or planned by municipalities or other housing agencies. Does not apply to privately owned dwellings.
[e]Also prohibits use of paints containing >1% lead on porches.
[f]Prohibits use of paints containing >1% lead on both interior and exterior surfaces accessible to children in all dwellings, whether publicly or privately owned. Requires proper maintenance of surfaces.
[g]Prohibits use of paints containing >1% of lead on interiors. "Exterior" requirement limited to flaking or peeling surfaces.

ing Code, and the fine for noncompliance is cumulative for each successive day of noncompliance after a grace period of approximately 4–6 weeks. Also, surfaces must be inspected after removal of the old paint before repainting is allowed. In New York City, under the 1970 ordinance, the city will itself remove old lead-based paint and recover the cost through a lien on the property if the owner fails to do so after proper notification. A number of the municipal ordinances (Table 4–2) require removal only from the residence in which the child with high blood lead concentration lives and from public access passages; other apartments and areas in multiple-unit buildings are not affected.

The Lead-Based Paint Poisoning Prevention Act (Public Law 91–695), signed into law on January 14, 1971, was to assist local governments in coping with the problem of lead poisoning in old, poorly maintained houses.[550] * The paint industry has complied with labeling provisions under the Federal Hazardous Substances (Labeling) Act (1960) and, even earlier, under ANSI Standard Z66.1. The hazard presented by lead-based paint is related both to the lead content of the paint and to poor maintenance of painted surfaces. It is easy for a child to pick and eat loose flakes from chipped and deteriorating painted surfaces. The lead content of such paint flakes is far in excess of the amount of lead likely to be inhaled, even in congested areas, so it seems clear that the direct ingestion of lead-containing paint chips is the principal environmental cause in clinical cases of lead poisoning in children. The question of the lead content of dusts as they may contribute to children's total oral intake of lead is considered later in this chapter.

Improperly Lead-Glazed Earthenware Vessels

Acidic foods and beverages—including tomatoes, tomato juice, most fruits and fruit juices, cola drinks, such alcoholic beverages as wine and cider, and pickles and relishes stored in vinegar or cider—can dissolve the lead in improperly lead-glazed earthenware (pottery) containers. Foods and beverages so contaminated have been responsible for fatal[309] and nonfatal[240] cases of human lead poisoning.

The many factors that influence the amount of lead that can be leached into food or beverage include the ratio of lead oxide to silica in the formulation of the frit, the presence of pigments and other

*Congress has appropriated $7.5 million for FY 1972.

constituents in the frit, the temperature at which the glaze is fired, the acidity and temperature of the food or beverage stored in the vessel, and the length of time the acidic food or beverage remains in contact with the improperly glazed vessel.[252,309] Extreme care is required to formulate and fuse a safe glaze on earthenware vessels. Of particular importance is the low temperature (less than 1150 C) used for firing earthenware pottery glazes. Safe conditions are not easily ensured by amateur potters. But stoneware is fired at 1200–1260 C and presents no hazard because the residual lead, after firing, is fused completely as an insoluble lead silicate glaze.

In one case, a man was found to be consuming 3.2 mg of lead per day in a chilled cola drink, which he drank nightly from a home-handicrafted earthenware mug.[240] In another case, apple juice stored in an earthenware pitcher was found to contain 157 mg/liter if stored in the pitcher for 3 hr and 1,300 mg/liter if stored for 3 days.[309] Klein et al.[309] tested 117 earthenware vessels purchased in Montreal, Canada, over the counter through retail outlets. Approximately 50% of the items tested had a "lead release" considered unsafe by current standards. These and other data are summarized in Table 4–3. The Canadian Department of Consumer and Corporate Affairs has confirmed these findings, especially in earthenware produced by studios and hobbyists and in imported items. Re-evaluation of current regulations, practices, and control measures is now under consideration in Canada and the United States to reduce this potential hazard to the general public. It is highly unlikely that hobbyists will ever be able to produce earthenware items that are consistently safe for use as food and beverage containers. Visual inspection of an item does not permit a purchaser to distinguish between glazed earthenware (which may not be safe) and stoneware (which is safe).[308]

Discarded Battery Casings

Discarded automobile battery casings made of wood[584] and vulcanite[197] have been used as fuel in wood-burning cookstoves and fireplaces during times of extreme economic distress among the poor. Fatal and nonfatal cases of lead poisoning, chiefly among young children, have been traced to this source. Such outbreaks have been controlled by halting the distribution of the casings to the poor and by institution of measures for the safe disposal of the casings.[197,584] Whether lead poisoning in these outbreaks resulted from inhalation of lead fume or dust or from ingestion of lead dust is not entirely

TABLE 4-3 Report of Lead Extractions from 264 Earthenware Glaze Surfaces[a]

Sample Group	No. Glaze Surfaces	Lead Extraction, ppm[b]						
		<0.5	0.5–7	7–20	20–100	>100	100–500	500–1,000
Group A[c]								
Imported pottery	29	9	5	6	6	3	–	–
Domestic commercial ware	48	17	7	4	15	5	–	–
Domestic handicraft	40	10	4	4	6	16	–	–
Totals	117	36	16	14	27	24		
Group B[d]	147	36	36	32	14	–	10	19

[a]Adapted from Klein et al. 309
[b]Standard room-temperature acetic acid test used; <7 ppm of lead considered safe for table use.
[c]Samples obtained over the counter from handicraft shops and department stores.
[d]Samples of identical size and clay composition treated with 49 different glaze compositions.

clear; however, Gillet[197] thought that ingestion was the major route of absorption. He noted that the maximal temperature obtainable in domestic cookstoves in use in Rotherham (1000 C) was not sufficient to volatilize lead and that almost all the cases of poisoning occurred in children of preschool age, the age group in which pica is most prevalent. Inhalation of lead dust by young children or contamination of food in these outbreaks might, however, result in a higher dose of lead per unit of body weight, compared with that to which adults were subjected, because of children's higher metabolism per unit of body weight.* The problem of the actual route of entry into the body (lung or gastrointestinal tract) remains unsolved in these battery-casing outbreaks; but in either case, the dose to the child would be higher. The burning of battery casings is the only nonindustrial type of potential respiratory exposure to lead that has been associated with actual human cases of lead poisoning.

Illicitly Distilled Whiskey

Lead is a common contaminant of the illicitly distilled whiskey (moonshine) manufactured in the United States. The reason is the method of construction of the stills. Automobile radiators are frequently used as condensers, with the other components connected by lead soldering. Thus, hot vapors and the liquor come into contact with metallic lead. Although the forms in which lead is present in the liquor have not been identified, it has been suggested that acetic acid in the distillate may react with lead to form lead acetate.[28] In any case, the concentration of lead in moonshine whiskey may exceed 1 mg/liter in 30% of samples (Table 4–4).

In contrast with moonshine, concentrations of lead in 20 brands of alcoholic beverages assayed by the Laboratory Services Branch of EPA at Cincinnati, Ohio, were found not to exceed 0.4 mg/liter; 12 of the brands contained less than 0.2 mg/liter.[171]

The use of moonshine whiskey is widespread. Figure 4–1 indicates

---

*Studies in respiratory physiology[515] indicate that oxygen consumption requires an intake of 5–6 m^3 of air per 1,000 cal metabolized. A 1-year-old child weighing 10 kg would metabolize 1,000 cal per day on the average and would inhale 5–6 m^3 of air. In conditions of comparable environmental exposure, a child would inhale two to three times as much of a given pollutant as would an adult per unit of body weight. The younger the infant, the higher the metabolic rate and the greater the difference in dose between adult and child on the basis of body weight.

TABLE 4-4 Lead Content of Illicitly Distilled Whiskey[a]

Study No., State, or Region	No. Samples Analyzed for Lead	No. Samples in Indicated Range				Max., mg/Liter
		<0.001 mg/Liter	0.001–0.999 mg/Liter	1–10 mg/Liter	>10 mg/Liter	
65	221	30	134	52	5	23.8
Nashville, Tenn., area	40	0	23	17	0	4.0
Southeast region	100	22	42	32	4	20.8
Southwest region	50	26	19	5	0	
Alabama	18	2	9	5	2	20.9
Florida	4	1	2	1	0	3.2
Georgia	30	4	15	10	1	16.4
Mississippi	17	3	10	3	1	20.5
North Carolina	35	12	15	7	1	38.5
South Carolina	265	29	154	70	12	86.4
Tennessee	11	2	8	1	0	2.2
Total	791	131 (16.6%)	431 (54.5%)	203 (25.7%)	26 (3.3%)	86.4

[a]Data from Alcohol, Tobacco and Firearms Division Laboratory, Internal Revenue Service, U.S. Treasury Department.

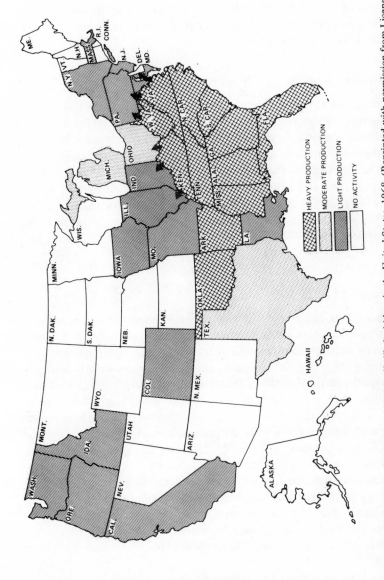

FIGURE 4–1 Production and distribution of illicitly distilled whiskey in the United States, 1968. (Reprinted with permission from Licensed Beverage Industries, Inc.[399])

83

the major areas of manufacture and distribution. Although the amounts produced are unknown, it was estimated in 1968 that more than 36 million gallons were produced.[399] The incidence of clinical poisoning by lead from moonshine is unknown; as is the case with many unusual illnesses, the frequency of diagnosis is directly related to physicians' awareness of the problem.

Miscellaneous Sources

Sporadic cases of classic human lead poisoning have been traced to lead-painted children's toys and furniture, lead toys and baubles eaten by children, lead nipple shields, home battery manufacture, artists' paint pigments (used in hand mixing), lead dust in shooting galleries (with the attendant at risk), soluble lead compounds conveyed in lead pipes, ashes and fumes of painted wood, some patented "medications," jewelers' wastes, and lead type in schools for the blind. Lead has been used in cosmetic products through the years; there is no information on whether it presents a significant hazard to health.

CLINICAL EFFECTS

Lead poisoning can give rise to several well-known but nonspecific clinical syndromes of illness in man, including anemia and the syndromes of acute abdominal colic, acute encephalopathy, chronic encephalopathy, peripheral neuropathy, and chronic or late lead nephropathy with or without secondary gout. Under conditions of prolonged or recurrent uncontrolled excessive exposure, the clinical picture in a given person is of recurrent episodes of acute lead poisoning on a background of slowly progressive renal insufficiency and cerebral incompetence.[19,78,169,394,524] Each of the syndromes of acute lead poisoning may abate spontaneously on cessation of the hazardous exposure. A single episode of acute encephalopathy in a young child may be followed by brain damage varying in severity from subtle learning deficits to profound mental deficiency. Clinical descriptions of lead poisoning may be found in the writings of Tanquerel[524] and Aub et al.,[19] in modern texts,[105,394] and in various reviews.[9,78,169]

It has long been thought that young children might be more susceptible than adults to the toxic effects of lead. Certainly, the clinical manifestations of a variety of diseases are more devastating in a very young child than in a mature adult. The observed differences in responses between children and adults may be attributed to children's rapid growth, which limits their capacity to respond to adverse agents. Factors associated with rapid growth may well limit a child's capacity to compensate for the absorption of increased amounts of lead, but this hypothesis has not been documented at the clinical level. The early symptoms of lead poisoning are subtle, subjective, and nonspecific and therefore not so readily recognized in children. Less severe signs and symptoms of lead poisoning, such as anemia and acute abdominal colic, are the clinical manifestations most often recognized in adults. In children, such mild symptoms are often either overlooked or attributed to other disease states, so that poisoning due to lead is more likely to be recognized first at a late or severe stage on the basis of nervous-system involvement (acute encephalopathy). Most adult lead poisoning is associated with occupational exposure, which is usually less severe than the types of exposure associated with childhood lead poisoning. The imbibers of lead-contaminated moonshine whiskey, who may be subject to very high doses, as are children, are usually first recognized clinically as having acute encephalopathy or late lead nephropathy. When the factor of dose is taken into account, the clinical response—particularly at high doses—appears to be comparable in children and adults. Clinical responses to moderate increases in soft-tissue lead content are ill-defined, particularly in very young children. Nevertheless, a rapidly growing child's response to moderately increased lead content may well differ from that of an adult, despite the current inability to perceive the response.

Anemia

Lead poisoning gives rise to a mild hypochromic and sometimes microcytic anemia. The anemia is also associated with shortened red-cell life-span, reticulocytosis, and the presence of basophilic stippled cells in the peripheral blood.[42,43,220,249,277,346,567,572] The symptoms of this anemia include pallor, waxy sallow complexion, easy fatigability, irritability, and headache. In young children unable to describe such symptoms, anemia may give rise to decreased play activity, and irritability may masquerade as a "behavior disturbance." Anemia due to lead poisoning has many morphologic features in common with the anemias of iron deficiency and thalassemia; hence, these three conditions are not always easily distinguished. Basophilic stippled cell counts may be influenced by the method of preparation of the smear[43] and by the presence or absence of anticoagulants. Bone marrow preparations in lead-poisoning anemia consistently show greatly increased numbers of sideroblasts, which distinguish the anemia due to lead poisoning from that due to iron-deficiency states. In the absence of iron deficiency, the iron content in serum and bone marrow may be increased in lead poisoning. The clinical symptoms of anemia due to lead are indistinguishable from those of chronic anemias with a variety of other causes. Anemia due to lead is often seen in association with acute abdominal colic.

Acute Abdominal Colic

In adults, acute abdominal colic due to lead poisoning is often preceded by headache and may be associated with generalized muscle aches. These are followed by constipation and, within a few days, attacks of crampy diffuse abdominal pain. When pain and constipation to the point of obstipation are severe, there may be vomiting, anorexia with associated weight loss and easy fatigability, and a complaint of a bad taste in the mouth. This sequence of events usually develops over a period of 1–2 weeks.[278] In patients without obvious exposure to lead, this syndrome may result in inappropriate laparotomy. In very young persons, acute abdominal colic due to lead poisoning finds its clinical expression in the form of anorexia, apathy, irritability, refusal to play, pugnaciousness, episodic vomiting, and constipation. These symptoms may abate spontaneously on cessation of the abnormal exposure to lead.

Acute Encephalopathy

Encephalopathy is the most severe acute clinical form of lead poisoning. It may arise precipitously with the onset of intractable seizures, followed by coma and cardiorespiratory arrest. Prodromal manifestations may or may not occur. In fatal cases, death usually occurs within 48 hr of the initial seizure, unless life is supported by artificial cardiopulmonary devices. This brief catastrophic sequence may also occur on a background of anemia and mild colic in patients who are under observation but are not thought to be very ill until the initial seizure. The fulminant form of encephalopathy usually develops within a week. Vomiting, which may have been sporadic previously, becomes increasingly frequent, persistent, and forceful. Apathy progresses to drowsiness and stupor, interspersed with lucidity or hyperirritability. In severe cases, these alterations in the state of consciousness progress rapidly to coma and convulsions during the final 48 hr.[9,105] About 20% of patients have a history of recent onset of clumsiness and show frank ataxia on examination. Other neurologic manifestations, such as paralysis and weakness, are usually found postictally. The prodroma of acute encephalopathy due to lead poisoning also include subtle changes in mental attitude, sluggishness, poor memory, inability to concentrate, restlessness, and hyperirritability. Adults may report mental depression, persistent headache, vertigo, and tremor shortly before the onset of convulsions.[19] Both the onset and the clinical course of acute encephalopathy are unpredictable. Symptoms may abate at any point in the sequence if the patient is removed from gross exposure to lead.

Two reports[101,106] indicate that one third to one half of children with acute encephalopathy due to lead poisoning may also manifest acute renal injury in the form of the Fanconi syndrome (generalized renal hyperaminoaciduria, glycosuria, and hyperphosphaturia in the presence of hypophosphatemia). In addition, patients with acute encephalopathy may also be oliguric. Pathologically, the most extensive neuronal injury is in the cerebellum, although there is diffuse injury to nerve cells throughout the brain. Vascular injury is the basic lesion responsible for diffuse severe cerebral edema and the pressure effects of acute encephalopathy. Factors that increase the risk of death include diagnostic lumbar puncture and diagnostic and therapeutic neurosurgical procedures during the acute phase. These and other important aspects of clinical diagnosis and management are discussed elsewhere.[9,106]

The division of encephalopathy into "severe" and "mild" groups is mainly of prognostic significance in terms of survival and the severity of neurologic sequelae. Patients whose condition is classified clinically as "severe" are those with either intractable seizures or coma or both for 24 hr or longer. Patients whose condition is classified clinically as "mild" encephalopathy include all those with the above features lasting less than 24 hr and those with less severe impairment of consciousness. Ataxic patients without impaired consciousness are sometimes included in groups classified as having "mild" encephalopathy and are sometimes grouped separately.[442]

Acute lead encephalopathy today is associated with the following types of exposure: ingestion of lead-pigment paint chips by children with pica, burning of discarded battery casings in homes for fuel, contamination of beverages by improperly lead-glazed earthenware vessels, and illicitly distilled whiskey containing lead.

Chronic Encephalopathy

Exposure to lead occasionally produces clear-cut progressive mental deterioration in children. They are usually over 3 years old. Their clinical history indicates normal development during the first 12–18 months of life or longer, followed by a steady loss of motor skills and loss of speech to the point of mutism. These children may also have severe hyperkinetic and aggressive behavior disorders and a poorly controlled convulsive disorder. There is often evidence of current excessive absorption of lead. Blood lead concentrations are in excess of 60 μg/100 g of whole blood, and x rays may show heavy multiple bands of increased density at the metaphyses of the growing long bones. These findings in older preschool children indicate prolonged increased absorption of lead. This clinical entity has been termed "chronic encephalopathy." Its etiology is not at all clear. It represents the final clinical expression of diffuse cerebral injury incurred during infancy and early childhood and may be due to a number of traumatic, toxic, viral, and bacterial agents. Such children also often have persistent pica, so that the evidence of current increased absorption of lead may be the result of pica superimposed on prior cerebral injury of a different cause. The diagnosis of acute lead encephalopathy can easily be missed repeatedly, and so this syndrome may also represent the sequel of prior episodes of acute lead encephalopathy and much higher blood lead concentrations in the past. The picture is also indistinguishable from the pattern seen after recurrent documented episodes of acute lead poisoning with or without acute encephalopathy, as described by Byers and Lord[78] and Perlstein and Attala.[442] The older medical literature[19,394] contains references to a similar picture of progressive premature dementia in adults in association with prolonged, grossly excessive occupational exposure to lead and a history of recurrent episodes of acute symptomatic lead poisoning. Fortunately, this is rare today, although it may conceivably occur in imbibers of lead-containing whiskey.

Peripheral Neuropathy

The distinguishing clinical feature of the peripheral neuropathy of lead poisoning is predominance of motor involvement, with minimal or absent sensory abnormalities. There is a tendency for the extensor muscles of the hands and feet to be involved. Three clinical forms are noted. In the first, patients with acute abdominal colic may also complain of very severe pain and tenderness in the trunk muscles, as well as pain in the muscles of the extremity. As the pain and tenderness subside, weakness may emerge, with very slow recovery over the ensuing several months. No epidemiologic data based on careful long-term follow-up are available to assess the frequency of this syndrome as a component of classic lead colic. In the second, more common form of peripheral neuropathy due to lead poisoning, the neuropathy is described as a painless peripheral extensor weakness occurring either after termination of excessive exposure or after long, moderately increased exposure. Emmerson[169] has described patients with pes cavus deformities resulting from old peripheral neuropathy. This suggests that neuropathy of sufficient severity may cause irreversible impairment of peripheral nerve function. The recent report of Catton et al.[94] concerning subclinical peripheral neuropathy in the absence of obvious clinical manifestations of lead poisoning suggests that the entire question of peripheral neuropathy needs re-evaluation. In the third form, neuropathic and myopathic features are almost indistinguishable. When muscle fasciculations and proximal girdle atrophy are present, the findings resemble those of amyotrophic lateral sclerosis.[503]

Late or Chronic Lead Nephropathy

The nephropathy seen in patients with a history of one or more episodes of acute lead intoxication is characterized by progressive and apparently irreversible renal insufficiency. Under the light microscope, renal biopsies and postmortem specimens show nonspecific interstitial fibrosis, tubular degeneration, and glomerular and vascular changes in small arteries and arterioles.[402,452] Under the electron microscope, characteristic tubular lesions similar to those in chronic experimental lead poisoning[211] may be found in humans.[193,452,453] Functionally and clinically, chronic lead nephropathy is characterized by progressive azotemia. In some patients, hyperuricemia with or without manifest gout may be associated with renal insufficiency.[29] The clinical differentiation between primary gout and lead gout is well described by Emmerson.[169] This clinical entity has, in recent years, been called "chronic lead nephropathy" by Richet et al.[193,452,453] in France, by Lilis et al.[354] in Rumania (in adults with chronic uncontrolled occupational exposure to lead), by Danilović[139] in Yugoslavia (in older children and adults consuming lead-contaminated flour), and by Morgan et al.[402] in the southeastern United States (in long-term imbibers of lead-contaminated illicitly distilled whiskey).

Nye,[427] in Queensland, Australia, was the first to note an association between chronic lead poisoning in childhood and delayed-onset chronic nephropathy. Because of the interval between the apparent termination of abnormal lead intake and the onset of clinical renal insufficiency and gout, the term "late" is sometimes applied to this lead nephropathy. As discussed by Lilis et al.,[354] there is considerable controversy in the literature as to the causative role of lead in progressive renal insufficiency with or without hypertension. Although Henderson[245] found a very high frequency of chronic nephritis among survivors of childhood lead poisoning in Queensland, Australia, Tepper[528] was unable to confirm this finding in Boston in young adults with a documented history of lead poisoning during early childhood. The apparent difference between the group studied by Tepper and the other groups is in the length of exposure. In the subjects studied by Tepper, acute lead poisoning occurred during the preschool years, whereas the other groups were subjected to prolonged uncontrolled exposure to lead for a period estimated at 10 years or longer.

At the time that the several groups of patients with chronic nephropathy underwent renal-function studies, spontaneous urinary lead excretion was normal, but the response to the CaEDTA mobilization test for lead was abnormal every time it was measured.[168,169,452] Emmerson[168] found this the most suitable measurement for differentiating between nephropathy apparently due to lead and other forms of chronic nephritis. His patients with lead nephropathy could be distinguished on the basis of bone-biopsy lead content, but not on the basis of spontaneous daily urinary lead output. Emmerson did not measure blood lead content; however, Richet et al.[453] reported minimally increased blood lead content in association with abnormal EDTA mobilization of lead in patients with renal injury attributed to the metal. Although the bulk of clinical evidence apparently points to prolonged and excessive absorption of lead as the central causative agent for this form of nephropathy, the possibility that other unrecognized factors play additive, synergistic, or modifying roles has not been adequately investigated and so cannot yet be excluded. For example, none of the reports includes measurements of other heavy metals. This topic is discussed in detail later in this chapter.

Relation between Symptoms of Acute Lead Poisoning and Lead Content of Blood

It is rarely possible in clinical situations to determine the amount of lead absorbed before the onset of symptoms of lead poisoning. In one case,[240] a man was estimated to have ingested approximately 3.2 mg/day for a period of 2 years before the onset of symptoms; however, no blood lead determination was made before treatment. The studies of Kehoe[298] in human adult volunteers who were fed known amounts of lead indicate that blood lead content may serve as an index of the degree of current and recent absorption of lead. Figure 4-2 shows the distribution of blood lead concentrations before treatment in relation to symptoms in 195 previously reported cases of childhood lead poisoning. Also shown are the concentrations from 98 fatal cases. The mean concentrations in fatal cases and in mild and severe cases of nonfatal acute encephalopathy were equivalent (approximately 330 μg/100 g of whole blood). All but one of 98 cases of fatal encephalopathy were associated with blood lead concentrations of 150 μg/100 g of whole blood or greater. Likewise, symptoms compatible with acute lead poisoning were, with few exceptions, found in children with concentrations greater than 100 μg/100 g of whole blood. Symptomatic lead poisoning has also been seen in persons with severe anemia in whom blood lead concentrations were less than 80 μg/100 g of whole blood. It cannot be stated unequivocally that the subjects classified in Figure 4-2 as asymptomatic were entirely asymptomatic; some had mild symptoms compatible with both mild lead poisoning and other disease states that were present at the time of examination. On the basis of clinical judgment, the symptoms were attributed to the acute infections found in the children, rather than to lead. Others[177,572] have reported comparable ranges of blood lead content for children with and without symptoms of lead poisoning.

The total urinary output of lead during 10 days of chelation therapy has been measured in nine children with acute encephalopathy. The data have been recalculated from a previous report[106] and are summarized in Table 4-5. The "chelatable lead" as determined by urinary output of lead does not represent the total body lead burden. Nevertheless, the values for chelatable lead shown in Table 4-5 exceed by a factor of 20 the estimates of total body lead burden based on postmortem analysis of tissues for lead by Barry and Mossman.[35] For normal children of comparable age and body weight, they estimated total body lead burden at 0.23 mg/kg of body weight (range,

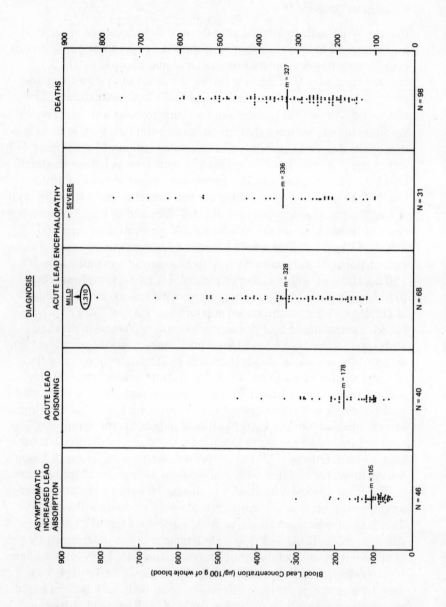

FIGURE 4-2   Relation between concentration of lead in blood and clinical symptoms in children with acute lead poisoning. The criteria for each of the diagnostic groups are as stated in Chisolm and Harrison,[110] except that spinal fluid examinations were not performed after 1956; after 1956, the minimal clinical criterion for the diagnosis of acute encephalopathy was the presence of drowsiness or stupor. The data presented in this figure have not been previously published. They are taken from the records of patients previously reported in Chisolm[101,106] and Chisolm and Harrison.[110]

Records of blood lead content before treatment were not available for 15 patients included in these reports, most of whom had asymptomatic increased lead absorption. Patients included in these reports who died are included in the death group. The data on deaths caused by lead-paint poisoning were obtained from the Baltimore City Health Department records. Records of blood lead content were available for 98 (1936–1970) of 132 reported deaths (1931–1970). Where blood lead content was not obtained during life, diagnosis is based on postmortem studies. A breakdown of deaths into 5-year periods (1936–1970) shows no significant variation in either distribution or mean of blood lead content in fatal cases. All blood lead analyses included in this figure were performed by the Baltimore City Health Department (dithizone method). The values shown are not corrected for deviation from normal hematocrit. Some of the children included in the group designated as "asymptomatic increased lead absorption" had mild symptoms that at the time of examination were attributed to other disease processes, rather than to lead. In such instances, the nonspecificity of mild clinical symptoms made differential diagnosis difficult.

Of considerable interest are the spread of values under each clinical category and the overlap of laboratory values from category to category. The relatively low concentrations of blood lead found in some of the children may be due, in part, to anemia, but they also suggest that a blood lead concentration may not always exclude lead as the cause of illness if it is not as high as is usually observed in illness. Blood lead concentrations greater than 60 μg/100 g in children are for all practical purposes compatible with the diagnosis of disease due to lead if there is clear evidence of impaired heme synthesis and the other clinical findings support the diagnosis.

93

TABLE 4-5 Excretion of Lead by Children with Acute Lead Encephalopathy under the Influence of Chelating Agents[a]

Patient	Age, Months	Lead Excretion, mg/10 Days[b]	Body Weight, kg	Lead Excretion, mg/kg Body Weight
R.S.	18	23.38	8.77	2.67
M.S.	18	40.24	9.0	4.47
W.K.	22	55.83	8.94	6.25
M.G.	24	51.04[c]	12.8	3.99
A.P.	25	30.82	9.0	3.42
C.R.	26	45.05	11.0	4.1
A.W.	26	70.37	14.5	4.85
K.LeC.	27	42.33[c]	13.5	3.13
R.N.	34	70.99	12.9	5.5
Mean			11.2	4.26
Median			11.0	4.1

[a]These data have not previously been published. Additional data on these patients were published by Chisolm.[106]
[b]Chelation therapy was given in two 5-day courses separated by an interval of 2–5 weeks.
[c]An estimated loss of 3 mg occurred during the second course of therapy. Loss excluded from recorded totals.

0.09–0.38 mg). Such comparisons suggest that acute encephalopathy is associated with 20-fold or greater increments in body lead burden.

In adults, Kehoe reports that clear-cut symptoms of acute lead poisoning[298] are associated with a blood content greater than 80 μg/100 g of whole blood, and most other clinical reports are in agreement. This clinical impression is based almost entirely on observations in occupationally exposed men who are otherwise healthy. Reports of some other investigators, however, have noted that symptoms and signs consistent with mild lead poisoning may be associated with blood lead concentrations of 50–80 μg/100 g of whole blood.[196,354,491] These reports are difficult to evaluate: In some instances, the affected adult has been separated from his occupational exposure for up to several weeks before the blood lead measurement; in other cases, the methods of analysis may not give results comparable with those obtained with the "USPHS" or comparable dithizone method. To these factors must be added the uncertainties in the clinical evaluation of the nonspecific symptoms that are compatible with mild lead poisoning. Adequate medical supervision of men occupationally exposed to lead requires not only serial determinations of blood lead concentration, urinary ALA concentration, and hemogram, but also repeated careful clinical evaluation by a physician familiar with each worker, his exposure, and his work habits. Such comprehensive medical supervision is essential in order to determine what component of any illness is attributable to the patient's occupational exposure to lead. This problem is discussed by Selander and Cramér.[490] Selander et al.[491] noted evidence of hepatocellular injury in some patients with symptoms of lead poisoning and blood lead content in the lower range. Inasmuch as hepatocellular injury is not usually observed in industrial lead poisoning, they suggested that the use of alcohol might modify a person's susceptibility to lead poisoning from the clinical viewpoint. It should be noted, also, that the hepatocellular injury may have been due to alcohol alone. Because acute lead poisoning and acute alcoholism induce many similar symptoms, the differential diagnosis may be exceedingly difficult and uncertain. Little is known of the influence of coexisting diseases that may modify one's response to lead.

Permanent Neurologic Sequelae

At least one fourth of young children who survive an attack of acute encephalopathy due to lead poisoning sustain severe permanent neurologic sequelae.[77,110,507] Chisolm and Harrison[110] reported and Byers[77] has confirmed the observation that the return of a child after a single known attack of acute encephalopathy to the same hazardous home environment increases his risk of severe permanent brain damage to almost 100%. Byers and Lord[78] and Byers[77] have delineated the nature of the central nervous system injury that follows symptomatic lead poisoning in early childhood. The injury does not differ qualitatively from what follows any diffuse cerebral injury incurred during early childhood (such as severe head trauma or viral or bacterial encephalitis or meningitis). In its most severe form, acute lead encephalopathy may be followed by cortical atrophy, hydrocephalus ex vacuo, severe convulsive disorder, idiocy, and blindness. Such a result is becoming increasingly rare, and subtle neurologic deficits and mental impairment are the more common outcomes. These include lack of sensory perception and perseverance, despite IQ scores of 80–100, or better, on verbally oriented intelligence tests. Form and proportion are distorted. Motor incoordination and lack of sensory perception severely impair learning ability. Often, the handicap is not recognized until after the child enters school. Such children also have short attention spans and are easily distracted. With respect to be-

TABLE 4-6 Sequelae of Lead Poisoning Classified by Mode of Onset in 425 Patients[a]

Sequelae	Mode of Onset												
	Encephalopathy		Seizures		Ataxia		Gastrointestinal Symptoms		Fever		Asymptomatic		Totals	
	No.	%	No.	%	No.	%	No.	%	No.	%	No.	%	No.	%
Mental retardation	23	39	14	33	5	29	43	19	3	19	5	9	93	22
Seizures	32	54	17	40	6	35	30	13	0	0	0	0	85	20
Cerebral palsy	8	14	0	0	1	6	0	0	0	0	0	0	9	2
Optic atrophy	4	7	0	0	1	6	0	0	0	0	0	0	5	1
Children with one or more of above sequelae[b]	48	81	29	67	10	59	73	31	3	19	5	9	168	40
Children with none of above sequelae[c]	11	19	14	33	7	41	159	69	13	81	53	91	257	60
Totals	59	100	43	100	17	100	232	100	16	100	58	100	425	100

[a] Adapted from Perlstein and Attala.442
[b] Multiple sequelae found in some patients.
[c] Patients who did not have symptoms suggestive of lead poisoning at initial visit, but were brought for other reasons; usually classified as asymptomatic increased lead absorption.

havioral aberration, it is difficult to determine how much is due to organic brain damage and how much represents the response of the affected child to the many facets of his total environmental deprivation. Nevertheless, many children with documented prior attacks of symptomatic lead poisoning develop hostile, aggressive, and destructive behavior patterns, which, in turn, may precipitate their exclusion from school and a demand for institutionalization. Although seizure disorder and behavioral abnormalities tend to abate during adolescence, mental incompetence is permanent (J. J. Chisolm, Jr., unpublished data, and Emmerson[169]).

Perlstein and Attala[442] studied 425 children 6 months to 10 years after the initial diagnosis of symptomatic lead poisoning or asymptomatic increased lead absorption was made. A total of 39% of the group showed one or more of the following: profound mental retardation, seizure disorder, paresis, or blindness. The severity of the sequelae appeared to be related to the severity of the acute episode. The findings are summarized in Table 4–6. Among the 59 children in the group who had had acute encephalopathy, 81% had one or more of the severe sequelae listed in the table. Of 43 who presented with seizures, 67% had one or more of the sequelae. Among the 232 who presented with acute abdominal colic, 31% had one or more of the sequelae. Among the 351 patients who presented with symptomatic lead poisoning but no fever, 24.2% were found at follow-up to have developed seizure disorder, which strongly suggests a causal relation between the seizure disorder and symptomatic acute lead poisoning. The mental retardation found in asymptomatic children is difficult to evaluate. Whether children without encephalopathy have long-continued excessive intake of lead with repeated but undiagnosed episodes of acute poisoning is not known, but it is probable, inasmuch as no definitive steps were taken to terminate the exposure and the initial age range at the time of diagnosis was 9 months to 8 years. Recurrent episodes of poisoning are mentioned in some patients. Similarly, Byers and Lord[78] noted permanent mental subnormality in 19 of 20 children who did not have clear-cut encephalopathy but who sustained recurrent bouts of acute poisoning during the preschool years. Because the true incidence of lead poisoning in young children is not known, the incidence of significant permanent injury to the central nervous system is also not known. Furthermore, all the studies just reviewed are retrospective. Whether asymptomatic increased lead abosorption can cause subtle but permanent impairment of nervous system function in young children is not now known.

Moncrieff et al.[397] reported minimally increased blood lead concentration (40–80 μg/100 g of whole blood) in almost half of a group of mentally retarded children. It is not possible on the basis of their data to determine whether there is any causal relation between the mental retardation and the observed increase in blood lead content. Many mentally subnormal children have persistent pica. Consequently, mental impairment with other causes might well have preceded the increased intake of lead; the final clinical picture would then represent the interaction of several etiologic factors.

The older medical literature refers to similar mental impairment,[19,394] encephalopathy, and seizures associated with uncontrolled occupational exposure to lead in adults.

Lead poisoning due to ingestion of lead-contaminated moonshine whiskey may give rise to a range of symptoms that spans the full clinical spectrum from the mild abdominal colic seen in industrially exposed workers to the acute encephalopathy seen in young children. This wide spectrum of clinical disease is apparently related to the wide range of lead content in various batches of moonshine. The following clinical observations are qualitative. Patients of all economic and social strata have been found. Examination of the military service records of some patients with lead poisoning from moonshine suggests that they formerly had jobs in military service that required personal initiative and reliability. At the time they were examined for lead poisoning they were incompetent. Inasmuch as the intellectual function of these patients has not been studied in detail and no epidemiologic studies have been performed to document these impressions, nor to separate the effects of lead from those of alcohol on nervous system function, this is suggested as an area for future research.

Clinical Diagnosis of Lead Poisoning

In the absence of a positive history of abnormal exposure to lead, the clinical diagnosis of lead poisoning is easily missed (e.g., in children with pica and imbibers of moonshine whiskey). The characteristic sequence of clinical events, with a positive history of known exposure, may alert the physician to the possibility. However, because the signs and symptoms of the syndromes of acute lead poisoning are shared by other diseases—particularly acute alcoholism and acute intermittent hepatic porphyria[134]—diagnosis may be overlooked. Likewise, physical examination rarely reveals findings specific for lead poisoning. The classic "lead line" on the gums requires the presence of poor dental hygiene and even then is seen only in persons with severe chronic exposure, as occurs in moonshine drinkers. The signs of acute encephalopathy are those of increased intracranial pressure from whatever cause. The signs of chronic encephalopathy may resemble the signs of a variety of cerebral degenerative diseases. Physical examination does not distinguish lead colic from a variety of acute surgical and nonsurgical conditions of the abdomen, especially peptic ulcer, pancreatitis, and acute intermittent porphyria. Lead neuropathy does show a predilection for motor weakness involving the most frequently used extremities, which may help to distinguish this form of peripheral neuropathy from other forms with more obvious sensory abnormalities. Lead myelopathy is difficult to distinguish from amyotrophic lateral sclerosis. Microscopic examination of the peripheral blood may reveal only the features of iron-deficiency anemia. On routine examination, the urine may be normal or may show the presence of minimal albuminuria, glycosuria, and nonspecific abnormalities. Basophilic stippling of red blood cells is an inconstant feature of gross lead poisoning and requires special techniques for consistent results. However, microscopic examination of aspirated bone marrow samples almost always reveals stippled sideroblasts in classic lead poisoning. Because of the nonspecificity of the clinical features, diagnosis requires a high index of suspicion, knowledge of the epidemiology of lead poisoning, and some specialized diagnostic tests, which are discussed later in this chapter. The principal pitfalls of clinical diagnosis are failure to obtain and establish an exposure history and failure to appreciate the rapidity with which classic lead poisoning may progress.

The clinical subtlety of lead poisoning is exemplified by the measures that may be necessary to establish the diagnosis when it is due to moonshine drinking.[401] If the patient has ingested lead-contaminated whiskey shortly before hospitalization, his blood and urinary concentrations of lead are usually increased. But if ingestion has been more remote, blood and urine levels may not be increased.[401] The severe anemia sometimes found in these patients must be taken into account in interpreting their blood lead concentrations.* The diagnosis of increased body burden of lead is sometimes possible only after administration of a chelating agent, such as CaEDTA, and measurement of the urinary excretion of lead. Observations on the 10

---

*Symptomatic lead poisoning has been seen in persons with severe anemia in whom blood lead concentrations were less than 80 μg %.

TABLE 4-7 Effects of Lead Poisoning Due to Chronic Ingestion of Illicitly
Distilled Whiskey on Selected Measurements for Assessing Lead Poisoning[a]

Patient	Blood Lead Content, μg/100 g[b]	Hematocrit Value	Base-line Urine Lead Content, μg/Liter[b]	Post-CaEDTA Urine Lead, μg/Liter[b,c]	Qualitative Urinary Coproporphyrin
1	80	21	180	2,200	positive
2	120	25	140	9,200	positive
3	130	35	–	1,300	positive
4	110	25	40	2,200	positive
5	80	24	180	2,700	positive
6	50	30	40	930	negative
7	60	29	30	2,100	positive
8	70	28	90	8,500	positive
9	50	28	50	2,000	not done
10	80	27		3,300	positive
	<40[d]		<70[d]	<450[e]	

[a]Unpublished data from H. H. Sandstead.
[b]Lead analysis performed by the Toxicology Laboratory, State of Tennessee Department of
Public Health. Urine collections were for 24 hr (8 a.m. to 8 a.m.).
[c]2 g CaEDTA was given intravenously over 6–8 hr starting at 8 a.m.
[d]From Goldwater and Hoover.[204]
[e]From Teisinger and Srbová.[526]

patients with overt lead poisoning shown in Table 4-7 illustrate this
fact.

METABOLIC AND FUNCTIONAL EFFECTS IN MAN

Lead is not known to be an essential trace element. No studies pertinent to this question have been reported. However, various segments
of the population do carry concentrations of lead in blood and urine
at which minimal changes in pyrrole metabolism can be detected.
The observed minimal metabolic changes are of the adverse type.
This section takes up the known adverse metabolic and functional
effects of increasing concentrations of lead on heme synthesis, the
kidney, the nervous system, and other organ systems in man. Observations in experimental models that complement, confirm, and
amplify observations in man with respect to the effects of lead on
heme synthesis, the kidney, and the nervous system are included.
The effects of lead that have been examined in experimental bio-

chemical systems, but not in intact man, are described later in this chapter.

Biosynthesis of Heme

Current knowledge of the biosynthesis of heme is based largely on experimental studies in avian erythrocytes and embryos, mammalian erythrocytes and liver, chloroplasts, and *Rhodopseudomonas spheroides*, a facultative anaerobic bacterium. These findings, which have been reviewed recently,[206,331] indicate that the metabolic pathway shown in Figure 4-3 is the common pathway in mammals and photosynthetic bacteria and plants for the formation of heme or chlorophyll. The necessary enzymes have been found widely distributed in mammalian tissues,[195,206,214,216,331,375] so it is highly probable that each cell synthesizes its own heme for the formation of its particular hemoproteins (hemoglobin, myoglobin, cytochromes, and catalases). A modified form of heme, the corrin moiety, is a major component of vitamin B_{12}. The intracellular organization of the pathway in animal tissues is apparently as follows: The initial step (formation of ALA*) and the final two steps (COPROGEN III → PROTO 9 and PROTO 9 + Fe → heme) are mediated by intramitochondrial enzymes, whereas the intermediate steps are mediated by soluble enzymes in the cytoplasm. Regulation is by negative feedback control through repression of ALAS formation and activity[206,331,416] by heme. There is some evidence that heme and PROTO 9 may also inhibit the activity of ALAD, the second enzyme in the pathway. This is an important consideration with respect to lead, in that PROTO 9 accumulates in lead poisoning. In liver and in chick embryos, some sex steroid metabolites and drugs in physiologic concentrations exert important modifying effects on the *de novo* production of ALAS.[215,289] Thus, some flexibility in response to the needs of the organism is apparent. Also, there is some evidence that globin synthesis is synchronized with heme synthesis.[363]

Lead clearly inhibits the formation of heme at several points, as shown in Figure 4-3.[43,104,195,220,226,275,277,351,473,546,567] Classic lead poisoning in both humans and experimental animals is characterized by accumulation of nonheme iron and PROTO 9 in red blood cells, accumulation of ALA in serum,[106,177,226] and the increased excretion of ALA and COPRO III (the oxidation product of COPROGEN III)

*See Glossary for abbreviations.

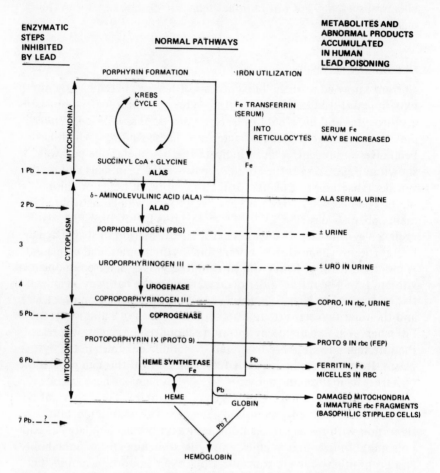

FIGURE 4-3 Lead interferes with the biosynthesis of heme at several enzymatic steps, with the utilization of iron, and, in erythrocytes, with globin synthesis. Inhibition of ALAD and heme synthetase (Steps 2 and 6), which are SH-dependent enzymes, is well documented, and accumulation of the substrates of these enzymes (ALA and PROTO 9) is characteristic of human lead poisoning. Inhibition of ALAS (Step 1) is based on experimental evidence only. Whether there is enzymatic inhibition or other factors operate at Step 5 is not clear; nevertheless, increased urinary excretion of COPRO is prominent in human lead poisoning. Minor increases in PBG and URO in urine are occasionally reported in severe lead poisoning. The utilization of iron is impaired; although the *in vivo* mechanisms are unclear, nonheme iron (ferritin and iron micelles) accumulates in red blood cells with damaged mitochondria and other fragments not found in normal mature erythrocytes. Serum iron may be increased in humans with lead poisoning, but without iron-deficiency states. Heme synthesis is reduced and, in red blood cells, globin synthesis is apparently impaired, although the mechanisms responsible for reduced globin synthesis remain unknown.

in urine. ALA and PROTO 9 are the substrates of SH-dependent enzymes,[104,106,195,216,331] but COPROGEN III apparently is not.

Increased excretion of PBG and URO in human lead poisoning has been reported only in more severely affected cases.[196,226] The transfer of iron from transferrin into human reticulocytes is only partially inhibited (20% inhibition at a lead concentration of 10^{-4} M);[275] however, electron microscopic studies reveal the accumulation of nonheme iron in developing red blood cells in the form of "ferruginous micelles," which are responsible for the ringed sideroblasts characteristic of lead poisoning and dense aggregations of ferritin in damaged mitochondria.[43,277,473] These accumulations of altered cytoplasmic and nuclear remnants (RNA and altered microsomal and mitochondrial fragments) are responsible for the basophilic stippling of red blood cells characteristic of human and experimental lead poisoning.[43,277,473] In vitro studies show that lead in man is tightly bound to red blood cells and not readily desorbed,[125,588] and electron microscopy shows lead deposited on the outer surface and within the membrane of red blood cells.[286] The localization of lead in red blood cells in vivo is not known. That the accumulation of porphyrins and metalloporphyrins within mitochondria may have physiologic significance is suggested by the experimental observation in mouse liver by Silverstein[502] that metalloporphyrins in concentrations of 10^{-5} M and 10^{-6} M may inhibit the activities of other intramitochondrial enzymes.

Waldron[567] has summarized the experimental studies on the overall effects of lead on heme and protoporphyrin formation in avian red blood cells when glycine is used as substrate—minimal inhibition at a lead concentration of 10^{-6} M, partial inhibition at 10^{-5} M, and complete inhibition at 10^{-3} and 10^{-4} M. In vitro observations show that inhibition by lead can be partially reversed by the addition of such SH reagents as glutathione (GSH), cysteine, BAL, and D-penicillamine.[104,195,216,351] Many studies indicate inhibition at some stage before the formation of ALA. For example, Morrow et al.[405] report that lead inhibits ALAS in in vitro preparations (12% inhibition at a lead concentration of 10^{-6} M, and 44% inhibition at 10^{-4} M). Although the intracellular distribution and concentrations of lead are largely unknown, the enzymatic inhibition demonstrable at 10^{-6} M in vitro is generally considered to be physiologically significant in the intact animal. The increased FEP and FEC in red blood cells, increased COPRO III in urine, and increased ALA in serum and urine indicate that these are the steps in heme biosynthesis most susceptible to inhibition by lead in man.

The inhibitory effect of lead on heme biosynthesis in organ systems other than hematopoietic tissue has received relatively little study.[104] That some of the ALA found in human urine may arise from tissues other than the hematopoietic system is suggested by the finding of measurable amounts of ALA in the absence of demonstrable erythropoiesis in urine in humans.[493] Gibson et al.[195] showed that lead ($10^{-3}M$) partially inhibited ALAD activity in beef liver. Recently, Millar et al.[391] reported that ALAD activity is inhibited in the blood, brain, and liver of lead-poisoned suckling rats. The inhibition in liver was 60% of that observed in blood, whereas the inhibition in brain was 80–90% of that in blood. However, in one experiment in which the lead intake in six suckling rats was sufficient to produce a mean blood lead concentration of 30 $\mu g/100$ g of whole blood, the degree of ALAD activity in brain was not significantly reduced, in comparison with the controls.[391] Further studies of heme synthesis in tissues other than erythrocytes (especially brain and kidney) are needed, because the quantitative aspects of the rate and regulation of heme synthesis in these tissues may well differ from those in the hematopoietic system.

The potential for significant interactions between lead and other heavy metals has received little attention. Passow et al.[436] point out the biologic complexities introduced by differences in membrane and intracellular distributions of various metals, the variety of ligands with which metals can interact, and the competition among metals for various types of binding sites. For example, in *Rhodopseudomonas spheroides*, lead, manganese, and cobalt increase the requirement for iron for the conversion of COPROGEN III to PROTO 9.[546] Similarly, Morrow et al.[405] have reported that ferrous iron in low concentration has a mild stimulatory effect on the activity of ALAS, whereas lead has an inhibitory effect in the same system. In beef liver, for example, copper, mercury, and silver are more effective inhibitors of ALAD *in vitro* than is lead,[195] but they are not known to be significant inhibitors of ALAD *in vivo* in man. This enjoins one to be cautious in the transfer of *in vitro* observations to *in vivo* situations. In occupationally exposed lead workers, Rubino et al.[463] reported a statistically significant positive correlation between rising concentrations of copper and PROTO 9 in red blood cells in the peripheral circulation. These preliminary experimental and clinical data strongly suggest that some of the important metabolic effects of lead may be modulated by competition between lead and other metals at various stages in the biosynthesis of heme. Clearly, potentially competitive metal-

metal interactions involving lead, such as those found in *Rhodopseu-domonas spheroides*, merit considerable study. In particular, inasmuch as lead can cause a functional impairment in the utilization of iron, persons with iron-deficiency states and persons with disorders characterized by functional impairment in iron utilization (such as copper deficiency, vitamin B_6 deficiency, and thalassemia) deserve study with respect to their susceptibility to given levels of lead absorption.

Only in some of the inborn errors of porphyrin metabolism and some toxic porphyrias are increases in pyrroles and ALA in the tissues and excreta comparable with those in classic lead poisoning in humans.[103,226,478] The pattern of pyrrole excretion found in lead poisoning differs from that found in acute intermittent porphyria and other hepatocellular disorders, as shown in Table 4-8. Erythropoietic protoporphyria is associated with very high concentrations of PROTO 9 in red blood cells. Deficiency and impaired utilization of iron are also associated with moderate increases in FEP of the same order of magnitude as those found in asymptomatic increased lead absorption.[226,351,473,572] Only classic lead poisoning is associated with FEP concentrations comparable with those in erythropoietic protoporphyria, an uncommon genetically determined disorder.

The adverse metabolic effect most specifically associated with lead is the inhibition of ALAD. When ALAD is inhibited, its substrate, ALA, accumulates; the accumulation is reflected by an increase of ALA in serum and urine. The increased excretion of ALA in urine in some porphyrias is the result of increased production of ALA and

TABLE 4-8 Patterns of Increased Pyrrole Excretion in Urine of Acutely Symptomatic Patients[a]

| Disease | Pyrroles[b] | | | |
	ALA	PBG[c]	URO	COPRO
Lead poisoning	+++	0	±	+++
Acute intermittent porphyria	++++	++++	+ to ++++	+ to +++
Acute hepatitis (toxic and infectious types)	0	0	0	+ to +++
Acute alcoholism	0	0	±	+ to +++

[a]Adapted from Chisolm.[107]
[b]0 = normal; + to ++++ = degree of increase; ALA = δ-aminolevulinic acid; PBG = porphobilinogen; URO = uroporphyrin; COPRO = coproporphyrin.
[c]Qualitative Watson-Schwartz test for PBG.

does not result from inhibition of ALAD.[158,206,215,289,414,478,544]
Several authors[57,145,247,351,391,415] using different *in vitro* techniques
have found that ALAD activity is inhibited in circulating red blood
cells in humans and that the degree of inhibition increases with the
concentration of lead in the blood. An approximately fourfold change
in the level of ALAD, as measured *in vitro*, is found in hemolysates
of peripheral blood from persons whose blood lead content is within
the normal range (i.e., 5–40 μg/100 g of whole blood).[145,247,391] In
humans, this effect is apparently specific for lead; ALAD activity is
not impaired in human iron-deficiency anemia.[351] Hernberg *et al.*[248]
report no relation between ALAD activity in hemolysates of blood
and the concentration of mercury in blood and urine in man. Nakao
et al.[415] report normal ALAD activity in blood from cases of arsenic
poisoning, carbon monoxide poisoning, acute intermittent porphyria,
several types of anemia, four cases of leukemia, and 46 cases of 21
different neurologic disorders. Only in acute alcoholic intoxication
has a transient decrease in ALAD activity in blood been reported—in
adult human volunteers who drank 300 ml of whiskey in 1 hr.[29]
Although a number of disease states remain to be evaluated, no other
exceptions have been reported to date. Haeger-Aronsen[226] found that
urinary ALA excretion was normal in human adults with a variety of
hepatic, hematologic, and neoplastic diseases. The available evidence
indicates, therefore, that the combination of inhibition of ALAD activity in blood and increasing excretion of ALA in urine is associated
in man only with increasing concentrations of lead; the only known
exception is the transitory effect of acute drunkenness.

Hernberg *et al.*[247,248] have suggested that impaired ALAD activity
in red blood cells is the earliest evidence of an adverse metabolic effect
of environmental exposure to increasing concentrations of lead. The
logarithm of the activity of ALAD in hemolysates of red blood cells
has an inverse linear relation with the concentration of lead in blood
when concentration is between 5 and 95 μg/100 g of whole blood
(Figure 4–4).[247] The interpretation of these *in vitro* findings is highly
pertinent to the question of airborne lead. However, the conditions
under which ALAD activity is measured must be considered. In all
the reported procedures, known amounts of ALA are added *in vitro*
to crude hemolysates of whole human blood, the hemolysate is incubated, and, after a suitable time, the amount of PBG formed is
measured. "Ghosts" or membrane fragments are not removed. Such
cofactors as GSH, which are present in blood in varying amounts and
which partially reverse inhibition due to lead in samples of blood

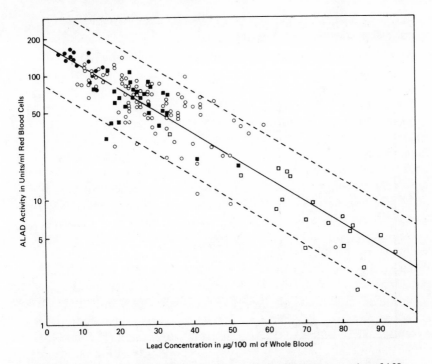

FIGURE 4-4 Correlation between ALAD activity and blood lead concentration of 158 persons representing different degrees of natural and occupational exposure to lead. Note logarithmic scale on ordinate. Solid circles, medical students; open circles, workers in print-shops; solid squares, automobile repair workers; open squares, lead smelters and shipscrappers. (Redrawn from Hernberg *et al.*[247])

from lead-poisoned subjects,[57,351] are not added in optimal amounts in the reported procedures. Because the chemical aspects of this *in vitro* assay are not completely understood, any conclusions concerning its *in vivo* significance should be considered tentative.

It is, however, clear that decreasing A L A D activity, as measured *in vitro* in human blood, is associated with increasing urinary excretion of A L A and increasing concentration of lead in blood. Nakao *et al.*[415] report a negative linear correlation between the logarithm of A L A D activity in blood and the excretion of A L A in urine as blood lead content rises from 40 to 165 μg/100 g of whole blood. Selander and Cramér[490] find a correlation between blood lead content and urinary A L A, when A L A in samples of urine collected for approximately 2½ hr in the morning is measured by the method of Mauzerall and Granick.[376] This method measures aminoacetone, a substance

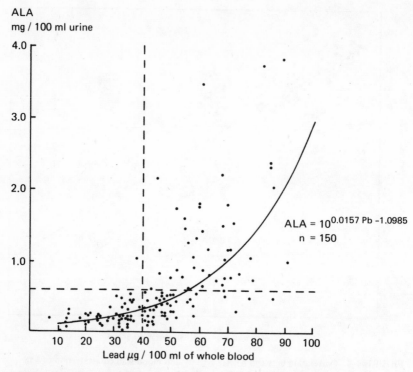

FIGURE 4-5 Values for ALA in urine plotted against those for lead in blood. The broken lines mark the upper normal limits. (Redrawn from Selander and Cramér.[490])

unrelated to lead, as well as ALA; although this does not affect the significance of the findings, it may obscure the location of the apparent threshold to some extent. Selander and Cramér's data (Figure 4–5)[490] indicate that there is an exponential relation between blood lead concentration and urinary ALA excretion. As blood lead concentration rises above 40 μg/100 g of whole blood, urinary ALA excretion rises at a progressively increasing rate. Considerable variation is seen in workers with blood lead concentrations between 40 and 59 μg/100 g of whole blood; 29 of the 33 workers with concentrations of 60 μg/100 g or higher have urinary ALA values that exceed the upper limit of normal ($\overline{m}$ + 2 SD) for the method of analysis used.[226] In a group of young children with blood lead concentrations between 25 and 75 μg/100 g of whole blood, an apparently similar curvilinear relation can be seen between the quantitative daily output of ALA in urine and blood lead concentration (Figure 4–6). However, in a group of adolescents who had lead poisoning at least 10 years

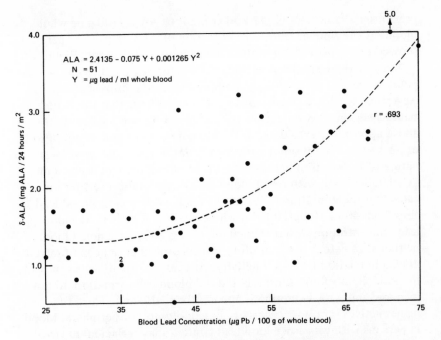

FIGURE 4-6   Relation between blood lead concentration and daily excretion of ALA in urine in a group of young children without clinically evident lead poisoning. The group consisted of 51 children between 1 and 5 years old drawn from an inner-city clinic population in Baltimore, Maryland. The range of blood lead concentration was 25-75 μg/100 g of whole blood. Whole blood samples for lead determination were drawn on admission to the hospital and analyzed by the laboratory of the Baltimore City Health Department by a dithizone technique. ALA output was measured in quantitatively collected 24-hr urine specimens by a method that excludes aminoacetone. Statistical analysis of the data indicates that ALA output is related to age and height but that it is best related to surface area in young children, in that the slope and regression between daily ALA output and surface area intersect at the origin. Therefore, expression of ALA output as mg/m^2 per 24 hr completely compensates for differences among the children due to age and body mass. A highly significant curvilinear relation is best fitted by the following quadratic equation: mg/m^2 per 24 hr = 2.4135 − 0.07500 (blood lead) + 0.001265 (blood lead)^2. For this fitted quadratic equation, $p < 0.01$, and the standard error of the fitted line is ± 0.6. A highly significant linear relation is also found in this group between blood lead concentration and the log of ALA excretion ($p < 0.001$). Within this narrow range of blood lead concentration (25-75 μg/100 g of whole blood), the data suggest that ALA excretion apparently increases only as blood lead concentration rises above approximately 40 μg/100 g of whole blood; however, the absence of a threshold for this relation cannot be excluded in these young children. Statistical analyses were performed by Dr. David E. Mellits, Department of Pediatrics, The Johns Hopkins University School of Medicine. These unpublished studies (J. J. Chisolm, Jr., personal communication) were supported by DHEW grant EC–R01–00201 from NIH, HSMHA study project 464, MCHS grant MC–R–240012–01–0, institutional research grant FR–53–78 to The Johns Hopkins University School of Medicine, and a grant from the Thomas Wilson Fund, Baltimore, Maryland. The studies were carried out on the Pediatric Clinical Research Unit of The Johns Hopkins University School of Medicine, which is supported by DHEW grant R–M01–00052.

previously and normal blood lead content (8–40 μg/100 g of whole blood) at the time of study, the excretion of ALA (mg/24 hr per m^2) showed no significant correlation with blood lead content (Figure 4-7).

None of these studies is entirely satisfactory by itself from the point of view of methodology, completeness, or groups studied. Nevertheless, all are consistent with the hypothesis that the exponential increase in ALA excretion associated with blood lead content above approximately 40 μg/100 g of whole blood signifies inhibition of ALAD that is physiologically significant *in vivo*. The curvilinear nature of the relation between ALAD in blood, ALA in urine, and "chelatable" lead with rising blood lead concentration further indicates that the inhibition of ALAD by lead accelerates as blood lead rises from 40 to 80 μg/100 g of whole blood and higher. At blood lead concentrations lower than about 35 μg/100 g of whole blood, neither stimulatory nor inhibitory effects of lead have been observed *in vivo* in relation to ALAD activity. At these "normal" levels of lead in blood, hemoglobin synthesis and red blood cell formation do not increase, and ALA excretion is apparently unaffected. Thus, the higher activities of ALAD activity in hemolysates of peripheral blood in persons with very low blood lead content may reflect an *in vitro* measure of "reserve enzyme capacity" that is not essential. Studies using more specific methods for the determination of ALA in urine, as well as studies of the factors that may influence ALAD activity *in vivo*, may in the future delineate more precisely the concentrations of lead in blood and soft tissues at which compensatory biologic mechanisms must be invoked.

Functional Effects of Lead on Red Blood Cells in Man

Hasan and Hernberg,[242] Waldron,[567] and Griggs[220] have summarized the *in vivo* effects of lead on red blood cells in man as follows: accumulation of lead, increased osmotic resistance, increased mechanical fragility, increased glucose consumption, increased loss of potassium at 37 C in a 2-hr incubation, decreased sodium and potassium ATPase activity in membrane fragments, decreased life-span, and increased proportion of immature red cells in the circulation (increased numbers of reticulocytes and basophilic stippled cells). For the most part, these represent effects on membrane functions. Hernberg *et al.*,[249] using tritiated diisopropyl fluorophosphonate, reported nonrandom shortening of human red blood cell life-span, which they interpreted as indicating a true shortening of life-span.

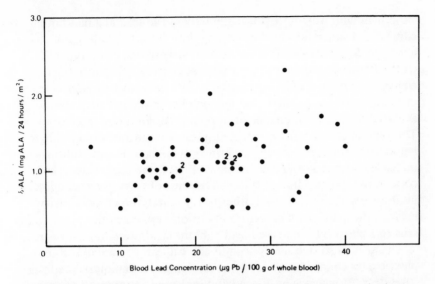

FIGURE 4-7 Relation between blood lead concentration and daily ALA excretion in urine in a group of adolescents with no known abnormal exposure to lead for 10 years or longer. The group consisted of 55 adolescents who had had acute lead poisoning as young children but no known unusual exposure to lead for at least 10 years before the studies shown here. Blood lead concentration was determined by a dithizone technique, and ALA was determined on quantitative 24-hr urine collections by a method that excludes aminoacetone.[561] ALA output is expressed as mg/m^2 per 24 hr to facilitate comparison with the data in Figure 4-6. Within the range of blood lead concentration in this group (8–40 $\mu g/$ 100 g of whole blood), no correlation was found between blood lead concentration and ALA excretion. This suggests that ALA excretion is low, constant, and independent of blood lead concentration when blood lead concentration is less than approximately 40 $\mu g/100$ g of whole blood in adolescents. These studies were supported by DHEW grant EC-R01-00201 from NIH. They were carried out in the Clinical Research Center of the Department of Medicine, The Johns Hopkins University School of Medicine, which is supported by DHEW grant 5-M01-RR-00032.

Significant reduction (to less than 105 days) was observed at blood lead concentrations greater than 80 $\mu g/100$ g of whole blood. In a patient with clinical lead poisoning, nonrandom destruction was also observed,[42] suggesting intravascular hemolysis, which is consistent with the jaundice sometimes seen in very severe acute lead poisoning. In Finnish adults occupationally exposed to lead, glucose consumption was increased, but three metabolic functions of red blood cells were not altered—lactate production, glucose-6-phosphate dehydrogenase (G6PDH) activity, and lactate dehydrogenase activity. However, in Italy, where a much higher incidence of G6PDH deficiency may be anticipated on a genetic basis, red blood cell preparations from men who were occupationally exposed to lead and had both clinical and subclinical lead poisoning showed statistically significant lowering of glutathione (GSH) content, glutathione stability, and G6PDH content, compared with normal controls.[462] G6PDH deficiency is a rather widely distributed genetic abnormality in persons of Mediterranean origin.[44] This enzyme lies in the pathway that is essential for the maintenance of normal GSH content in the tissues. The genetic defect renders affected persons peculiarly susceptible to hemolytic crises on exposure to primaquine, naphthalene, sulfonamides, and other substances. In view of the rather large reserve of GSH in red blood cells and the effectiveness of GSH in reversing the inhibitory effect of lead and other heavy metals on ALAD activity *in vitro*, the question of susceptibility of otherwise healthy primaquine-sensitive persons to increased lead content is, at present, unanswered.

The anemia so frequently seen in clinical lead poisoning is complex. Under conditions of severe acute exposure, hemolysis predominates,[42,44,567] whereas prolonged and increased exposure of the sort usually associated with clinically evident lead poisoning leads ultimately to erythroid hypoplasia and marked morphologic changes in the bone marrow. The usual picture is of a mild to moderately compensated hemolytic anemia with hemoglobin concentrations rarely less than 10 g/100 g blood. The hemolytic component is small in most circumstances. Impaired heme synthesis is the major cause of the anemia. The degree of reduced red cell life-span correlates most closely with the reticulocyte count.[249] As the lead content in the hematopoietic tissues increases, the compensatory mechanism becomes inadequate and anemia follows. Frank anemia is usually not apparent until sustained blood lead concentrations exceed about 80 μg/100 g of whole blood. Even in the absence of frank anemia, various somewhat less serious degrees of lead exposure may be associated with abnormalities in membrane functions, maturation, metabolism of red blood cells, and biosynthesis of heme.[242]

Kidneys

At the histologic level, the unique intranuclear inclusion bodies have long been considered pathognomonic of severe lead poisoning in man. They are readily reproduced in experimental lead poisoning in rats, and there is some evidence that they represent an inert lead–protein complex.[91,208-210,212] Goyer *et al.*[212] have proposed that inclusion bodies represent a storage mechanism by which renal cells can maintain lower cytoplasmic concentrations of lead. This provocative hypothesis remains to be proved. Experimental evidence and human autopsy and biopsy specimens of Goyer *et al.*,[210] Galle and Morel-Maroger,[193] and Richet *et al.*[453] indicate that lead has adverse metabolic effects on enzymes in the mitochondria and other cell organelles.

At the functional level, renal glycosuria has long been recognized as a concomitant of clinical lead poisoning. More recently, hyperaminoaciduria (of the generalized renal type) has been reported in asymptomatic men occupationally exposed to inorganic lead[124] and in children with acute symptomatic lead poisoning.[101, 106, 108, 587] For the most part, clinical investigators have used rather insensitive semiquantitative techniques. Clearer delineation of any threshold for hyperaminoaciduria would require the use of clearance techniques and ion-exchange chromatography. Experience in other disease states affecting the kidney indicates that aminoaciduria of the generalized renal type is a most sensitive, nonspecific index of functional injury to proximal renal tubular cells and that the biologic significance of this type of aminoaciduria is not nutritional (i.e., the loss of nutrients in the form of glucose and amino acids is inconsequential). In children, it is associated with clinical illness and blood lead concentrations greater than 80 μg/100 g of whole blood, and it is reversible on termination of exposure.[101] Studies in rats with high doses of lead demonstrate that hyperaminoaciduria is correlated with alterations in mitochondrial structure and function. In addition, fructosuria and citraturia have been reported in children with acute lead poisoning, but the significance of these observations remains entirely unexplained.[101]

In children with acute encephalopathy and blood lead concentrations greater than 150 μg/100 g of whole blood, the full Fanconi triad (hyperaminoaciduria, glycosuria, and hypophosphatemia in the presence of hyperphosphaturia) has been reported and is estimated to occur in approximately one third of patients with acute encephalopathy caused by exposure to lead. The significance of the hypophosphatemia in this triad is that it in turn can result in demineralization of bone.[338] The Fanconi triad is evidence of severe injury of proximal renal tubular cells and can be caused by many agents, including lead and such other heavy metals as cadmium and uranium. In children with severe lead poisoning, this injury to the renal cells is also reversible after treatment and cessation of gross lead intake. It may be tentatively concluded that the full Fanconi triad is associated only with severe clinical lead poisoning. It may also be tentatively concluded that hyperaminoaciduria alone is a manifestation of severe overexposure to lead; it has been reported in severe occupational exposure, and it is highly unlikely that exposure to lead in the ambient air alone can cause hyperaminoaciduria. This belief is buttressed by observations in children with clear-cut symptomatic lead poisoning who do not exhibit hyperaminoaciduria, as measured by semiquantitative paper chromatographic techniques. That even the acute Fanconi triad is reversible is not surprising, in view of the regenerative capacity of renal tubular cells. Similarly, clinical investigative experience indicates that profound injury to proximal tubular cells is the prerequisite of hypophosphatemia and demineralization of bone and is associated only with severe forms of lead poisoning.

Observations in men who have drunk lead-contaminated whiskey suggest that high levels of lead intake or long-continued exposure to lead from this source may be associated with impairment of other renal tubular transport mechanisms.

Renal tubular acidification may be impaired, as, apparently, may the ability of patients to conserve sodium when they are fed a diet low in sodium.[469] The latter suggestion is based on observation of men who had drunk illicitly distilled whiskey. Similar observations have not been reported in patients with less complicated conditions or in experimental animals. Therefore, an effect of lead on renal sodium conservation must be considered tentative. Another function of the kidney that may be impaired by lead is the secretion of renin by the juxtaglomerular complex in response to sodium deprivation.[378,469] The physiologic variables that stimulate this complex to secrete renin are not entirely understood. Inasmuch as it is composed of cells of the distal convoluted tubule (macula densa) and of juxtaglomerular cells, which are epithelioid cells in the wall of the afferent glomerular arterioles, it seems possible for lead to affect either component of the complex. However, because renal tubular cells appear particularly susceptible to the effects of lead, for the present it is reasonable to assume that the effect of lead on the juxtaglomerular complex is mediated primarily through the cells of the macula densa. In any case, the effect has been found reversible after treatment of patients with CaEDTA.[378]

An interesting consequence of the chronic renal injury due to lead is the syndrome of saturnine gout.[169] Lead interferes with the secretion of urates by the renal tubules.[29] Hence, although uric acid is not overproduced (as in other forms of gout), the body pool of urates increases, and crystals are deposited in the joint spaces, resulting in the classic gouty diathesis. In contrast with other forms of gout, the

frequency of disease is the same in both men and women. In addition, according to the experience of Emmerson[169] and Morgan et al.,[402]
saturnine gout is almost always associated with impaired renal function.

Nervous System

Information on the adverse effects of lead on the function of the
nervous system in man is limited almost entirely to clinical and postmortem observations. The pathologic studies of Pentschew[440] and
Pentschew and Garro[441] on the brains of children dying from acute
encephalopathy and observations in experimental animals indicate
that the most severe tissue injury is found in the cerebellum and in
capillary endothelial cells.

Recent experimental studies, particularly those of Lampert and
Schochet[324] and Fullerton,[190, 191] have shed some new light on the
peripheral neuropathy of lead poisoning. Their findings indicate
that chronic feeding of relatively high doses of lead is necessary
to produce the lesions. Electron microscopic studies show that
segmental demyelination was associated with injury to the Schwann
cell (including injury to its mitochondria), that regeneration can occur, and that eventual "onion bulb" formation and scarring of the
nerve fiber result from chronic poisoning. These observations are consistent with observations in humans that peripheral neuropathy associated with lead is associated with high-level chronic and uncontrolled
exposure (usually occupational). However, Catton et al.[94] report
finding minimal electrophysiologic abnormalities in peripheral nerve
conduction in a few occupationally exposed workmen whose blood
lead concentrations were 70–80 $\mu g/100$ g of whole blood and who
were considered otherwise clinically asymptomatic. This is the only
report of clinical investigation concerning the relation between peripheral nerve conduction and low exposure to lead. Similarly, the
interesting report of Simpson et al.[503] concerning an acetylene burner
(for 20 years) with a complex neuropathy resembling progressive
muscular atrophy (amyotrophic lateral sclerosis) points to chronic
high-level exposure to lead as the etiologic agent. Although the available but scanty evidence indicates that neuropathy in humans is associated with chronic high-level exposure, the cases just cited suggest
that the question of peripheral nerve function, especially as it may be
related to the occupational type of exposure, needs re-examination
with the newer electrophysiologic techniques. It is most unlikely that
lead in ambient air alone can cause sufficient absorption of lead to
produce this kind of injury. The effects of lead on behavior and per-

formance in man and experimental animals are discussed later in this chapter.

Other Organ Systems

In addition to the well-documented effects on the hematopoietic system, kidneys, and nervous system, some reports suggest that patients with clinical lead poisoning, and often some complicating intercurrent disease, may also exhibit adverse effects in other organ systems. The following observations are presented here in the hope that they will stimulate research to establish more clearly whether these effects are concomitants of classic lead poisoning and, if so, to establish the soft-tissue concentrations of lead at which they become evident.

The effect of lead on the endocrine and reproductive systems has received relatively little attention. Its impairment of thyroid function both *in vitro*[506] and *in vivo* in rats[468,595] and in man[396,471] has been reported. *In vitro* observations on thyroid slices[506] have shown that lead, like other heavy metals, impairs uptake of iodine by the gland. In the intact lead-poisoned rat,[468,595] uptake of iodine-131 and conversion of iodine to protein-bound iodine are retarded, females being more severely affected than males. In lead-poisoned man,[396,471] the 24-hr uptake of iodine-131 is sometimes decreased. Administration of thyroid-stimulating hormone will usually overcome the effect. The various studies indicate that lead may injure the pituitary–thyroid axis, at the level of the thyroid, the anterior pituitary, and possibly the hypothalamus. A second effect of lead on the hypothalamus and/or anterior pituitary is a decrease in secretion of pituitary gonadotropic hormones observed in some patients.[450,470] It appears that lead may also impair function of the pituitary–adrenal axis.[470] Some patients with nonfulminant or severe lead poisoning due to ingestion of illicitly distilled whiskey have been shown to have a decreased responsiveness to an inhibitor (metapyrone) of 11-beta hydroxylation in the synthesis of cortisol. Urinary secretion of 17-hydroxycorticosteroids and plasma concentrations of cortisol and immunoreactive ACTH have been found decreased in response to this test. Some patients also do not have an appropriate increase in plasma cortisol when made hypoglycemic with insulin. Most of those tested with exogenous ACTH responded normally. At present, it is suggested that lead, and not some other constituent of illicitly distilled whiskey, is the toxicant responsible for the decreased functional reserve of the pituitary and possibly the adrenal gland of these patients. Support for this opinion comes from two studies[409,444] carried out with methods less definitive than would be desirable. In one, involving 25 persons with chronic tetraethyl lead poisoning, many were found to have a decreased pituitary reserve, but they were normally responsive to exogenous ACTH. In the second, workers occupationally exposed to organic lead also revealed evidence of impaired pituitary–adrenal function.

Concerning the human adrenal cortex, according to Makotchenko,[370] the responsiveness of the zona fasciculata to exogenous ACTH may sometimes be suppressed in lead-poisoned persons—a finding also observed in a few men with lead poisoning due to illicitly distilled whiskey.[470] Function of the zona glomerulosa (aldosterone secretion) has also been found suppressed in some men with lead poisoning due to illicitly distilled whiskey.[469]

The effect of lead on human reproduction has not been studied in detail in recent times. It was recognized 75 years ago that lead poisoning in women industrial workers resulted in decreased fertility and an increased abortion rate.[228] Exposure of women to concentrations of lead similar to those prevalent in industry at the turn of the century no longer occurs, and the effect of lead on human reproduction is primarily of historical importance. However, lead is known to cross the placenta,[32] and ingestion of lead-contaminated whiskey during the first trimester of pregnancy might occasionally cause fetal injury.[433] Excessive exposure to lead during pregnancy has resulted in neurologic disorders in children.[14]

In children[189,501] and adults[413,451] with acute lead poisoning, cardiac arrhythmias have been found by electrocardiography. Alterations in cardiac conduction have been noted consistent with a diagnosis of myocarditis and were responsive to treatment with CaEDTA. In two adult cases, the abnormalities recurred on renewal of excessive exposure but were again responsive to treatment with CaEDTA. The mechanism of this effect is unknown, but the clinical circumstances strongly suggest an association with acute lead poisoning. In view of the myopathy that has been reported in skeletal musculature,[503] these findings cannot be overlooked; on the contrary, they call for research.

EVALUATION OF BODY BURDEN

Clarification of the relations between lead and human health requires that human subjects be evaluated by measurements of both the degree of lead absorption and its storage and of some adverse metabolic and functional effects attributable to increased concentrations of lead in soft tissues. In addition, the evaluation should take into consideration the recency and duration of excessive absorption of lead.

Types of Measurement

Blood lead concentration and, in the presence of normal renal function, endogenous urinary lead excretion are the most widely used indices of recent and current absorption of lead. In "healthy" adults[204,298,554] and children[457] without undue exposure to lead (such as industrial exposure or paint ingestion by children), blood lead concentration ranges between approximately 10 and 40 μg/100 g of whole blood. In acute lead poisoning, blood lead concentration is usually grossly increased (greater than 100 μg/100 g of whole blood) in association with current excessive absorption (see Figure 4–2). The following factors must be taken into account in interpreting a given blood lead concentration: proper collection of whole blood sample and reliability of laboratory performing the analysis (see Appendixes B and D), hematocrit value, current or recent administration of chelating agents that temporarily decrease blood lead content, presence of hemolytic anemia, and period since termination of undue exposure.[102] Long-term continuous administration of a chelating agent, such as D-penicillamine, suppresses blood lead content to the normal range during the diuresis of lead,[106,198] and intermittent chelation therapy is associated with fluctuating blood lead content.

Marked changes in the mass of circulating red blood cells may influence whole-blood lead content, in that 90% or more of the lead in blood is attached to the red cells.[141,457] In persons with moderate to severe anemia, clinical evaluation of the significance of a given blood lead content may be facilitated by correcting the observed concentration to the approximate value that would be expected if the patient's packed red cell volume (hematocrit) were within the normal range.* The relevance of such corrections must, however, be assessed further

---

*This correction may be made according to the following simple calculation:

$$\text{expected blood lead} = \frac{\text{observed blood lead}}{\text{observed hematocrit}} \times \text{hematocrit normal for age and sex.}$$

This correction should be made in subjects with moderate or severe anemia due to lead or other causes but probably is not warranted in persons with minor deviations from normal hematocrit.

through the use of other indices of lead absorption and adverse effects (e.g., response to chelating agents and ALA excretion). Subjects whose high-level exposure has terminated several months to several years previously may still have evidence of increased body lead burden, as measured by the CaEDTA mobilization test and blood lead concentrations that are minimally to moderately increased.[106,354,448,452]

Endogenous (spontaneous) urinary lead excretion may be defined as the excretion of lead that occurs normally in the absence of chelating agents. It is best estimated by quantitative measurements of the daily 24-hr output of lead to minimize diurnal variations[395] in the excretion of lead, as well as variations in the overall concentrations of solutes in urine. However, most of the available data in adults are based on measurements of the concentration of lead (in micrograms per liter) in morning or random samples of urine. In adults without undue lead exposure, the concentration of lead in such samples is generally less than 80 μg/liter.[204,298,554] In young children, the concentration of lead in random samples of urine is of little diagnostic use; quantitative 24-hr collections are required, and normal concentrations (less than 55 μg/24 hr) may be found in severe acute lead poisoning.[79] In men occupationally exposed to lead who appear to be in good health, the concentration of lead in urine (in micrograms per liter) is increased. However, in persons with chronic lead nephropathy or other forms of renal insufficiency, endogenous urinary lead excretion (in micrograms per 24 hr) may be within the normal range in the presence of increased body lead burden.[125,168,354,402,452] In subjects remotely occupationally exposed to lead and in moonshine drinkers, endogenous urinary lead excretion may also be normal (see Table 4–7).[448,453] Although the measurement of endogenous urinary lead excretion in timed collections of urine from healthy adults may be suitable for epidemiologic purposes, it is clearly inappropriate in patients with renal impairment from whatever cause.

Body lead burden may be estimated by direct measurement of lead content in bone biopsies, but that has rarely been done in the living.[246,577] Due account should be taken of differences between flat bone (rib, skull) and dense tubular bone (femur, humerus)[35] if results are expressed as micrograms per gram of fresh tissue. No difference is apparent (except for teeth) if results are expressed as micrograms per gram of ash. The lead content of shed deciduous teeth may provide an index of past gross lead absorption.[8] Such measurements in bony tissues do not, however, give an estimate of the fraction of "exchangeable" lead in bone, which can be rapidly mobilized.

Emmerson[168] showed that increased bone lead concentration is positively correlated with the increased output of lead in urine that is
provoked by the administration of calcium EDTA. (This technique is
commonly known as the CaEDTA mobilization test for lead.) This
finding is consistent with experimental observations that a large fraction of the lead mobilized by CaEDTA is derived from bone. Various
investigators[106,168,402,448,452,453] have shown that an abnormal response
to the CaEDTA mobilization test is the most reliable way (short of
bone biopsy) to demonstrate an increased body lead burden when
high-level exposure took place much earlier and particularly in subjects with renal insufficiency. Heavy reliance on this test is also attributable, in large measure, to the widespread unavailability of accurate
blood and endogenous urine lead analyses. According to Emmerson,[168]
the CaEDTA mobilization test may differentiate between nephropathy due to lead and renal insufficiency due to other causes (Figure
4–8). In subjects with renal insufficiency, urine must be collected
quantitatively for 4 days after a single intravenous infusion of 1 g of
CaEDTA.[168] The technique of the test may affect the result. According to Emmerson's technique, the upper limit in healthy adult subjects is less than 600 μg of lead excreted during 4 days. Teisinger and
Srbová[526] use a different technique; their results are shown in Table
4–9. If renal function is normal, a 24-hr urine collection is adequate.
In conditions of current and recent exposure, the CaEDTA or
D-penicillamine mobilization test is correlated with the excretion of
heme precursors and hence provides an index of the "metabolically
active" lead, which is thought to represent the fraction of the total
body lead that is responsible for adverse metabolic effects.[106,109,131]
Thus, the CaEDTA mobilization test is currently the most widely
used procedure for estimating both current and remote absorption of
increased amounts of lead. Although this test serves as one of the important current criteria for the diagnosis of nephropathy due to lead
in adults, it cannot be used to make a positive retrospective diagnosis
of acute lead encephalopathy in subjects with permanent brain damage. Children who have sustained permanent brain damage as a result
of acute encephalopathy may not have a persistently increased residual
"mobile" fraction of the body lead burden, as measured by the
CaEDTA mobilization test. These and other data relative to the metabolism of bone in children and adults suggest that the CaEDTA
mobilization test has as yet undefined limits as an index of high levels
of lead absorption and storage in earlier years.

Because of its usefulness in diagnosis and in studies of dose-response

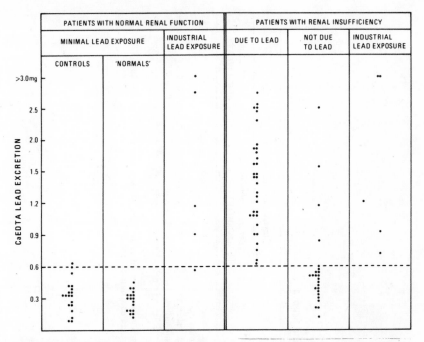

FIGURE 4-8 Values for CaEDTA lead excretion in relation to previous lead exposure and disease. Method of administration of CaEDTA: 1 g of CaEDTA in 250 ml of a 5% aqueous solution of glucose was administered by intravenous infusion over the course of 1 hr. Urine was then quantitatively collected for 4 days. (Redrawn from Emmerson.[168])

relations, there is urgent need for the standardization of procedures for administering the CaEDTA mobilization test. Standardization would greatly facilitate both comparisons and interpretation of results from different laboratories. Experimental observations show unequivocally that oral administration of CaEDTA can increase the absorption of lead present in the gut; consequently, oral CaEDTA tests may give misleading estimates of the "mobile" fraction of the body lead burden, in that the amount of lead measured in the urine may include that absorbed from the gut owing to oral administration of the drug. Untoward reactions to CaEDTA are apparently related to both dose and rate of parenteral administration. The lower dose (1 g) and its longer infusion time (1 hr) used by Emmerson[168] provide both an adequate margin of safety and meaningful data. No untoward reactions have been reported by Emmerson, even in adults with renal insufficiency, and a comparable technique has also been used in children without untoward reaction (25 mg/kg of body weight administered

TABLE 4-9 CaEDTA Mobilization Test—Technique of Teisinger and Srbova[a]

Group	No. Cases		Urinary Lead Excretion in 24 hr, mg	
			Before Injection of CaEDTA	After Injection of CaEDTA[b]
Normal	50	99% confidence limits of average value	$0.031 < \overline{X} < 0.043$	$0.143 < \overline{X} < 0.153$
		Extreme values	0.016, 0.099	0.058, 0.352
Exposed	47	99% confidence limits of average value	$0.067 < \overline{X} < 0.082$	$0.612 < \overline{X} < 0.629$
		Extreme values	0.012, 0.268	0.166, 3.212

[a] Adapted from Teisinger and Srbova.[526]
[b] Method of administration of CaEDTA: each patient was given a single intravenous injection of 15 ml of a 20% solution of calcium disodium ethylenediaminetetraacetate (2.8 g of anhydrous substance), and urine was collected quantitatively for 24 hr.

intramuscularly to a maximal dose of 1 g). (For intramuscular injection, procaine is added.) Urine should be collected quantitatively for 24 hr (4 days in persons with renal insufficiency). This test should not be used in symptomatic patients or those with blood lead content greater than 100 μg/100 g of whole blood, because the dosage may be insufficient to meet their therapeutic needs. Clinical judgment is clearly required in the use of this test in persons with high blood lead content, but no significant reactions have been reported in persons with normal or slightly increased blood lead content. Selander[487] has used D-penicillamine in a standard routine way with other drug support. With impaired renal function, the use of CaEDTA or D-penicillamine should be approached with caution, particularly when they are used therapeutically.

The measurement of heme precursors (PROTO, COPRO, ALA) provides the most sensitive index of current and recent absorption of inorganic lead salts. Normal values in "healthy" subjects and those with overt clinical lead poisoning are listed in Table 4–10.

Increases in urinary ALA and COPRO precede the appearance of clinical symptoms, and the values decrease when abnormal absorption is terminated. Measurement of urinary COPRO apparently is relatively insensitive to increments in occupational exposure to airborne lead. Various workers agree that, among urine tests, urinary ALA provides the best index of the level of absorption of lead[131,146,226,491] (see Figure 4–5). In persons with blood lead content over 40 μg/100 g of whole blood, arithmetic increases in blood lead concentration are apparently associated with exponential increases in urinary ALA and COPRO excretion, as well as exponential increases in the "mobile" or "metabolically active" lead in the tissues, as measured by the CaEDTA mobilization test.

Most of the analytic procedures currently in use for measuring ALA in urine are based on the method of Mauzerall and Granick.[376] Haeger-Aronsen[225] has recently reported that the method of Grabecki et al.,[213] which does not require chromatography, gives comparable results. These methods, as noted by Mauzerall and Granick,[376] also measure aminoacetone, an aminoketone that apparently fluctuates with food intake.[160,373] Aminoacetone excretion is not influenced by lead,[106,160] but such methods may still be suitable for the control of exposure of industrial workers. However, more specific methods[373,561] that exclude aminoacetone are indicated in studies designed to measure normal and minimally increased urinary excretion of ALA. Measurement of ALA in random urine samples in children is not

TABLE 4–10 Heme Precursors in Blood and Urine in "Healthy" and Lead-Poisoned Humans

Heme Precursor	Healthy Subjects (Mean ± 1 SD and/or Range)	Lead Poisoning and Increased Lead Absorption (Mean and/or Range)[a]	Type of Subjects	References
FEP, μg/100 ml packed red cells	m=28; r=12–45 (N=9)	m=2,475; r=1,040–6,620 (N=13)	Children	572
	r=25–125 (N=21)	–	Children	589
	m=30; r=16–52 (N=20)	–	Adult males	485, 589
	m=37; r=18–51 (N=20)	–	Adult females	485, 589
	–	r=570–2,516 (N=6)	Children	418
	m=27	r=252–1,068 (N=31)	Exposed adults	473
FEC, μg/100 ml packed red cells	m=1.6	r=0–26	Exposed adults	473
	m=0.8	–	Children	589
	r=0.5–1.5	–	?	485
Plasma PROTO, μg/100 ml	m=1.0	r=0–60	Exposed adults	473
Plasma COPRO, μg/100 ml	m=0.3	r=0–5.3	Exposed adults	473
Plasma PORPHYRIN, μg/100 ml	m=0.8; r=0.4–1.5	–	–	589
Plasma or serum ALAD, μg/100 ml	m=19 ± 4 (N=50)	m=> 27 (N=12 of 34)	Exposed adults	226
	m=11 ± 5 (N=13)	m=37; r=21–77 (N=16)	Children	177
	m=5.6 ± 1.9 (N=18)	r=20–140 (N=28)	Children	103

	Normal values	Abnormal values[a]	Population	Ref.
ALAD activity assay				
Units of activity/ml red cells	—	100; ALAD=2.274-0.018 × blood Pb(µg/100 ml) for blood Pb r=5-95	Adults	247
nM PBG/hr per 10^{10} red cells	r=405-635 (N=57)	10; ALAD=0.0436 × blood Pb(µg/100 ml) + 6.7685 (N=57)	Children	391
	r=419-651 (N=20)		Adults	391
Urine ALAD,				
µg/100 ml[b]	r=10-570	r=0-5,000	Exposed adults	226
µg/24 hr[b]	m=2,130 ± 420	r=5,000-68,000	Exposed adults	226
µg/24 hr per kg body wt[b]	m=80 (N=339)		Children with the following blood Pb data: m=21; r=7-55 mg Pb/100 g whole blood	31
µg/24 hr[b]	m=1,610 95% r=80-4,390			
µg/24 hr[c]	r=810-1,800 (N=7)	r=6,500-73,000 (N=8)	Children	103
Urine COPRO				
µg/100 ml	m=7 ± 0.9 (N=100)	r=150-1,220	Adults	226
µg/24 hr	r=100-250		Exposed adults	226
µg/24 hr			Adults	485
µg/24 hr	m=38.5 ± 17.9 (N=12)		Boys 41-61 lb	263
µg/24 hr	m=66.2 ± 32.8 (N=21)		Boys 121-170 lb	263
µg/24 hr		r=450-3,420 (N=6)		109

[a] All abnormal values for children are for clinical lead poisoning; all abnormal values for adults are for occupational exposure to lead, in some cases with mild symptoms.
[b] By the method of Mauzerall and Granick.[376]
[c] By the method of Urata and Granick.[561]

suited for the early detection of increased lead absorption.[48] Owing to the wide variation in the concentration of ALA in random samples of urine from young children, large proportions of both false-negative and false-positive results have been encountered in attempts to adapt this test for mass screening. Because of this variation, the test seems relatively insensitive in children with blood lead concentrations of less than about 80–90 μg/100 g of whole blood. This is in contrast with experience in the medical supervision of industrially exposed workers, in whom serial measurements may be made under rather standardized conditions. In such persons, it is the trend of frequently repeated measurements that is most useful to the industrial physician. In industry, urinary ALA is one of several indices of the level of absorption that may be used serially in evaluating individual workers. This is quite different from the situation among children, in whom the attempt has been made to use a single determination of the ALA concentration in random samples of urine as the sole diagnostic test. ALA is stable in acid urine, but not in neutral or alkaline urine.[106,226] Hydrochloric acid, refrigeration, and protection from light may be used for preservation until analysis.

Critical factors in the analysis of FEP and FEC in blood and COPRO in urine are discussed by Schwartz *et al.*[485,486] and Wranne.[589] Among the important factors are use of dilute iodine as the oxidant in the analysis,[485] avoidance of ether (it may contain peroxides),[486] stabilization of COPRO in urine by addition of alkali (sodium carbonate)[485] and sulfanilamide, and protection from light. The use of ethyl acetate in place of ethyl ether is safer and minimizes interference due to peroxides. Although the quantitative determination of porphyrins in blood is limited largely to research, a simple rapid technique for estimating the proportion of fluorescent erythrocytes (due to PROTO) by fluorescence microscopy is reported to correlate well with CaEDTA mobilization test results in the case of high-level current exposure.[418]

Diagnostic Criteria

The various types and degrees of adverse metabolic, functional, and clinical effects attributable to increasing concentrations of lead in the tissues may be related to the concentration of lead in blood and, to a limited extent, to endogenous urinary lead excretion. This is shown schematically in Table 4–11, in which much of the information presented earlier in this chapter is summarized. The table is based on the concept that the rates of absorption, excretion, and storage of lead are interdependent. When the rate of absorption exceeds the rates of excretion and storage, the concentration of lead in the soft tissues rises. As soft-tissue concentration rises, adverse metabolic effects begin to appear, and these are followed by adverse functional and clinical effects. Some of the functional and clinical effects are reversible. The concentrations of lead in blood shown in the table have not been corrected for deviations in hematocrit from normal. The overlapping values reflect, therefore, the effects of anemia and the uncertainty of clinical diagnosis, particularly in persons with mild symptoms and other disease states associated with symptoms similar to those of lead poisoning.

In persons with blood lead concentrations lower than approximately 40 μg/100 g of whole blood, no adverse effects related to current exposure have been demonstrated *in vivo*, although changes in the level of ALAD activity in hemolysates of human blood have been demonstrated *in vitro*. These may be classified diagnostically as normal or "healthy" persons. Epidemiologic data indicate that most of the general population is in this category.[204,554] Blood lead concentrations in this range may be found in persons whose excessive exposures have been remote in time. Level II in Table 4–11 designates persons with a minimal increase in urinary ALA excretion only and is associated with blood lead concentrations between approximately 40 and approximately 60 μg/100 g of whole blood. Epidemiologic data[204,298,554] indicate that some groups residing or working in congested urban areas might be expected to show a minimal increase in urinary ALA if it were measured. Mean blood lead concentrations between 40 and 60 μg/100 g of whole blood have been reported in two studies of urban children.[49,62] With respect to ambient airborne lead, all population groups so far reported are in Levels I and II, as defined in Table 4–11.

The term "asymptomatic increased lead absorption" is used to designate persons with evidence of increased lead absorption and storage and increased concentrations of ALA and pyrroles in blood and urine, but without evidence of renal impairment, anemia due to lead, or other symptoms compatible with acute lead poisoning. The hematologic disturbance is compensated by increased red blood cell production. Alterations in the properties of red blood cells may be demonstrable *in vitro* in this group. It also appears that some may have abnormalities in peripheral nerve conduction. It is rare to find subjects with blood lead concentrations greater than 60 μg/100 g of

TABLE 4-11 Level and Types of Effects of Inorganic Lead Salts as Related to Estimates of Various Levels of Absorption—Recent and Remote

Type of Effects	Level I: No Demonstrable in vivo Effect	Level II: Minimal Subclinical Metabolic Effect	Level III: Compensatory Biologic Mechanisms Invoked	Level IV: Acute Lead Poisoning		Level V: Late Effects of Chronic or Recurrent Acute Lead Poisoning
				Mild	Severe	
Metabolic (accumulation and excretion of heme precursors)	Changing ALAD[a]	Slight increase in urinary ALA may be present	ALA, UCP, FEP progressively increased	ALA, UCP, FEP increased 5- to 100 fold		Increased if excessive exposure recent, but may not be increased if excessive exposure remote
Functional injury: Hematopoiesis	None	None known	Shortened red-cell life-span, reticulocytosis (±) (reversible)	Shortened red-cell life-span and reticulocytosis with or without anemia (reversible)		Anemia (±) (reversible)
Kidney (renal tubular function)	None	None known	?	Aminoaciduria, glycosuria (±) (reversible)	Fanconi syndrome (reversible)	Chronic nephropathy[b] (permanent)

128

Central nervous system	None	None known	?	Mild injury (??? reversible)	Severe injury (permanent)	Severe injury[b] (permanent)
Peripheral nerves	None	None known	?	Rare	Rare	Impaired conduction (wrist, foot drop usually improve slowly, but may be permanent)
Clinical effects	None	None known	Nonspecific mild symptoms (may be due in part to coexisting diseases)	Colic, irritability, vomiting	Ataxia, stupor, coma, convulsions	Mental deficiency (may be profound), seizure disorder, renal insufficiency (gout) (permanent)
Index of level of recent or current absorption:						
Blood lead, μg/100 g of whole blood	<40	40–60	50–100+	>80 With anemia, intercurrent disease: 50–100+	>80	May be normal
Urine lead (adults only), μg/liter	—	<80	<130	>130 (May be less in severe illness)	>130	Spontaneous excretion may be normal

[a]See p. 106 for discussion of changing levels of ALAD.
[b]CaEDTA mobilization test in chronic nephropathy is positive; may or may not be positive in permanent central nervous system injury.

whole blood who have not had some exposure to lead, in addition to that found in normal diet and ambient air in urban areas. With respect to children, the term "asymptomatic increased lead absorption" has been defined in a few cities for legal purposes as a confirmed blood lead concentration greater than 60 μg/100 g of whole blood. It has been recommended recently that this limit be revised downward.[102] Table 4–11 indicates considerable overlap in blood lead concentrations between Level III (compensatory biologic mechanisms invoked) and Level IV (acute lead poisoning). For example (Figure 4–5), there may be much variation in urinary ALA, as well as in the excretion of other heme precursors at blood lead concentrations between 40 and 80 μg/100 g of whole blood. Sustained blood lead concentrations above approximately 80 or 90 μg/100 g of whole blood are uniformly associated with deranged heme synthesis, as well as other clinical manifestations of lead poisoning.

The diagnosis of acute lead poisoning is based on a full consideration of metabolic, functional, and clinical factors. Classic acute lead poisoning has been defined as the presence of lead-related anemia, symptoms exclusive of central nervous system manifestations, or both. In the presence of anemia due to other causes, severe anemia due to lead poisoning, or other diseases (such as renal insufficiency and sickle cell disease) that may modify a subject's response to increased lead content in the tissues, symptomatic lead poisoning may be associated with blood lead concentration as low as approximately 50 or 60 μg/100 g of whole blood. If inorganic lead contributes to the symptom complex in such patients, either heme precursors (e.g., ALA in urine) will be greatly increased, the response to the CaEDTA mobilization test will be abnormal, or both. In view of the nonspecificity of mild symptoms of acute lead poisoning and the ease with which they may be confused with acute alcoholism, acute intermittent prophyria, and various surgical and nonsurgical abdominal conditions, a thorough laboratory evaluation with respect to lead is essential, and even then, differential diagnosis may be difficult.

Acute lead encephalopathy is almost always associated with blood lead concentrations greater than 120 μg/100 g of whole blood (Figure 4–2), marked diuresis of lead in response to chelation therapy, and the clinical findings described earlier in this chapter. According to present criteria, the diagnosis of chronic lead nephropathy requires the demonstration of an increased body lead burden by the CaEDTA mobilization test (or bone biopsy) and the presence of functional renal impairment, as previously described. Permanent residual effects of acute central nervous system injury after acute lead encephalopathy are not necessarily associated with the persistence of an increased body lead burden, as measured by the CaEDTA mobilization test.

All reported instances of permanent injury to the nervous system and kidneys in man that have been attributed to lead have been associated with a history of single episodes of acute lead encephalopathy, recurrent episodes of symptomatic lead poisoning, or prolonged absorption of greatly increased amounts of lead. The exposure to lead of persons with permanent renal or neurologic injury caused by lead must have been, at some time, greatly in excess of the exposure that can be attributed to lead in the ambient air. Whether persons who meet the above criteria for asymptomatic increased lead absorption may also manifest subtle impairment in renal and nervous system function—or, for that matter, endocrinologic function—as they do in heme synthesis and various other hematologic indices, is not known; as indicated in Table 4–11, no data are available from which such estimates can be made.

Summary

Blood lead concentration, spontaneous urinary lead excretion, and the CaEDTA mobilization test may be used to measure current and recent levels of exposure to lead. Spontaneous urinary lead output, as determined either quantitatively or qualitatively, may not be increased in persons who have an increase in the mobile fraction of body lead burden but who also have renal insufficiency. In the presence of renal insufficiency, urinary lead output should be measured quantitatively for 4 days after the parenteral administration of CaEDTA. The available data indicate that the CaEDTA mobilization test provides an estimate of the mobile fraction of the total body lead burden, and experiments in animals suggest that most of the mobile fraction is derived from bone. However, it appears that only a fraction of the lead in bone is mobilized by chelating agents. Autopsy analyses indicate that bone biopsy is required for estimation of total body lead burden, but this has rarely been done in the living. However, it is the mobile fraction of the total body lead burden that is apparently responsible for the adverse immediate effects of lead. The CaEDTA mobilization test may not necessarily provide an index of irreversible tissue injury that has resulted in tissue scarring in the very remote past.

The concentrations of heme precursors in body fluids and urine provide the best understood metabolic indices of the adverse effects of lead. Of these, ALAD activity in hemolysates of blood and ALA in urine have been most extensively studied with respect to various degrees of absorption of lead. FEP has been studied in normal populations and in persons with overt lead poisoning, but not at intermediate subclinical levels of increased lead absorption. Studies of UCP at intermediate levels of increased lead absorption are limited. Nevertheless, the pattern of increase for all these heme precursors appears to be similar.

Arithmetic increases in the lead content in blood above 40 μg/100g of whole blood are associated with exponential increases in urinary ALA output, urinary COPRO output, and urinary output of lead after administration of CaEDTA (or D-penicillamine). Significant correlations are also found between the chelatable lead and the excretion of heme precursors and suggest that urinary ALA and UCP provide an index of the "metabolically active" or toxic fraction of the total body lead burden. For the clinician, the curvilinear relation between blood lead content and ALAD, ALA, UCP, and chelatable lead indicates that arithmetic increases in blood lead concentration are associated with an exponentially decreasing margin of safety. For example, an increase in blood lead content from 40 to 60 μg/100 g of whole blood may be associated with relatively little change in health status, whereas an increase from 60 to 80 μg/100 g of whole blood markedly increases the risk of symptomatic illness. The diagnostic evaluation of human subjects may be based on the concept of exponentially increasing risk that attends arithmetic increments in blood lead content. It is possible that increments in spontaneous urinary lead output may follow a similar pattern, although the available data do not show this clearly.

EPIDEMIOLOGY

Children

Today in the United States, lead poisoning in children is believed to be due almost entirely to the repetitive eating of leaded house paint.[358] Most of the available data are based on retrospective analyses of small groups of cases from cities in which childhood lead poisoning is a reportable disease and in which the municipal health departments have active programs—namely, New York City, Chicago,

Philadelphia, and Baltimore. Although the nationwide incidence of
the disease in children is unknown, some epidemiologic features are
well established: prevalence of pica in preschool children, seasonal
variation, age distribution of cases, association with dilapidated and
deteriorating housing, race, and sex.

The term "pica" has been defined as the repetitive ingestion of
things that are not food (e.g., string, dirt, paper, putty, paint, clay,
and cigarette butts). It is important in a variety of accidental poisonings in preschool children.[513] The behavioral and biologic factors
responsible for this age-related activity are not understood. Lourie
and his associates[364,392] have stressed disturbed parent–child relations
as a factor that can intensify pica in the child, whereas Neumann[420]
has suggested that it may be a vestigial instinct. Lourie and associates[364,392] and Sobel[513] found that the habit begins at the age of
about 12 months, that it may persist until the age of 3–5 years, and
that it occurs in at least 50% of children in both middle-class and
poverty groups. Thus, pica is apparently a rather common behavioral
activity in normal preschool children, and it may become intensified
in response to stress.

The well-recognized association between childhood lead poisoning
and old housing[49,122,221,271,273,358,484,583] has been discussed earlier in
this chapter. No differences related to sex have been found. The vast
majority of reported cases are found in Negro and Puerto Rican children. This concentration of cases is apparently related to the high
concentration of such children in deteriorating urban housing and not
to any known genetic, racial, or ethnic factors.

The seasonal distribution of the fatal and nonfatal cases for which
blood lead concentrations are given in Figure 4–2 is shown in Figure
4–9. This is characteristic of the seasonal distribution reported
throughout the United States.[49,122,271,273,358,583] Between 85 and 90%
of all fatal and nonfatal symptomatic cases are recognized during the
months of May through October. Blanksma et al.[49] reported data that
suggest that seasonal factors are also operative, even in "normal" circumstances. In a group of 746 control children under 6 years old
without undue exposure to lead, the mean blood lead content for the
entire year was $23.5 \pm 7.8 \ \mu g/100$ g of whole blood. However, within
this group, the mean peak blood lead content by month of testing
was found in June (mean, approximately 36 $\mu g/100$ g of whole blood),
with a secondary peak in February. This observation requires confirmation.

Within the preschool age range, 80–85% of all reported fatal and

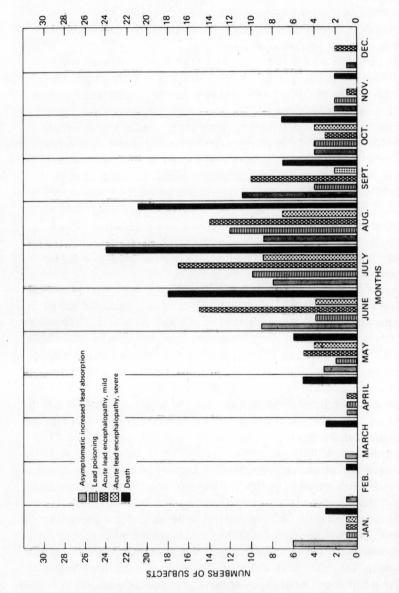

FIGURE 4–9 Seasonal distribution by month of report of diagnosis of fatal and nonfatal cases of lead poisoning and increased lead absorption (same cases shown in Figure 4–2).

nonfatal cases occur in children 12-35 months old[122,271,273,514,583] (Figure 4-10). After a survey of 103 children from the metropolitan Philadelphia area who did not have anemia, a history of pica, or signs suggestive of poisoning, Robinson et al.[457] report that blood lead content is constant between the ages of 6 months and 13 years (median, 27 μg/100 g of whole blood; middle 90% range, 15-40 μg/100 g of whole blood). This may be contrasted with the findings in 1953-1954 in a metropolitan pediatric clinic serving children who lived exclusively in dilapidated housing. The findings in 333 children distributed by age and blood lead content are shown in Table 4-12. Among 219 children 10-36 months old, 106 (48.4%) had blood lead concentrations of 50 μg/100 g of whole blood or higher, and eight (3.7%) had blood lead concentrations of at least 100 μg/100 g of whole blood, the point above which the risk of encephalopathy becomes significant. Localized concentrations of cases in the very worst housing areas have been noted in other cities in 1- and 2-year-olds.[221,271,514] Although age-related data are not given, Blanksma et al.[49] noted differences between various geographic areas within Chicago in the incidence of blood lead concentrations over 50 μg/100 g of whole blood (Table 4-13). However, there are no published data on blood lead content in healthy children who live in modern safe housing.

Estimates of the incidence of leaded-paint poisoning and the prevalence of blood lead concentrations that may be associated with adverse health effects can be made only on the most tenuous grounds. With the exception of a few of the larger cities, it is not a reportable disease. For the most part, recognition is based on the case-finding approach, which in turn depends on the level of awareness in the local medical community and the availability of diagnostic laboratory facilities. Only in Chicago (since October 1966) and in New York City (since January 1970) are prospective mass-screening programs currently in operation for young children. The Chicago program is concentrated in nine areas in the city and includes the operation of an ambulatory treatment center. About 68,800 children under 5 years old in these areas (47% of that segment of the population) were tested in 1967 and 1968 (Table 4-13). Of these, 3,935 (5.7%) had blood lead concentrations of 50 μg/100 g of whole blood or higher.[49] An additional 48,000 children were tested in 1969. The numbers and percentages of children found each year to have blood lead concentrations of 50 μg/100 g of whole blood or higher were 2,379 (8.5%) in 1967, 1,556 (3.8%) in 1968, and 1,172 (2.4%) in 1969. During 1967 and 1968, 1,154 (1.68%) of the children tested were treated as

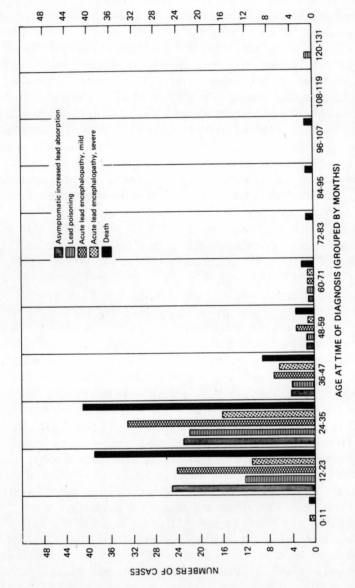

FIGURE 4-10 Numbers of cases for each diagnostic classification, grouped by month of age at time of diagnosis (same cases shown in Figure 4–2).

TABLE 4-12 Distribution of Children According to Blood Lead Content and Age[a]

Blood Lead, Concentration, μg/100 g of Whole Blood	Age, Months							
	7-10	10-18	18-24	24-30	30-36	36-42	42-48	48-60
19 or less	0	1	0	0	0	0	0	0
20-29	8	9	4	2	2	3	2	3
30-39	8	14	9	11	4	3	6	7
40-49	5	20	10	17	10	8	3	14
50-59	0	16	6	16	7	3	3	11
60-69	0	5	11	7	10	4	4	4
70-79	0	2	7	1	3	5	1	0
80-89	0	2	1	1	2	1	1	2
90-99	0	0	1	0	0	0	0	0
100 or higher	0	0	1	4	3	1	1	0

[a]Adapted from Bradley et al.[62]

cases of poisoning, and in 1969, 456 (0.95%) were treated as cases of poisoning. This decrease after the first year (1967) in the numbers of reported cases may be attributed to the backlog of previously unrecognized cases, first identified at the inception of the screening program. A "steady state" may be anticipated when a backlog of older children is finally reduced and new cases are confined to the 1- to 2-year-old group representing the annual input of new births. A continued input of new cases at a steady rate may be anticipated so long as the hazard in old housing exists and the number of deteriorating dwellings containing lead-based paints remains unchanged.

In New York City, during the first 7 months of 1970, 64,644 blood specimens were analyzed for lead by the Health Department; 2,070 children with blood lead concentrations of 60 μg/100 g of whole blood or greater were found, and two deaths attributable to lead poisoning were reported.[514] The distribution of blood lead concentrations indicates a mean of approximately 20 μg/100 g of whole blood, with 11% greater than 50 μg/100 g and 0.2% 110 μg/100 g or greater in children 1–6 years old.[514] The epidemiologic data cited above are, in general, limited, in that only children with blood lead concentrations greater than 50 or 60 μg/100 g of whole blood are identified. The percentage of children in these groups with concentrations greater than 40 μg/100 g of whole blood is clearly much higher. Elsewhere in this chapter, evidence is presented that urinary ALA excretion in-

TABLE 4-13 Data of Survey Areas for Chicago Blood Lead Screening Program, 1967–1968[a]

Urban Area	(A) No. Children under 5 Years Old (1960 Census)[b]	1967 (B) Children tested No.[b]	% of A	1967 Children with High Lead[c] No.	% of B	1968 (C) Children Tested No.[b]	% of A	1968 Children with High Lead[c] No.	% of C	Totals for 1967–1968 (D) Children Tested No.[b]	% of A	Totals Children with High Lead[c] No.	% of D
1	10,000	2,500	25	157	6.3	3,100	31	53	1.7	5,600	56	210	3.8
2	15,100	1,700	11	73	4.3	1,800	12	56	3.1	3,500	23	129	3.7
3	22,000	2,000	9	262	13.1	3,000	14	166	5.5	5,000	23	428	8.6
4	22,300	5,200	23	509	9.8	5,500	25	270	4.9	10,700	48	779	7.3
5	13,700	4,100	30	316	7.7	4,900	36	142	2.9	9,000	66	458	5.1
6	24,500	6,600	27	393	6.0	7,700	31	277	3.6	14,300	58	670	4.7
7	20,500	3,400	17	432	12.7	7,000	34	356	5.1	10,400	51	788	7.6
8	15,300	2,200	14	218	9.9	6,100	40	227	3.7	8,300	54	445	5.4
9	4,500	300	7	19	6.3	1,700	38	9	0.5	2,000	44	28	1.4
Totals	147,900	28,000	19	2,379	8.5	40,800	28	1,556	3.8	68,800	47	3,935	5.7

[a] Adapted from Blanksma et al.[49]
[b] Figures given to nearest hundred.
[c] 50 µg/100 g of whole blood or higher.

creases as blood lead content rises above 40 μg/100 g of whole blood and that increasing urinary ALA excretion represents metabolic interference due to lead in the biosynthetic pathway for the synthesis of heme.

Street dust is a potential source of ingested lead, especially in children. Monthly dustfall samples were collected in 77 midwestern cities in 1968.[266,499] The mean lead concentration in dust from various sectors of each city was calculated after averaging the results for all the cities as follows: residential, 1,636 μg/g of dust; commercial, 2,413 μg/g of dust; and industrial, 1,512 μg/g of dust. The swallowing of as much as 1 g of such dust could result in the oral intake of an amount of lead that exceeds by a factor of 10 or more the estimated mean daily intake of lead from normal food and drink in nonexposed young children (130 μg/day excreted in feces).[33,110] Although the available data on the distribution of blood lead concentrations and other epidemiologic data clearly indicate that this *alone* does not account for clinical lead poisoning in children, the swallowing of lead-contaminated dusts may well account, in large part, for the higher mean blood lead content in urban children[49,62,457] and the rather large fraction whose blood lead content falls in the range of 40–60 μg/100 g of whole blood, thereby bringing them into the range in which increased urinary excretion of ALA may be observed. For a child with pica for paint, the combination of the ingestion of a few chips of paint and an increased intake of lead from contaminated dusts would provide a total lead intake sufficient to cause symptomatic illness.

In summary, adequate epidemiologic data, based on proven methods of lead analysis (dithizone technique), on the distribution of blood lead concentrations in young children without undue exposure to lead are not available. The problem is complicated by the prevalence of pica in young children. The few data that are available are based largely on samples of children in metropolitan areas. In these groups, mean blood lead concentrations are somewhat higher than those found in adults, but in one report the range did not exceed 15–40 μg/100 g of whole blood. One unpublished report showed that rural and suburban children have lower blood lead content than adults in similar environments. However, large-scale screening programs in urban areas suggest that perhaps 5–10% of young children who live in deteriorating old housing have concentrations of lead in their blood that may be associated with adverse metabolic effects, at the very least; and 1–2% may have evidence of lead poisoning. Where active screening programs are in operation, the numbers of reported cases increase, while the numbers of reported deaths decrease to well under 1% of reported cases. Season, age, pica, and housing are the identified epidemiologic determinants of childhood lead poisoning in the United States today.

The extent to which airborne lead in congested urban areas contributes to increased lead absorption and lead poisoning in children is not clearly defined. With respect to young children, it is not a matter exclusively of inhalation and particle size, inasmuch as young children mouth and actually eat things that are not food rather indiscriminately. Airborne lead wastes from such sources as automotive emissions and the weathering and demolition of old buildings can be expected to have a significant additive effect on the total intake. This would be sufficient to evoke compensatory metabolic responses that are now considered subclinical (such as increased urinary A L A), at the very least. It may be estimated that dustfall from airborne lead, if swallowed, can make a significant contribution to a small child's total lead intake and thereby contribute to the occurrence of lead poisoning, especially in urban areas. Even so, the direct ingestion of lead-pigment paints is clearly the principal environmental source in cases of severe acute lead poisoning in young children.

Adults

In studying diseases due to a single environmental agent, such as lead, three main stages in man's state of knowledge may be distinguished. The first is the recognition of the disease state, without appreciation of the nature of the causative agent. It is at this stage of man's knowledge that Paul of Aegina and Avicenna described patients suffering from "colicky affections" accompanied by paralysis, which may well represent lead poisoning; but by the second century B.C., some writers had already entered the second stage of man's knowledge of the biologic effects of lead, with the recording of unequivocal evidence linking the disease to the causative agent, lead. At that time, Nikander wrote his "Alexipharmaca," describing both colic and paralysis as the result of ingesting litharge (lead oxide). The third stage of knowledge of the biologic action of an agent, such as lead, comes with the demonstration that the severity of the effect produced is directly related to the amount of the agent. This third stage is often delayed, because only severe disease produced by massive doses is recognized at first, and more subtle effects are missed. Such situations are illustrated by the sporadic and usually accidental lead exposures reported after 1500, at about which time the development of printing made the dissemination of such reports easier and their preservation more certain.

In 1572, an epidemic of lead poisoning occurred in the French province of Poitou, owing to drinking wine adulterated with litharge; from then on, repeated epidemics of lead poisoning due to intentional or accidental adulteration of cider,[504] rum,[382] or food[241] or to drinking water conveyed in lead pipes[330,383] were reported. More recently, there have been outbreaks of lead poisoning presumably due to airborne lead particles from the burning of old automobile batteries to provide domestic heating.[218,584]

It is with the beginning of the Industrial Revolution, with the splitting of the manufacturing process into discrete operations performed by separate groups of workers with different degrees of lead exposure, that it becomes possible to study sickness rates and relate them to the amount of lead in the workers' environment.

One of the first studies that clearly showed a relation between degree of lead exposure and amount and severity of the sickness produced was that of Duckering in 1908.[161] As a result of his measurements of the amount of lead in the air breathed by workmen in a number of British factories and his records of the number of men with signs of lead intoxication, Legge and Goadby suggested in 1912 that

if the amount of lead present in the air breathed contains less than 5 milligrammes per 10 cubic metres of air, cases of encephalopathy and paralysis would never, and cases of colic very rarely, occur. And this figure is a quite practical one in any process amenable to locally-applied exhaust ventilation. Somewhere about 2 milligrammes, or 0.002 gramme, of lead we regard as the lowest daily dose which, inhaled as fume or dust in the air, may, in the course of years, set up chronic plumbism.[342]

With the demonstration that exposure to a specific amount of lead caused a specific biologic response and that the clinical response became less as the dose of absorbed lead diminished, the prevention of the disease depended increasingly on the ability of engineers to control the amount of lead in workmen's environment. This ability to control lead poisoning by a combined medical and engineering approach backed by government regulations is illustrated by the figures for notified cases of lead poisoning in Great Britain, which decreased from 1,058 in 1900 to 239 in 1928.[341] Similar studies in the United States[159,218] confirmed that the number of cases of plumbism was

TABLE 4-14   Cases of Lead Poisoning among Battery Workers in Areas Having Different Lead Exposures[a]

Atmospheric Lead Concentration, mg/m³ of Air	No. Men Exposed	Men with Early Plumbism	
		No.	%
0–0.074	97	4	4.1
0.075–0.14	84	6	7.1
0.15–0.29	168	50	29.8
⩾0.3	125	67	53.6

[a]Adapted from Dreessen et al.[159]

positively correlated with the amount of lead in the air, as shown in Table 4-14.*

Because the major route of entry for lead in an industrial worker is the lungs, information from the study of industrial populations commonly relates the clinical or biochemical findings to the concentration of lead in the air. But similar relations between the amount of lead absorbed and the biologic effect produced have been found for ingested lead[298] and for lead injected intravenously as a therapeutic agent.[40] It has also been found that the degree of exposure to lead is reflected in the concentrations of lead in the blood and urine of exposed persons. Such relations may vary considerably when the values from different persons are compared, but the variation is much less when the average or median values for groups of persons are studied. The values in Table 4-15 should be used only to show a general tendency for increasing exposure to be reflected in increased blood lead concentrations, inasmuch as the exposure to lead is not completely described in terms of particle size, which is known to play an important part in the deposition and absorption of lead in lungs. Another factor that tends to reduce the degree of correlation between the lead concentration in blood and that in the air in the study summarized in Table 4-15 is the medical control exerted by the physicians in charge of the workers. This control removed many of the men in the high-exposure group and placed them in areas of lower exposure; they appear in Table 4-15 under the heading "Exposure Changed."

*For reasons given in the discussion of Table 4-15, such data as those for Table 4-14 can be used to show qualitative relations only, and no conclusions as to allowable limits for the concentration of lead in the air should be drawn from this information alone.

A more recent study[585] that illustrates the relation between lead exposure and urine and blood lead concentrations yielded the data in Table 4–16. In this study, by Williams *et al.*, although the number of men observed (39) was not large, the use of personal air samplers and the number of observations made make the results more valuable than usual. From these data, Williams *et al.* calculated correlation coefficients (γ) and regressions of the biochemical value (Y) with the mean 8-hr lead-in-air concentration (X). The results are shown below:

	γ	Y	X
Blood lead	0.90	$30.1 + 201X$	$-0.0975 + 0.00399Y$
Urine lead	0.82	$45.5 + 486X$	$-0.0277 + 0.00138Y$

Experimental exposures of human beings to known concentrations of airborne or ingested lead have provided graphic data describing the

TABLE 4–15 Average and Median Blood Lead Content (Dithizone Method) in mg/100 g of Blood in Storage-Battery Workers, by Exposure and Duration of Employment[a]

Duration of Lead Exposure, Years	Exposure not De-finable	Exposure Changed	Air Lead Content, mg/m^3			
			0–0.074	0.075–0.14	0.15–0.29	$\geqslant$0.3
0–4						
Number	26	12	17	16	32	20
Average	0.0352	0.0368	0.0187	0.0316	0.0378	0.0463
Median	0.024	0.040	0.021	0.030	0.038	0.050
5–9						
Number	30	46	10	13	40	24
Average	0.0352	0.0475	0.0278	0.0405	0.0501	0.0505
Median	0.033	0.046	0.033	0.040	0.043	0.050
10–14						
Number	5	22	23	24	30	32
Average	0.0508	0.0344	0.0198	0.0375	0.0502	0.0481
Median	0.036	0.037	0.018	0.038	0.046	0.048
15+						
Number	7	26	44	30	59	45
Average	0.0341	0.0520	0.0293	0.0407	0.0457	0.0493
Median	0.027	0.054	0.023	0.036	0.045	0.045

[a]Adapted from Dreessen *et al.*[159]

TABLE 4-16 Departmental Means and Standard Errors of 8-hr Lead-in-Air, Blood, and Urine Lead Concentrations of Workers in Various Departments of Electric-Storage-Battery Plant[a]

Job	No. Workers	Air Lead Concentration, mg/m³		Blood Lead Concentration, μg/100 g Blood		Urine Lead Concentration, μg/Liter	
		Mean	SE	Mean	SE	Mean	SE
Machine pasting	6	0.218	0.025	74.2	4.7	163.8	21.2
Hand pasting	8	0.150	0.029	63.2	9.2	111.3	14.1
Forming	9	0.134	0.013	63.0	2.7	114.0	7.2
Casting	6	0.052	0.003	–	–	87.9	6.8
Plastics department A	5	0.012	0.0008	27.2	1.4	34.5	3.2
Plastics department B	5	0.009	0.0008	29.1	1.6	34.8	2.0

[a]Adapted from Williams et al.[585]

relation between degree of exposure and blood and urine lead concentrations.[298]

All the information so far discussed deals with occupational or experimental exposure, but a similar correlation between lead concentrations in air and blood has been found at air lead concentrations above 2 μg/m³ in the urban environment.[202] There have been no cases of characteristic lead poisoning due to lead as a community air pollutant. Therefore, from this point on, attention will be centered on studies of health effects of lead other than classic lead poisoning. Three main epidemiologic approaches have been used in seeking such health effects: to compare the health of occupational groups with documented lead exposures with the health of groups not so exposed, to study persons with a given disease and compare their tissue concentrations of lead with those of persons who do not suffer from the disease but are otherwise similar, and to study the geographic distribution of a given disease and compare it with the geographic distribution of a type of lead exposure.

HEALTH EFFECTS

The first method, if properly carried out, probably offers the chance of the greatest precision, but it suffers from some limitations inherent in the nature of an employed population, such as restrictions in age range and initial state of health. In the case of the lead industries, it is also likely to be a predominantly male group.

There have been very few epidemiologic studies of groups occupationally exposed to lead in which a large number of factors were documented and the results in different exposure groups compared. One of the earliest of such studies to use modern epidemiologic methods was of persons exposed to lead arsenate as a result of its use as an insecticide. As in most epidemiologic studies, which may be looked upon as naturally occurring experiments in which the investigator has little or no control over the experimental design, this study[417] of the orchardists in the Wenatchee area of Washington State was complicated (as far as this discussion is concerned) by the fact that it dealt with exposure to lead arsenate. This raises the question of the relative importance of the lead, compared with the arsenical, portion of the lead arsenate molecule in the overall toxicity of the compound. An attempt to answer this was made by special studies in animals. It was found that the greater toxicity of the molecule is to be attributed to the lead radical, rather than to the arsenic; no synergistic action of lead and arsenic was found.[174]

The lead concentrations, shown in Table 4-17, are not as high as

TABLE 4-17 Urine and Blood Lead Content of Persons in Wenatchee Study, by Severity of Exposure[a]

Group	Urine Lead Content			Blood Lead Content		
	No. Analyses	Average, μg/Liter	SD, μg/Liter	No. Analyses	Average, μg/100 g	SD, μg/100 g
Low exposure						
Men	146	35	21	148	26	11
Women	123	28	19	124	26	10
Intermediate exposure						
Men	102	43	30	108	30	11
Women	25	27	15	27	22	10
High exposure						
Men	386	88	60	329	44	16
Women	61	46	25	58	34	13
Children under 15						
Boys	81	53	39	17	37	15
Girls	65	54	40	14	36	10

[a]Adapted from Neal et al.[417]

those sometimes seen in other industrial exposures, but that makes them particularly important, because the urine lead concentrations range from slightly higher than commonly found in urban communties to the same as in moderate lead exposures in industry.

Among the factors studied in assessing the health of the orchardists were weight, blood pressure, diseases of the cardiovascular system, skin disorders, eye irritation, chronic nervous diseases, blood dyscrasias, kidney disease, pulmonary tuberculosis, visual acuity, syphilis, neoplastic disease, and fertility. Each was studied to find out whether it had been modified by the lead arsenate exposure. Insofar as comparative data for other populations were available, no evidence was found that any of these factors was altered by the exposure. Special attention was given to medical examination of children, because in the Wenatchee area, where orchards surrounded the communities or the houses in which they lived, there were unusual opportunities for children to be exposed to lead arsenate insecticide sprays and spray residues on branches, leaves, and grass, in addition to residues ingested on apples. In only one respect did these children differ from children in other districts: their urinary lead and arsenic concentrations were nearly twice as high as those of a group of 18 children measured at the same time in Washington, D.C. (who had a mean urine lead content of 0.026 mg/liter; SD, 0.0128). There was no indication of adverse effects of lead arsenate exposure on the health of the Wenatchee children.

Although the study of persons exposed to lead arsenate has many deficiencies as a source of information on the possible biologic effects of lead as an urban air pollutant, it is particularly important for two reasons: It is one of the few modern studies that include a substantial number of women of childbearing age, and it is one of the few studies that include children exposed to lead in a form other than paint.

The study (previously referred to)[159] of storage-battery workers whose blood lead concentrations were shown in Table 4–15 also looked for effects of exposure to lead on the incidence of diseases other than plumbism. Of the 766 men studied, 75% had been employed in electric-storage-battery plants for more than 5 years, and about 12% for 20 years or more. In this study, the incidence of disease in the high-exposure group (exposed to 0.15 mg/m³ or more) was compared with the incidence in the low-exposure group (exposed to less than 0.15 mg/m³). The prevalence of arteriosclerotic–hypertensive heart disease did not increase with increasing atmospheric lead concentration. In the age range 45–54, which covers the period when degenerative cardiovascular disease is making its appearance, 53 workers were exposed to atmospheric lead concentrations below 0.15 mg/m³, and 32% were found to have arteriosclerotic–hypertensive heart disease, as defined in the study. Of the 66 workers in the same age range exposed to concentrations in excess of 0.15 mg/m³, 32% had this type of heart disease. Unfortunately, there was no cohort study.

Another type of statistical treatment, shown in detail in Table 4–18, is to use the population exposed to less than 0.15 mg/m³ as a basis for predicting the number of cases that would be expected if the same incidence prevailed in all age groups of the more heavily exposed populations. If this assumption were correct, one would expect to find 35 cases of heart diseases of the arteriosclerotic–hypertensive group in 263 workers 25–64 years old exposed to atmospheric lead concentrations in excess of 0.15 mg/m³. Making allowance for the differences in age distribution, the 37 cases found agree closely with the expected number. The agreement is even closer for the 102 workers who changed jobs within 5 years of the time of study: 13.7 expected cases; 14 observed. Thus, it may be concluded that an increase in lead exposure was not accompanied by any increase in the prevalence of this group of diseases of the cardiovascular system.

When lead-affected workers are compared in the same way as before with workers exposed to less than 0.15 mg/m³ of air, one would expect to find 27.3 cases of arteriosclerotic–hypertensive heart disease in the 169 lead-affected workers 25–64 years old. Actually, there were 34 cases, but, considering the standard deviation (4.78) attached to that estimate, the difference is not statistically significant. Application of a chi-square test confirms this conclusion.

Response to a standard exercise test was as good in men exposed to lead concentrations of 0.15 mg/m³ or more as in men of comparable age exposed to lower concentrations. Men who had changed jobs during the preceding 5 years also, as a class, had equally satisfactory returns to pre-exercise pulse rates and systolic and diastolic blood pressure. Blood pressures, measured with a mercury sphygmomanometer, agree closely with the average values for 6,667 industrial workers in nine other industries studied by the Public Health Service.[66] As an additional check, a tabulation was made of men with pre-exercise blood pressures in excess of 150 mm Hg. The number and percentage with higher systolic pressures, for storage-battery workers compared with other industrial workers,[66] agree closely, showing that hyper-

TABLE 4-18 Computation Sheet, Showing Number of Cases of Arteriosclerotic–Hypertensive Heart Disease Expected in Workers Relatively Heavily Exposed to Lead, Assuming Age Incidence To Be Same as in Relatively Lightly Exposed Workers

Years (a)	Exposed to Less Than 0.15 mg/m³			Exposed to 0.15 mg/m³ or More			Exposure Changed		
	No. Exposed (b)	No. Cases (c)	% Affected (d)	No. Exposed (e)	No. Expected Cases (d) × (e)	No. Observed Cases (f)	No. Exposed (g)	No. Expected Cases (d) × (g)	No. Observed Cases (h)
25–34	31	1	3.2	94	3.0	3	31	1.0	0
35–44	51	3	5.9	84	4.9	5	38	2.2	4
45–54	53	17	32.1	66	21.2	21	22	7.0	5
55–64	19	6	31.6	19	6.0	8	11	3.5	5
Total					35.1	37		13.7	14

148

tension of this degree is no more prevalent in the storage-battery industry than in other industries.

Information on the effect of exposure to lead on the cardiovascular system has been given in some detail because many earlier writers thought this system was affected by lead. However, after reviewing those authors, Aub[19] (p. 121) concluded that,

although the general clinical opinion holds that arteriosclerosis is a result of chronic plumbism, this idea is based entirely on the occurrence of this condition in many post mortem examinations. That arteriosclerosis is much more frequent in those exposed to lead than in other individuals of the same age, however, needs much more statistical proof before it can be accepted.

Some 20 years later, Cantarow and Trumper, in their book[84] on lead poisoning, claimed that lead at such high concentrations that lead poisoning has occurred or is likely to occur may be associated with degenerative vascular disease.

Support for the view that lead at high concentrations may be linked to degenerative vascular disease is found in a British study of battery workers,[154] in which three exposure grades were defined as: Grade A, no exposure; Grade B, negligible exposure; and Grade C, exposure represented for the last 20 years by a mean urine lead content of 0.100–0.250 mg/liter (in the past, these have frequently exceeded 0.250 mg/liter). The mean exposure periods for the pensioners in Grades B and C were 35.3 and 32.3 years, respectively; for men who died while employed, the mean exposure periods for Grades B and C were 26.8 and 21.8 years, respectively. There was found to be a significant excess of deaths from all causes among the pensioners in Grade C, but not in either of the other grades. When the deaths attributed to vascular lesions are studied in this series, a highly significant excess of deaths due to cerebrovascular catastrophes was found among Grade C pensioners. As can be seen in Table 4–19, although the deaths of pensioners before 1951 showed an excess of observed over expected in both Grades B and C, after 1950 only Grade C shows an excess of deaths. This suggests that improvements in hygienic standards, with a consequent decrease in lead exposure, may have resulted in the observed improvement in mortality experience. It is unfortunate that this study, initiated to learn the incidence of cancer among battery workers, did not yield more information on the physiologic status of the men; for instance, the incidence of hypertension in the various exposure groups would have been most interesting.

TABLE 4-19 Expected and Observed Deaths from Cerebral Hemorrhage, Cerebral Thrombosis, and Cerebral Arteriosclerosis in Pensioners, 1926–1961, and in Employed Men, 1946–1961

| | | Grade of Exposure[a] | | | | | |
| | | A | | B | | C | |
Group	Year of Death	No. Deaths Expected	No. Deaths Observed	No. Deaths Expected	No. Deaths Observed	No. Deaths Expected	No. Deaths Observed
Pensioners	1926–1950	0.7	0	0.2	3	0.8	5
	1951–1961	7.2	6	3.2	3	8.5	19
	1926–1961	7.9	6	3.4	6	9.3	24[b]
Employed	1946–1961	3.2	3	3.1	3	5.6	9

[a] See text.
[b] $p < 0.001$; chi square, 21.7.

The apparent difference between the experiences of European and North American investigators studying the effect of lead on the blood vessels is thought by Lane[329] to reflect the working conditions on the two sides of the Atlantic, although he points out that the study of Dreessen et al.[159] included only 12% of men with more than 20 years of exposure and that there has been no adequate study of U.S. workers exposed to high concentrations of lead for one or two decades. The study of Cramér and Dahlberg[130] supports the view that lead workers in carefully supervised plants do not, even after long exposure, have a higher risk of hypertension than nonlead workers. They studied 364 workers, of whom 82 had been employed for more than 20 years and 265 for more than 10 years. The incidence of hypertension in various age and exposure groups was studied and compared within groups and with data gathered in an extensive Norwegian study of men not exposed to lead. In none of these comparisons was there any evidence of an effect of lead exposure, in terms of either duration or severity, on the incidence of hypertension.

The same confusion of claims and counterclaims regarding the effects of lead surrounds the subject of kidney disease and hypertension. Views on these conditions, as on arteriosclerosis, appear to depend on the characteristics of the lead exposure of the workers studied. The earlier observers saw many more cases of heavy prolonged exposure to lead than is possible today and were convinced that chronic kidney disease and hypertension were direct, although delayed, consequences of exposure to lead. The extensive literature on this matter has been reviewed by Radošević et al.[449] Browning[68] points out that no actual undue rise in blood pressure of workers in the electric-storage-battery industry was demonstrated by Belknap,[38] Dreessen et al.,[159] or Lane,[328] that the absence of significant change shows that the exposure had not reached a dangerous level, and that the relative absence of chronic renal disease in lead workers is probably due to the improvement of conditions in modern lead industries.

It appears that modern lead workers in well-supervised plants, although still absorbing more lead than other workers, do not run a risk of arteriosclerosis, hypertension, or kidney disease due to exposure to lead. This conclusion is supported by the Wenatchee study,[417] with its generally moderate level of lead exposure, and the studies of Baader[21] and Vigliani.[565] The epidemiologic experience with groups of persons exposed to lead and other materials through their consumption of illicitly distilled whiskey is dealt with elsewhere in this report, but, in general, it may be said that the kidney disease seen in such groups is associated with high lead absorption.[402]

SUSCEPTIBILITY DIFFERENCES

It is important to raise the question of whether some groups of workers are more susceptible than others to the effect of lead. As in every question of biologic effects of lead, the degree of exposure must be considered. Differences in susceptibility might show up in conditions of severe lead exposure that would not be common in the general population; it is also possible that some persons are unusually susceptible to "normal" degrees of exposure to lead. On balance, the available evidence favors the former, rather than the latter, situation.

Two groups have been the main subjects of concern, controversy, and legislation with regard to exposure to lead: women and children. The controversy over whether they are more susceptible than men to lead poisoning involves many of the problems that were touched on in discussing the relation of lead to kidney disease. An additional factor in the case of women and children that makes resolution of the controversy difficult is the banning of both groups from the lead trades in most western countries for the last 50–70 years. Thus, the only available occupational data pertain to a period when severe and prolonged exposure to lead was common and the criterion of a lead effect was clinical lead poisoning. Oliver[428] said in 1902:

So far as occupational exposure to lead is concerned, my opinion is (1) that women are more susceptible than men; (2) that while female liability is greatest between the ages of 18 and 23 years, that of men is later; and (3) that while females rapidly break down in health under the influence of lead, men can work a longer time in the factory without suffering, their resistance apparently being greater.

However, German authors at about the same time felt that the apparent susceptibility of women to lead poisoning was explained, not by their sex, but by the fact that they were usually more poverty-stricken than the men, undernourished, and obliged to do work for their families in addition to their factory work. Also, women's skirts and hair collected the lead dust, so that they carried it home with them after work.[52] Support for this view is presented by Hamilton[227] for the U.S. battery industry around the beginning of the century. In areas where men belonged to strong unions, they enjoyed good pay and living conditions, while the nonunionized women were underpaid, poorly housed, poorly fed, and subject to the worry and strain of supporting dependents on low wages. In these conditions, a much larger proportion of women than of men suffered from lead poisoning. In the nonunionized pottery industry, in which both men and women were making low wages and were subject to poor conditions, the incidence of lead poisoning was slightly greater among men.

Information supporting the greater susceptibility of women to lead is given by Lane,[328] who quotes a British departmental committee report on the dangers attending the use of lead in the manufacture of earthenware and china. The report makes it possible to compare the incidence of lead poisoning in men and women engaged in the same work—ware cleaners, dippers, and dipping assistants. The incidence of lead poisoning in females was shown to be 2–3 times that in males. Of course, such factors as work habits, labor turnover, and general health might influence these statistics, but the reporting committee was sufficiently impressed with the data to express its belief that women are more susceptible to lead poisoning than men.

If the statistics on relative susceptibility of men and women leave much to be desired, there is even less information on whether lead poisoning produces significantly different clinical pictures in men and women. In one of the few comparisons undertaken, there is a suggestion of such a difference. Prendergast[446] found the following incidences of various expressions of lead poisoning among 640 cases of plumbism in the Staffordshire potteries:

| | Incidence, % | |
	Men	Women
Colic	77.6	69.8
Paralysis	57.0	30.0
Convulsions	15.0	34.9
Blindness (total)	2.3	7.7
Blindness (partial)	3.5	10.2

These admittedly sketchy data suggest that, when there has been sufficient exposure to lead to cause clinical poisoning, women are more likely to have central nervous system manifestations, and men, peripheral nervous system manifestations. This finding might be related to the greater likelihood that men will be engaged in heavy work, and the amount and type of physical effort have been thought to affect the incidence and location of muscular paralysis.

In the study of the earthenware and china workers previously referred to, the committee found that the incidence of miscarriage per 100 women was almost 3 times as great among those who continued to work with lead after marriage than among those not occupationally exposed to lead. In a review of the effect of lead on reproductive capacity, Lund[367] concluded, on the basis of studies conducted before 1920, that, "even when the mortality of that time is taken into account, the number of productive pregnancies is abnormally small" (in mothers occupationally exposed to lead). The earlier writers— Hamilton, Oliver, Legge, Cantarow and Trumper—were unanimous in their view that lead in high concentrations affected the reproductive capacity of women and that, in the light of the poor hygienic conditions in the lead trades at that time, women should not work in these trades. As a result of these views, legislation was enacted in many countries barring women from occupations in which they would be exposed to lead. Therefore, there are almost no data on the effect of the generally much lower concentrations of lead now prevailing in these industries on reproductive capacity. The Wenatchee study[417] remains as the only source of evidence, and that study found no effect on fertility. In summarizing their study of the fertility of men and women in the Wenatchee study, the authors concluded that

the instances reported in the literature of an effect of lead on human fertility appear to be limited to men and women who were far more heavily and much more regularly exposed to lead than the residents of Wenatchee. It would appear that a clinical state approaching that of frank lead poisoning is necessary before the fertility of men or women is affected.

Most of the early writers on the health of lead workers have remarked on the individual variability shown by persons exposed to high levels of lead—some men become poisoned within a few weeks, whereas others can work for years in the same surroundings without apparent harm. Undoubtedly, some of this variation in response was due to differences in working habits, and even today similar variations can be found, although now it is more likely to be confined to a difference in the amount of lead absorbed, rather than to variations in overt toxicity. For instance, there is a good correlation between blood and air lead concentrations with relatively little variation from man to man when the major portion of the lead exposure is from the air; but when the work involves such jobs as hand pasting of battery plates, with a much greater chance of "local" lead contamination, the variability of lead absorption between men is as much as fourfold.[585] Therefore, it is probable that at least some of the apparent individual resistance to lead poisoning seen by the earlier writers reflects variations in working habits and, therefore, in lead absorption.

There remains, however, a likelihood that different persons respond differently to a given dose of lead. It seems unlikely that this difference would be of any practical importance at the degrees of lead exposure now found in the general population,[15] but this merits further study. Such studies should first consider persons who are known to have biochemical defects in systems of the body that are recognized as influenced by lead, such as sickle cell anemia, glucose-6-phosphate dehydrogenase deficiency, the porphyrias, thalassemia, and gout.

RELATION OF TISSUE CONCENTRATIONS OF LEAD TO DISEASE

Although studying the tissue levels of lead in various diseases and looking for a congruence between disease distribution and lead exposure are attractive concepts, when the results are positive, the investigator is faced with a formidable task in dealing with the question: Did lead cause the disease under study? This problem of deciding whether two variables are merely associated or causally related is dealt with by Bradford Hill.[253] Among the aspects to be considered in deciding for or against a causal relation between two variables, Hill suggests strength of association, consistency, specificity, temporal relation of association, dose-response curve, biologic plausibility, coherence with known facts, experimental evidence, and judgment by analogy.

Tissue lead concentrations have been studied in two diseases other than classic lead poisoning: renal disease in Queensland, Australia, and multiple sclerosis in England. The Queensland study of bone lead content in renal disease[246] showed 160 cases of Bright's disease (chronic renal disease) in 866 autopsies. Of those 20–49 years old at the time of death, 63% had no known cause for their renal disease, and the remainder suffered from diseases recognized as involving the kidneys. The bone lead concentrations of the persons with renal disease of known causation were significantly lower than those of the persons with renal disease of unknown causation; this lends support to the belief that longstanding absorption of lead in sufficient quantity can cause chronic renal disease. The source of the lead in the Australian cases was childhood ingestion of exterior house paint. The authors of the study suggest that surveys of the lead content of tissues taken from persons who die of renal disease of unknown cause might be useful in providing diagnostic clues to the cause. Their conclusions have been supported by Emmerson,[168] who was able to show, in a group of Australian patients with renal disease of undetermined origin, that the mobilization of lead from bone by a standardized infusion of CaEDTA gave evidence of a significant past exposure to high concentrations of lead in 12 of 16 cases, which suggested that lead played a part in the causation of the renal disease.

Campbell *et al.*[82] reported that teeth from patients with multiple sclerosis contained, on the average, significantly higher concentrations of lead than teeth from normal, healthy persons. This observation was followed up by Butler,[74] who observed that physiologic changes accompanying chronic diseases may promote the deposition of metals in the skeleton, as illustrated by the increased deposition of zinc in teeth in tuberculosis. Butler analyzed urine, blood, cerebrospinal fluid, and bone in 31 patients with multiple sclerosis and in 54 persons with other neurologic disease. Lead concentrations in the two series did not differ significantly from commonly accepted normal values. Examination of necropsy tissue, including brain and spinal cord, from patients in whom the diagnosis of multiple sclerosis was confirmed histologically did not show significantly increased lead content. Butler concluded that his study did not support the view that lead plays a part in the etiology of multiple sclerosis.

GEOGRAPHIC DISTRIBUTION

The final epidemiologic relation to be explored is that of geographic distribution of a disease to some index of exposure to lead. Two diseases have been considered in this light: multiple sclerosis and cancer. Warren[569] has drawn attention to the great variation in the incidence of multiple sclerosis in different geographic areas of Norway, Scotland, Sweden, England, and Canada; some of those areas with a high incidence of the disease have lead-bearing rocks. There are many reasons for not accepting this as a causal relation. It is difficult to obtain adequate statistics on the true incidence of a disease whose prevalence is normally between 30 and 60 per 100,000 of population; if deaths are the basis of the reporting, mortality rates of the disease may vary from zero to 4 per 100,000. In the areas reported as having a high incidence, such as the Orkney and Shetland Islands of Scotland, with a total population of around 36,000, the addition of a single case of a disease that is particularly difficult to diagnose with certainty can increase the overall prevalence by as much as 25%. Additional impediments to accepting a causal relation are the strong North–South gradient in prevalence;[321] the lack of recognition of multiple sclerosis as a sequela of industrial exposure to lead; the failure to show increased lead content in the brain, blood, or urine of multiple sclerosis patients;[74] and the evidence that multiple sclerosis is probably an autoimmune disease or possibly related to an earlier viral infection.[500]

The epidemiologic evidence that lead can cause cancer in man is mentioned more because of the seriousness of the disease than because of the strength of the evidence. Warren[569] points out that, if variations in cancer mortality rates are plotted on a geographic basis, striking differences appear among some circumscribed areas. Allen-Price,[6] on the basis of a survey in Devon, England, claims that the incidence of cancer is higher in persons living on the highly mineralized Devonian geologic formation than in persons living on the adjoining carboniferous and granite formations. Warren states that in some cases rocks containing more than 1,000 ppm of lead can be correlated with some of the high-cancer areas encountered by Allen-Price, but this was not a consistent finding. Warren mentions two other rather tenuous examples and suggests that further studies be carried out. Apart from the difficulties, mentioned earlier, of obtaining reliable mortality statistics for small geographic areas, the even larger problem of the reliability of the information on which the cause of death is based is a well-recognized epidemiologic problem. Although it is known that lead at concentrations of 1% or more in the diet causes renal cancer in rats, there is no evidence that this happens in other species, including man. Lane's study[329] of lead workers was undertaken specifically to examine the incidence of cancer in this occupational group; no increase in the incidence was found. Although many human diseases have been alleged to be caused by lead, cancer is not one of them; even in the days of heavy and prolonged exposure to lead sufficient to cause renal disease, lead was not thought by clinicians to be linked to cancer.

BEHAVIORAL EFFECTS

Behavioral Effects in Man

OVERT AND ACUTE BEHAVIORAL CHANGES

Lead poisoning is characterized by a range of overt symptoms already described in detail in previous sections of this chapter. Among the changes in man associated with higher nervous system function are severe headaches, depression, insomnia, and irritability.

Sensory effects have also been commonly described. These are usually abnormal sensations and excessive sensitivity. Especially prominent have been visual disturbances ranging from mild, transitory changes to partial or complete blindness. Motor effects include paralysis, which usually develops slowly and varies in severity; muscular twitching and tremors; and epileptiform seizures.

Lead poisoning from gasoline-sniffing by adolescents has been reported, as well as one extreme case in an adult who developed lead encephalopathy.[336] Hallucinations, excitability, impairment of recent memory, and a slightly ataxic gait were associated with increased blood lead content. Ordinarily, gasoline-sniffing would not produce lead poisoning, owing to the comparatively low volatility of tetraethyl lead, as discussed more extensively in Chapter 6.

INSIDIOUS BEHAVIORAL CHANGES

Biochemical changes occur at blood lead concentrations well below those defining industrial toxicity and are perhaps the correlates of insidious changes. For example, interference with heme biosynthesis is the earliest evidence detected as the blood lead content rises above 40 μg/100 g of blood. Lane[327] has pointed out that only the lead worker undergoing some toxic episode comes to medical attention. The worker who has become slowly and insidiously poisoned, who is "below par" but without acute manifestations, appears to be well, because he presents no overt health problems. However, he may be subject later to chronic nephritis and cerebral hemorrhage.[327] As Hardy[238] points out,

nonspecificity of sign and symptom, delayed diagnosable damage because of the body's incredible margin of safety, and more than one insult acting like lead or with lead require sophisticated attention to the potential effect of low doses of lead—in much the same manner as low levels of ionizing radiation have been studied since the use of atomic energy for military purposes in 1945.

If the notion of "insidious poisoning" is valid, one might expect that workers exposed to lead concentrations below those which produce overt symptoms of toxicity would also undergo behavioral changes similar to the sensory, motor, and other alterations characteristic of frank lead poisoning, but to a lesser degree. However, no investigations of this have been reported. Nonetheless, a responsible company physician in sufficient contact with his workers is in a position to evaluate the early behavioral changes resulting from low-level poisoning. Given a familiarity with the base-line behavior of a worker, the physician can be alerted by the frequency of changes in some symptom categories that are otherwise difficult to interpret—irritability, lassitude, constipation, headaches, insomnia, abdominal cramps, and other diffuse complaints—as well as any increase in accident rates.

In experimental administration of lead to human subjects for long periods, blood concentrations rose and then remained fairly constant.[294,297] However, while the blood remained in a steady state with regard to lead content, the body lead burden slowly increased as a small difference between lead intake and lead output persisted. This picture of positive lead balance should be viewed against the clinical background of lead poisoning in making a decision about the possible effects of low levels of exposure to lead:

The symptoms of lead poisoning are, initially at least, rather vague; irritability and other mood changes predominate in the early stages, frank psychosis and encephalopathy later. The long biologic half-life results in so slow a buildup of toxic levels in the body that no connection may seem evident between the beginning of exposure to a chronically noxious environment and the development and progression of the symptoms of lead poisoning.[203]

LATE BEHAVIORAL EFFECTS OF EARLY EXPOSURE

At least 25% of those who survive acute encephalopathy from lead poisoning in early childhood have permanent central nervous system injury.[442] The nature of the residual behavioral deficit cannot be easily characterized as "mental retardation," inasmuch as most studies report the majority of the intelligence-test scores as in or above the "dull normal" level. For example, Thurston et al.,[537] in a 5- to 10-year study of 11 cases of lead poisoning in young children, found no Stanford-Binet intelligence-test scores lower than dull normal. However, more specialized tests of visual–motor function (Graham and Kendall test, Bender Gestalt test) yielded results very similar to those seen in children with brain damage due to birth injuries or cerebral anoxia. Although the initial hyperactivity syndrome disappeared by the time the later tests were administered, only three of the children were doing satisfactory schoolwork. Similar results have been reported by Byers and Lord,[78] Bradley and Baumgartner,[61] Mellins and Jenkins,[388] and Jenkins and Mellins.[276]

The damaging effects of lead poisoning associated with frank encephalopathy seem well substantiated, but an intriguing question remains: whether excessive lead ingestion in young children produces permanent central nervous system and behavioral deficits if the magnitude of ingestion is not sufficient to result in demonstrable encephalopathy. Habitual ingestion of lead paint can increase the body lead burden and result in a chronic hyperkinetic–aggressive behavior disorder. Whether this condition, which lacks the features of acute encephalopathy, nonetheless produces neurologic damage via chronic derangements of metabolism is important to determine, because pica for lead paint often implies protracted, recurrent episodes.[111]

Byers and Lord[78] studied 20 schoolchildren who had been hospitalized for lead poisoning in early childhood. None had shown evidence of encephalopathy, and they were judged, at the time of hospitalization, to have made complete recoveries. Only one made satisfactory progress in school, the others having various intellectual and emotional difficulties. However, by current standards, many of these cases would be judged as mild encephalopathy. In a recent review of this area, Wiener[581] concluded that, although most studies report behavioral impairment due to lead poisoning, none satisfies the demands of statistical control. There are also problems with respect to sampling bias and the application of various diagnostic procedures and definitions.

The evidence with respect to the special effects of early exposure to a relatively small increment in lead concentration, particularly in its implications for later behavior, remains unclear. However, existing studies, if not definitive, nevertheless afford some presumptive evidence of central nervous system dysfunction.

Behavioral Effects in Experimental Animals

TOXIC BEHAVIORAL EFFECTS

Although the nascent subdiscipline of behavioral pharmacology has developed rapidly over the last 10–15 years,[150,306,535] behavioral toxicology is much younger in this country.[575] Consequently, only a few experimental studies are available that deal with the behaviorally toxic properties of lead.

Using a water T-maze, in which an animal must swim into the correct arm of the T to escape from the situation, Bullock et al.[72] found that administration of tetraethyl lead (TEL) had little effect on the performance measured. Rats were given TEL intraperitoneally for 8 days to a total dose of 15 mg/kg of body weight. Four days after the last dose, maze training was begun. Escape times differed only slightly between control and experimental groups, and swimming times not at all. Other animals were given TEL injections after training had started. There were no performance differences between experimental and control groups. All TEL-treated rats showed tremor, ataxia, fighting, and, after a few days, convulsions and death. The water T-maze is apparently a rather insensitive instrument for evaluating TEL toxicity; nor has it proved suitable for evaluating other pharmacologic agents.

Using a classically conditioned motor response in rats, Gusev[222] reported finding behavioral impairment when animals were exposed to high and low atmospheric concentrations of lead oxide for 6 hr daily for 6 months. The actual number of exposure days, excepting the off-days, was 148–150 days. Using force and latency-of-response measures, no impairment was seen at an average air concentration of 1.13 $\mu g/m^3$ of lead. At the higher dose level (11 $\mu g/m^3$), disturbed reflexes began to occur about 1.5–2 months after the start of exposure and increased in severity over the exposure period; base-line conditioned-reflex activity was re-established 10–23 days after lead exposure was discontinued. As exposure time increased, differential reactions to strong (bell) and weak (light) conditioned stimuli were often disrupted, and positive reactions to a negative conditioned stimulus (buzzer) also occurred. No changes in the formed elements of the blood were seen in any of the experimental animals. Histopathologic changes in the central nervous system were noted in rats and rabbits exposed to about 11 $\mu g/m^3$ of lead oxide, and the rat bone lead content was 10 times as high as that in either control animals or those exposed to the lower dose. The author did not discuss the probable contribution to the total lead intake produced by grooming of the fur.

In an experiment using the same methods as Gusev,[222] Shalamberidze[494] found that a lead sulfide concentration of 48.3 $\mu g/m^3$ (calculated as metallic lead) produced disturbed conditioned reflexes in rats exposed to ore dust inhalation 6 hr daily for 6 months.

Novakova,[423] using similar classic conditioning techniques, reported that combined chronic doses of arsenic (0.0025 mg/kg) and lead (0.005 mg/kg) were additive in their effects and disrupted the acquisition of conditioned reflexes. These behavioral tests were administered between the fourth and eighth months of chronic dosing.

Only two studies in this country of the behavioral effects of low-level exposure to lead were found. Goldfish were given shock avoidance training and then exposed to specific concentrations of lead nitrate for 48 hr.[574] Tests after 24 and 48 hr of exposure, with different groups being exposed to different lead concentrations, yielded significant behavioral impairment at concentrations as low as 0.07 ppm. This is only 1/857 of the concentration that is lethal to 1% of the animals, and it approximates the concentration in potable water. Mercury was more toxic than lead, and arsenic and selenium were less toxic. Impairments were found at 0.003, 0.1, and 0.25 ppm, respectively. In the light of Russian experiments on the behavioral toxicity of atmospheric lead, it is interesting to note that these results show impairment at a similar exposure.

Using a spatial escape response in fish, Jones[280] showed that the three-spined stickleback (*Gasterosteus*) would escape from lead nitrate solutions as dilute as 1 ppm, whereas the threshold for minnows (*Phoxinus phoxinus*) was 0.4 ppm.

All the drugs commonly associated with the production of physical dependence (amphetamines, barbiturates, morphine, alcohol) also suppress the paradoxic, or rapid-eye-movement (REM), phase of sleep. They also produce a long rebound of the REM phase on withdrawal of the drug.[429] In the light of this sensitivity of the REM phase of sleep to drugs, it is interesting that the chronic absorption of lead also affects REM sleep.[592] Rats given lead acetate (1.5 mg/ml) in their drinking water showed altered REM-phase patterning. This could be related to the fact that an early sign of lead poisoning is insomnia.[84]

DEVELOPMENTAL EFFECTS OF EARLY EXPOSURE

If the developmental processes of the fetus or immature organism are subject to pathologic alteration by exposure to lead, such pathologic changes will necessarily have behavioral implications. If rats nursing their young are fed diets containing either 1% or 4% lead carbonate, lead appears in the milk and affects the neonates.[441,460] The young show evidence of lead poisoning, faulty growth, and various neurologic changes, including paraplegia, changes in the cerebellum and striatum, and blood–brain barrier dysfunction.

Although various lead salts administered (at 50 mg/kg) to hamsters on day 7, 8, or 9 of gestation produced skeletal malformations in sacral and tail vertebrae,[178] recent evidence reveals a low degree of teratogenic effects in rats and mice.[381] Little radioactive lead was found to cross the placenta. However, Barltrop[32] cites evidence of placental penetration by lead in rats and presents evidence suggesting maternofetal blood-lead equilibrium in women.

Suggested Lines of Behavioral Investigation

Perhaps the most controversial and also the most pressing aspect of the lead-exposure problem is the effect of chronic exposure to low concentrations of lead in the environment. The extent to which such chronic exposure influences behavior needs to be evaluated with reference to well-understood behavioral base lines. Long-term studies, similar to those undertaken by the Russian investigators, but using operant conditioning as well as other methods, need to be instituted. There is no substitute for the chronic exposure of organisms to various dosages and the consequent delineation of dose-response functions. Demonstrations that some dosage "has an effect" on behavior provide an insufficient base from which to proceed toward the study of behavioral mechanisms of action. The lessons afforded by behavioral pharmacology in this regard are well worth noting.

Some areas of investigation could be used to illuminate the particular effects lead may be suspected of having at low dosages. Inasmuch as lead poisoning produces peripheral neuropathy[190,191] and muscular changes[84] and lead ions produce preganglionic transmission block,[315] the effects of chronic exposure to lead on motor-control tasks[176] might yield early indications of the behavioral toxicity of lead.

Lead poisoning also produces various visual disturbances. These might be evaluated not only by acuity and flicker-fusion determinations, but by the use of the evoked-response technique. Promising investigations along this line have been instituted by Xintaras et al.[591] In evaluating the effect of lead on sleep patterns, Xintaras et al.[592] have opened the area of complex, natural behavioral sequences to behavioral toxicology. The study of complex learned-behavior schedules[179] is likely to prove indispensable, but the effects of lead exposure on the patterning of REM phases, thresholds of aggression,[269] and food–fluid intake patterns should also receive attention. And ethologic studies of courtship and parental sequences should not be neglected, because they may provide early indications of wildlife problems not likely to be discovered in laboratory studies.

In studying the toxicology of lead, it is imperative for investigators to use well-known agents in the research program as reference standards to validate their experimental arrangements. Thus, Xintaras et al.[591] used the well-known effects of pentobarbital on the evoked response to validate their evoked-response preparation before studying the lesser-known effects of carbon monoxide and ozone.

Lead is not the only toxic substance to which an organism might be subjected at a particular time, so investigators should also consider the effects of lead combined with other pollutants (such as carbon monoxide) or probable vehicles (such as ethanol). The possible synergistic effects of various pollutants are largely unknown;[541] but the not uncommon combination of alcoholism and lead poisoning is known to be a medical problem.[97,237]

Finally, the relative sensitivity of the fetus, neonate, child, and adult to chronic, low-level exposure to lead needs investigation, as do the reversibility of toxic effects and the evaluation of residual effects. The possibility of specific susceptibility of the developing brain at various fetal and juvenile stages should be evaluated most carefully. Some of these studies could be done on lower organisms, particularly primates, but, in light of the serious suspicions that lead may produce some unknown fraction of the mental retardation and perceptual disorders found in children exposed to this element in their environment,[111,581] epidemiologic and other correlational and clinical studies of this problem should be encouraged.

OBSERVATIONS IN EXPERIMENTAL ANIMAL SYSTEMS

Biochemistry

Lead has a strong affinity for some biochemical ligands, including the epsilonamino group of lysine, the carboxyl group of glutamic and aspartic acids, the sulfhydryl groups of cysteine, the phenoxy group of tyrosine, and imidazole residues. Consequently, it may displace metals from enzymes, modify tertiary structure of enzymes, and block enzyme substrate interactions. When lead is so concentrated as to exceed the ability of the numerous reactive sites in and on cells to receive it, metabolic consequences ensue that are manifested by lead poisoning. However, as in deficiency disease, poisoning may be recognized clinically somewhat later, because of insensitivity of the usual clinical methods of diagnosis.

An understanding of the evolution of poisoning at the cellular level is essential to an understanding of clinical lead poisoning and the possible effects of ambient lead. Rothstein[461] has suggested that enzymes associated with the cell envelope may be among the most sensitive to lead. He pointed out that the envelope is the first point of contact between the cell and lead in the interstitial fluid. Some of the apparent effects of lead on membrane transport in the erythrocyte and renal tubule support his hypothesis. Rothstein believes that the internal milieu of the cell may dilute low amounts of lead that pass the external membrane. Some organelles within the cell seem particularly susceptible to lead, including mitochondria,[210] nuclei,[91,212] and microsomes.[91] Their sensitivity to lead and apparent accumulation of the metal, as demonstrated by lead-210 tracer studies,[91] extend Rothstein's[461] hypothesis, that cell membranes are particularly susceptible to lead, to include intracellular membranous structures and their enzymes. Inasmuch as the cell envelope is not a static barrier between the interior of the cell and the external environment, but rather is a membrane across which many metabolites travel, both actively and passively, entry of lead into the cell, perhaps in place of calcium, and its subsequent attachment to ligands on the membranes of organelles are not in conflict with the Rothstein hypothesis.

Effects of lead bound to mitochondria have been evaluated in the renal tubule of the rat.[208,212] Isolated mitochondria demonstrate impaired oxidative phosphorylation, in addition to defective structure of their membranes. Ultrastructural transformation is inhibited, and mitochondria that do transform have labile membranes[209] and decreased ability to phosphorylate ADP (adenosine diphosphate) in pyruvate–malate substrate. Mitochondria that do not transform from the condensed to the orthodox form in the presence of pyruvate-malate substrate are thought to have impaired electron transport. Of interest in terms of the effects of lead on mitochondrial enzymes is its inhibition of intramitochondrial aspects of heme synthesis.

The observations of Goyer and co-workers on mitochondrial respiration and phosphorylation are of particular interest in view of the recent *in vitro* studies by Ulmer and Vallee[546] on the dithiol enzyme, lipoamide dehydrogenase. This enzyme is part of the macromolecular complex of enzymes that synthesize acetyl coenzyme A and succinyl coenzyme A from pyruvate and a-ketoglutarate, respectively. Lead, at concentrations of 6.5×10^{-6} M, will inhibit its action. Studies on a second dithiol molecule in the enzyme–lipoic acid complex, similar to those done on lipoamide dehydrogenase, have apparently not been reported. It is of interest, however, that DL-a-lipoic acid did not protect mice from a lethal dose of lead.[518] Inhibition of lipoamide dehydrogenase by lead is probably representative of the effects of lead on many dithiol enzymes. Because the studies were *in vitro*, their direct application to man is not possible. They simply lend support to the concept that very small concentrations of lead can inhibit critical enzyme systems.

Evidence that lead may also suppress protein synthesis through alteration of the tertiary structure of RNA or inhibition of reactions in which it participates has come from the finding that RNA from lead-intoxicated experimental animals contains considerable lead[546] and from the *in vivo* concentration of lead-210 by liver microsomes.[91] According to Sroczynski *et al.*,[517] lead poisoning in rabbits does impair protein synthesis. Phosphorus-32 tracer studies suggest that RNA synthesis may also be inhibited.[410] At concentrations of 10^{-5} M, lead causes hydrolysis of *Escherichia coli* RNA.[546] Whether this occurs *in vivo* at lower concentrations is unknown. If transfer RNA were hydrolyzed by lead, incorporation of amino acids into peptides would be suppressed. Lead at 10^{-4} M suppresses the activity of enzymes involved in the incorporation of [^{14}C] leucine into transfer RNA of *E. coli*. It is thought that this is due to inhibition of the sulfhydryl enzyme aminoacyl synthetase. Because 10^{-4} M is a greater concentration of lead than usually found in intact mammalian systems, it is most improbable that these observations would have any bearing in man.

Lead is also concentrated by cell nuclei, as documented in liver and kidney[91,212] and implied by the chromosomal abnormalities present in leukocytes from lead-poisoned mice[410] and lymphocytes from lead-poisoned men[344] and by the bizarre mitotic figures sometimes found in bone marrow smears taken from lead-intoxicated men. The intranuclear inclusions in liver and kidney are currently thought to be inert lead–protein complexes, and they may well represent a protective storage mechanism.[211] The mechanism of lead's effect on chromosomes is unknown. However, because the abnormalities produced are of the "gap-break" type and are not paired between chromatids, it is thought that they occur after DNA replication. Considering that activation of DNase from liposomes will apparently damage chromosomes[7] and that DNase activity is markedly increased in urine from lead-poisoned rats,[319] Muro and Goyer[410] have speculated that increased DNase activity in lead-poisoned cells may produce these chromosomal effects. The significance of these observations for human health is unknown. It seems clear that the concentrations of lead necessary to produce these abnormalities are much greater than those found in the environment. For the present, these studies may be viewed as interesting laboratory phenomena with no known genetic implications.

Of the enzymes associated with the cell envelope, those involved in sodium–potassium transport appear susceptible to lead at concentrations found in lead-poisoned man. Hasan *et al.*[243] have reported that erythrocyte sodium–potassium adenosine triphosphatase activity is lower in lead-intoxicated men than in controls (4.42 ± 1.23 × 10⁻¹³ versus 6.34 ± 1.29 × 10⁻¹³). Their finding is consistent with the earlier finding of Joyce et al.[285] and with their own studies, which indicate that potassium leaks from and sodium enters lead-poisoned erythrocytes incubated in vitro. Again, the implications of these findings are unknown. Some workers[291] are of the opinion that the sodium–potassium ATPase enzyme system may be of major importance in maintaining the correct internal milieu in the cell. Whether significant alterations in the internal milieu occur in vivo as a consequence of lead seems not to have been reported. Of interest in this regard is the apparently decreased renal sodium-retaining ability in some men with lead poisoning due to ingestion of illicitly distilled whiskey.[469] This has not been investigated in experimental animals in controlled conditions; therefore, the minimal dose of lead necessary to produce the effect has not been determined. In addition, the effect seems to have been related to long, heavy exposure; therefore, it seems unlikely to be of significance with regard to ambient lead.

Physiology

Absorption of lead from the gastrointestinal tract appears to be regulated by some of the same physiologic mechanisms as control the absorption of calcium and phosphorus. Increased dietary calcium and phosphorus will, in fact, decrease the absorption of lead, and decreased dietary intake of calcium appears to increase lead absorption.[495] It has been shown in rats given lead in their drinking water (at 200 μg/ml) that low dietary calcium will greatly increase the severity of anemia and biochemical indices of lead poisoning. Bone lead content is higher and bone calcium content is lower than those in rats given the same amount of lead in their drinking water and a normal calcium diet intake.[505] It appears that vitamin D will also enhance the absorption of lead from the gastrointestinal tract.[511] The mechanism of action is as yet undefined.

The composition of the diet apparently may influence the occurrence of lead poisoning. Baernstein and Grand[22] reported that a 20% casein diet would protect rats from lead chloride (1½%) in the diet to a greater extent than a 6% or 13% casein diet. Addition of methionine or cysteine to the 6% casein diet decreased the mortality and improved the weight gain of both lead-fed and control rats. These studies are supported by the work of Gontzea et al.[205] Recently, it has been shown that cysteine *in vitro* will protect activity of A L A D in rabbit liver from lead.[144] The apparent protective effects of some diets against poisoning by lead shot in ducks are discussed in Chapter 5.

It has been suggested that synthesis of nicotinic acid from tryptophan is impaired in experimental lead poisoning.[439] Experimentally, it appears that nicotinic acid may decrease porphyrinuria in lead-poisoned rabbits,[41,466] but this finding has not been confirmed in rats.[2] In support of the suggestion that lead produces abnormalities in tryptophan metabolism, xanthurenic acid excretion in the urine has been found to increase.[439] However, when Tenconi and Acocella[527] carried out tryptophan loading tests in rats, they did not find an increase in xanthurenic acid excretion. At present, there is no evidence that nicotinic acid has therapeutic value in lead poisoning.

It appears that chromium may have a protective effect on survival of rats given low doses of lead for long periods.[482] The data suggest that chromium deficiency makes rats more susceptible to lead. Implications of these observations for man are as yet unclear.

Other Effects

Because many factors are suspected of influencing both the severity and the clinical manifestations of lead toxicity, it would seem useful to be able to recognize common denominators. The common mode of action of a number of the factors discussed is the effect of mobilizing lead into a transportable or diffusible form. Little is known presently about the biochemical nature of diffusible lead.

Likewise, the toxicology of lead at the cellular or molecular level is ubiquitous and probably entails a number of mechanisms, depending on the physiologic or biochemical process involved. What is known about these reactions is discussed in detail elsewhere and only briefly mentioned here. A summary of the toxicologic indices of lead poisoning from the published literature is presented in Appendix E.

Lead is known to interact with some enzymes; those concerned with heme synthesis, particularly A L A D, are the best studied and have been discussed in detail earlier. Lead ions also impair the oxidative and phosphorylative functions of mitochondria,[209] and it is also suggested that it interferes with transmission of impulses at preganglionic nerve endings by reducing the output of acetylcholine.[315] *In vitro* studies have shown that lead may impair protein synthesis by polyribosome disaggregation.[573] In spite of the sophistication of these studies, knowledge of these effects of lead is not complete enough to identify a common physicochemical property of the lead ion.

Understanding of synergistic and antagonistic factors in lead toxicity will be greatly improved when more basic knowledge of the metabolism of lead is available.

The possibility that lead at physiologically significant concentrations affects mutation in plant or animal cells has no firm experimental evidence. The effect of high concentrations of lead on plant cells has been discussed in Chapter 2. Novick and Roth[424] have reported in *Staphylococcus aureus* a mutational transfer of resistance to lead (as well as to penicillin, cadmium, and mercury); these results are not yet confirmed. The chromosomal damage found in experimental lead poisoning by Muro and Goyer[410] has also been mentioned earlier. In all investigations cited, lead was introduced at higher concentrations than the organism would normally encounter or, in fact, could survive for long. It is not known whether low concentrations of lead may have an effect on somatic mutations that very likely contribute to the aging process.

Although epidemiologic studies have not shown any relation between lead exposure and the incidence of cancer, several investigators have been able to show that lead experimentally administered in very high doses is carcinogenic. The first observation of neoplasia induced by lead was reported by Zollinger,[597] who injected lead phosphate subcutaneously into rats and observed renal adenomas and adenocarcinomas. Similar results were obtained by other workers with oral or parenteral lead phosphate, lead acetate, or basic lead acetate in rats[60,244,371,458,542,563] and in mice.[562] Tumors of testis, adrenal, thyroid, pituitary, prostate, and lung have arisen in the course of long-term dietary administration of lead acetate to rats.[594] In a study of cerebral gliomas induced in rats by various agents, Oyasu *et al.*[432] obtained the highest yield with lead subacetate; coadministration of 2-acetylaminofluorene did not increase the incidence of gliomas.

Beginning with the classic account by Weller[576] of the "blastophthoric" effect of chronic lead poisoning in man and animals, the evidence has accumulated of a teratogenic action of high concentrations of lead salts. Results with the chick embryo[76,93,290] have supplemented an earlier study of intravenously administered lead in the rabbit.[45] Ferm and Carpenter[178] have reported developmental malformations in the golden hamster, resulting from intravenous administration of a lead salt at a dosage of 50 mg/kg on day 7, 8, or 9 of pregnancy.

Despite the accumulated evidence in laboratory animals on very high dosage, teratogenic effects of lead have not been seen in cattle or sheep.[274,498]

SUMMARY

Body Lead Burden

Postmortem analysis of tissues for lead indicates that approximately 95% of the total body lead burden in man is stored in bone. Although the concentration of lead in bone appears to increase during life until at least 40 years of age, the concentrations of lead in the various soft tissues, excluding aorta, normally remain low and relatively stable throughout adult life. Limited age-related data in adults without known industrial or other unusual exposure to lead indicate that blood lead content also remains constant and within the "normal" range throughout life. These observations are consistent with the hypothesis that the total body lead burden may be divided into two major pools: a small "mobile" fraction found primarily in the soft tissues and a much larger, but relatively "nondiffusible" fraction, which is apparently tightly bound in matrix of bone. In man, increments in the "mobile" fraction of the total body lead burden are associated with the known acute toxic effects of lead. Blood lead content and the "chelatable" lead* provide an index of this small "mobile" fraction of the total body lead burden. In persons with normal renal function, spontaneous urinary lead excretion (which has long been used as a measure of current and recent absorption of lead) may provide similar information, but this point has not been clearly documented. Current evidence concerning the contribution of the nondiffusible fraction to the soft-tissue pool is incomplete. In general, it is sequestered in bone and is therefore not likely to be associated with adverse health effects. Concentrations of lead in bone are usually greater in persons from industrialized countries than in those from the less developed countries.

Effects of Lead on Biosynthesis of Heme

Studies in experimental models and in severe acute lead poisoning in man indicate that lead can inhibit the biosynthesis of heme and the

*That is, the quantity of lead excreted in urine in response to a standardized dose of a chelating agent, such as CaEDTA or D-penicillamine.

utilization of iron. Acute lead poisoning in man is characterized by a decrease in ALAD activity *in vitro* in blood, an increase in ALA in serum and urine, an increase in UCP, and an increase in FEP.*

Significant relations have been found in man between blood lead content and (1) the *in vitro* assay of ALAD activity in hemolysates of peripheral blood, (2) urinary excretion of ALA, and (3) "chelatable" lead, as measured by the CaEDTA mobilization test. There is an inverse linear relation between the logarithm of ALAD activity *in vitro* in hemolysates of blood and the concentration of lead in blood when blood lead content is between 5 and 95 μg/100 g of whole blood (or more). Throughout the "normal" range of blood lead concentration (5–40 μg/100 g of whole blood), ALAD activity in blood, as measured *in vitro*, decreases by about 75%. Some studies, however, indicate that the excretion of ALA (the substrate of ALAD) in urine remains constant and low in adults and adolescents with blood lead content less than approximately 40 μg/100 g of whole blood. (This observation has not been confirmed in young children; no children with blood lead content less than 25 μg/100 g of whole blood have been studied for this.) But arithmetic increases in blood lead content above approximately 40 μg/100 g of whole blood are correlated with a continuing exponential decrease in ALAD activity in hemolysates of peripheral blood, an exponential increase in urinary ALA excretion, and an exponential increase in "chelatable" lead. When blood lead content exceeds 60 μg/100 g of whole blood, it appears that most persons may be expected to show an increase in urinary ALA excretion. The Panel reached this conclusion on the basis of evaluation of several studies, none of which by itself could be considered adequate to support the conclusion. When all the available data are considered together, they are consistent with the hypothesis that the inhibition of ALAD activity *in vivo* in intact man becomes physiologically significant as blood lead content rises above approximately 40 μg/100 g of whole blood and that the partial inhibition observed is reflected by an increasing rate of excretion of its substrate (ALA)

---

*UCP and FEP levels have been studied in relation to toxic concentrations of lead in man, but not extensively in relation to minimal increases in tissue lead content and in subclinical lead poisoning. UCP is affected also by hepatic injury, and increased FEP content is associated with both deficient supply and impaired utilization of iron. In man, inhibition of ALAD activity in hemolysates of peripheral blood and increased ALA in serum and urine apparently represent a specific response to rising lead content in soft tissues. The only reported exception is transient impairment of ALAD activity in the blood of men with acute alcoholic intoxication.

in urine. As sustained blood lead content exceeds approximately 80 μg/100 g of whole blood, impairment in the biosynthesis of heme in the hematopoietic tissue can no longer be compensated by an increased rate of production. Failure of this compensatory mechanism is, in turn, followed by frank anemia.

The biosynthesis of heme is probably also impaired in other tissues; however, the level at which significant impairment in the biosynthesis of heme may occur in other tissues has not been defined. The biologic significance of declining ALAD activity *in vitro* in red blood cells in persons with blood lead concentrations less than 40 μg/100 g of whole blood is not presently understood. It may be tentatively suggested that, in such persons, this *in vitro* phenomenon represents a nonessential "reserve enzyme capacity," insofar as red blood cell formation is concerned. Asymptomatic persons with blood lead concentrations between 40 and 80 μg/100 g of whole blood are apparently able to compensate by increasing their rate of red cell production. However, lead poisoning is associated also with impaired utilization of iron, so that persons with iron-deficiency states, disorders associated with impaired utilization of iron, hemolytic anemias, chronic infectious diseases, severe liver disease, or renal failure may not be able to compensate as well for soft-tissue or "mobile" lead concentrations associated with blood lead concentrations in the range of 40–80 μg/100 g of whole blood. Such population groups have not been adequately examined in this regard.

Clinical Effects and Epidemiologic Considerations

Studies of the clinical effects of increased tissue lead content are based almost entirely on the clinical evaluation of industrial workers in the lead trades, children in urban areas, and imbibers of lead-contaminated illicitly distilled whiskey. These sources of exposure to inorganic lead salts constitute the major health hazards associated with lead in the United States today. The other potential environmental sources of lead listed early in this chapter have been responsible for sporadic cases and minor outbreaks of clinical lead poisoning. Occupational health supervision and the institution of measures to minimize exposure of workers have greatly reduced the occurrence and incidence of severe lead poisoning in the lead trades since the early 1900's. Today, estimates of the magnitude of the industrial health problem posed by exposure to lead are fragmentary, because adequate incidence data are not available. The principal occupational problem probably lies in small shops, whose owners do not provide

adequate medical surveillance and lead-exposure control programs, as
are usually maintained by large corporations. (Hazards due to exposure to lead alkyls are limited to a very small number of closely supervised workers employed in the manufacture of tetraethyl and
tetramethyl lead.) As with occupational exposure, epidemiologic
data concerning the incidence of lead poisoning in children are also
inadequate. The available data do suggest, however, that 5–10% of
preschool children residing in deteriorating urban housing consume
sufficient lead to have "increased lead absorption," as judged by
blood lead concentrations, and that approximately 1% may be found
to have symptoms compatible with the diagnosis of clinical lead poisoning. The extent to which lead-bearing dust in urban areas may
contribute to the problem is not known. Also unknown is the magnitude of the problem in moonshine-whiskey drinkers, but it is suspected that it may be significant, especially in the southeastern part
of the United States. Today, it is generally true that clinically evident
lead poisoning most frequently results from the absorption of lead
through the gastrointestinal, rather than the respiratory, tract. To
place the question of lead in the ambient air in proper perspective, it
may be stated that clinically evident disease due to inhalation of inorganic lead salts does not usually occur unless the concentration in
the air exceeds 0.5 mg/m^3—roughly 100 times the maximal concentration reported in the ambient air in urban areas and 1,000 times
that reported in rural ambient air.

Clinical studies indicate that clear-cut clinical signs and symptoms
of acute lead poisoning are related to the degree of current and recent
absorption of lead and, in the absence of severe anemia, are almost
always associated with blood lead concentrations greater than 80
μg/100 g of whole blood. At higher concentrations, the severity of
acute clinical manifestations is not closely associated with and cannot be precisely predicted from blood lead concentration. It can be
stated only that derangement of heme synthesis is always evident and
that the risk of symptomatic illness increases markedly as blood lead
content rises above 80 μg/100 g of whole blood. The factors that may
precipitate acute lead poisoning are not clearly understood. Whether
symptoms compatible with acute lead poisoning may, in fact, be
attributed to lead in persons with blood lead content between 50 and
80 μg/100 g of whole blood is controversial. In part, the controversy
arises because of the subtle and nonspecific nature of the early symptoms of lead poisoning. Not only is clinical diagnosis difficult in lead-
poisoned persons, but the general unavailability of adequate laboratory diagnostic facilities limits their clinical evaluation. At present, it

is unlikely that the biologic significance of blood lead concentrations between 50 and 80 $\mu g/100$ g of whole blood can be resolved on the basis of routine clinical evaluation alone. The clinical interpretation of observed blood lead content can be greatly facilitated in the presence of moderate to severe anemia if it is corrected for low hematocrit values. This correction is not indicated for mild deviations from expected hematocrit. Although there is no scientific basis for correction of hematocrit, available clinical reports indicate that patients with moderately severe anemia, clear-cut symptoms of poisoning, and blood lead content of less than 80 $\mu g/100$ g of whole blood will usually be found to have a corrected blood lead content of over 80 $\mu g/100$ g if the correction is made. Clinical evaluation of difficult cases may be facilitated by use of the CaEDTA mobilization test.

The acute toxic effects of lead on the hematopoietic system, kidneys, and nervous system are summarized in Table 4–11. Whereas the toxic effects of lead on hematopoiesis (anemia) and the kidneys are apparently reversible, injury to the central nervous system might not be. Indeed, at least 25% of the survivors of acute lead encephalopathy are said to sustain permanent brain damage. Chronic lead nephropathy and nervous system sequelae (even in the absence of known encephalopathy), as recognized clinically today, are apparently associated with long-continued abnormal exposure to lead and recurrent symptomatic episodes of poisoning. The occurrence of central nervous system sequelae in at least 25% of children after acute encephalopathy appears a reasonable estimate. However, the frequency of residual central nervous system deficits attributable to less severe lead poisoning in children cannot be accurately estimated from the published clinical material. Epidemiologic studies in adults occupationally exposed to lead have revealed no evidence of an association between lead and cancer or multiple sclerosis and no evidence of increased mortality due to degenerative cardiovascular disease. Workers under today's careful medical supervision in plants with adequate exposure control programs have not been found to have an increased incidence of hypertension. Past occurrences of hypertension, renal insufficiency, and fetal wastage in occupationally exposed adults were associated with uncontrolled protracted exposure.

Biochemical and Functional Considerations

There is no evidence that lead is an essential trace element, although the hypothesis that minute amounts may serve some essential function in metabolism has not been examined. On the contrary, all experimental data obtained both *in vitro* and *in vivo* show that the metabolic effects of lead in concentrations as low as 10^{-6} M are of the inhibitory or adverse type. At the enzymatic level, the inhibitory effect of lead on sulfhydryl-dependent enzymes is well documented *in vitro*; sulfhydryl-dependent enzymes clearly inhibited by lead include two in the biosynthetic pathway for heme formation (ALAD and heme synthetase) and lipoamide dehydrogenase, an essential component in the pyruvate and a-ketoglutarate decarboxylase systems. It seems clear that lead forms ligands with groups other than disulfide and sulfhydryl in biologic systems, but this area has received only cursory attention. At the cellular level, the formation of respiratory pigments (heme and cytochrome), energy production, and some membrane functions appear to be the aspects of metabolism most susceptible to the adverse effects of lead. Although the effects of lead on the biosynthesis of heme in red blood cells are reasonably well delineated, gaps in knowledge remain and little is known of its effect on heme synthesis in other tissues.

Evidence obtained from red blood cells and rat kidney indicates that the structure and function of the mitochondria are altered by lead. In the kidney, the most sensitive consequence of this impairment of mitochondrial function appears to be aminoaciduria. Aminoaciduria apparently represents a response to the high soft-tissue concentrations of lead associated with severe acute poisoning in man; the question has not been examined subclinically.

With regard to membrane functions, the significance of the finding of decreased sodium–potassium ATPase activity *in vitro* in red cell fragments in men with increased lead exposure is unknown. Whether significant alterations occur *in vivo* in man as a consequence of this particular *in vitro* effect of lead is not known. It is, however, possible that the apparently decreased renal sodium-retaining ability of some men with lead poisoning due to ingestion of illicitly distilled whiskey may result from a comparable impairment in membrane transport in the kidney. This question has not been examined in experimental animals in controlled conditions, so the minimal dose of lead necessary to produce the renal effect has not been determined. Inasmuch as the effect appears to be related to long and heavy exposure to lead in illicitly distilled lead-contaminated whiskey, it is unlikely to be important with regard to lead in ambient air and a normal diet.

From the limited experimental data, it can only be surmised that interactions between lead and other metals—such as iron, manganese, and cadmium—may be important. Similarly, factors that apparently affect absorption, storage, and excretion of lead in experimental conditions—such as heat, dehydration, vitamin D deficiency, and dietary calcium and phosphorus imbalances—have not been examined in sufficient detail to estimate their significance for intact man. The possible effects of increased lead content in the soft tissues on integrated nervous system function (behavior and performance) have received scant attention. It is suspected that these effects, when studied in intact experimental animals, might be best approached in nonhuman primates.

The alterations in endocrine function observed in men with lead poisoning due to the ingestion of illicitly distilled whiskey are incompletely understood. The adverse effect on thyroid function appears clearly due to lead; similar effects have been produced by feeding lead to rats. Because the other endocrine abnormalities described have not been reproduced in animals or described in patients with lead poisoning due to industrial exposure (with the exception of adverse effects on renin secretion), the presence of other contributing factors in moonshine has not been ruled out.

The significance of intranuclear inclusions in proximal renal tubules of man and animals with lead intoxication is incompletely understood. Goyer's suggestion that they represent inert lead–protein complexes and that they may serve as a protective storage mechanism in liver and kidney is provocative. It is noteworthy that these inclusions have not been described in other organs. There is scant knowledge with respect to the biologic binding and intracellular localization of lead: it appears to bind to mitochondria, microsomes, or nuclei. The physiologic implication of this binding is a subject for further investigation. The significance of the many experimental studies for intact man is unknown, particularly because most of the studies have been based on high dosages of lead without attention to dose-response relations.

Subclinical Effects

The uncertainties concerning the threshold at which the biologic effects of lead become clinically manifest are reflected in Table 4–11. This table includes the concept that physiologic mechanisms may be able to compensate—at least temporarily—for increases in the "mobile" fraction of the total body lead burden. In the case of the hematopoietic system, biologic compensation is apparently accomplished by increasing the rate of red blood cell production when blood lead content is 50–80 μg/100 g of whole blood. For renal and nervous system function, the thresholds for clinical correlation with the biochemical effects of lead are not known. Present knowledge suggests that significant uncompensated impairment of renal and nervous system function is unlikely in persons whose blood lead content does not exceed about 50 or 60 μg/100 g of whole blood. In patients with sustained higher blood lead content, it appears likely that thresholds for adverse functional effects in these organs will be exceeded. The long-term consequences of sustained small increases in soft-tissue lead content are not known. Available epidemiologic information suggests that clinically obvious and severe adverse effects do not occur in such conditions. The degree of subclinical effect is an area in which research is urgently needed; reliance should be placed on clues provided by experimental biochemical studies in approaching this problem in man.

5

Biologic Effects of Lead in Domestic and Wild Animals

DOMESTIC ANIMALS

It generally is recognized that lead is the most common cause of accidental poisoning in domestic animals. The condition is diagnosed most frequently in cattle and dogs. It should be kept in mind that a discussion of lead poisoning in domestic animals must differ from the approach taken for man. Whereas subtle, subclinical effects of lead are highly relevant and important for man, similar considerations regarding animals are not practical. Lead poisoning in animals usually is recognized only when overt clinical signs of poisoning are apparent.

The natural curiosity and licking habits of cattle make any available lead-containing material a potential source of poisoning. Some of the sources incriminated are lead-base paint (either from discarded paint cans or from paint peeling from walls), used motor oil, discarded oil filters, storage batteries, some types of greases and putty, and linoleum.[71, 236] These sources can be found in the vicinity of farm buildings and in dumps in pastures. It is noteworthy that these sources are rarely incriminated in lead poisoning of horses. Horses are much more selective in their eating habits than cattle. They usually do not lick old paint cans, storage batteries, or peeling paint, nor do they find the taste of motor oil attractive.

178

Histories of exposure in dogs commonly include chewing on objects painted with lead-base paints (e.g., when home remodeling entails scraping of plaster and old paint), eating linoleum, or ingesting lead materials, such as lead slugs and curtain weights.[599] Dogs less than 6 months old are affected more commonly than older dogs, but this may be related to the almost completely indiscriminate eating habits of younger dogs.

Several outbreaks of lead poisoning in domestic animals have been recorded in which the apparent source of metal was contamination of pasture or crops by industrial lead operations. These outbreaks differ from the more common cases of lead poisoning described previously, in that several animals may be involved. Some of the areas involved in North America are St. Paul, Minnesota;[232] Belleville, Pennsylvania;[316] Trail, British Columbia;[479] and Benecia, California.[431] Deaths of horses attributable to lead poisoning have been noted in the Benecia area since the early 1900's. It is reported that the presence of lead and arsenic has made it impossible to raise horses near smelters in East Helena, Montana, for several decades.[207]

Pastures and crops are contaminated by fumes and dusts that are emitted by lead industries and settle on the surrounding countryside. Animals that eat this vegetation can accumulate sufficient lead to produce clinical signs of lead poisoning. A number of studies have been made to determine whether the lead found in vegetation is of direct airborne origin or due to translocation from soil.[165] These studies have been reviewed recently by Mueller and Stanley,[408] who conclude that translocation from soil does not contribute more than 15 μg of lead per gram (dry weight) of forage, even when plants are grown in soil containing about 700–3,000 μg/g. Thus, amounts of lead in excess of 15 μg/g most likely are due to direct aerial fallout. The extent to which contamination can occur is illustrated by concentrations of 3,200 μg/g (dry weight) found in corn leaves 75 yards from a lead smelter.[232]

It has been estimated that 6–7 mg/kg per day constitutes a minimal cumulative fatal dosage of lead for cattle.[232] This intake represents a concentration of about 300 ppm in the total diet. The cattle studied were approximately 2 miles from a smelter but were fed lead-contaminated hay and corn silage grown in fields adjacent to the smelter. A fatal case of lead poisoning occurred after approximately 2 months on this diet, and an intake of approximately half this dosage had no observed effect on cows at another farm in the previous winter. In this connection, it is of interest that dosages of 5–6 mg/kg per day were fed to cattle for a period of 2 years with no observable clinical effects,[3] but that longer intake at this rate may be fatal.[4]

There is some evidence that horses are more susceptible than cattle to the chronic ingestion of lead. Whereas horses contracted lead poisoning on pastures adjacent to a lead smelter in the Trail area, cattle grazing in the same area appeared healthy.[479] At one farm adjacent to the St. Paul smelter, horses succumbed to lead poisoning in March after a winter lead intake in their hay estimated at 2.4 mg/kg per day.[232] It was not possible to determine the lead intake from pasture grazing in the previous summer. However, inasmuch as cows and horses had similar pasture that summer and the winter ration for the horses contained appreciably less lead than that for the cows, it would seem that cumulative toxicity occurred somewhat more readily in horses. It is of interest to consider that pasture grass containing over 80 μg of lead per gram (dry weight) was toxic to horses in the Benecia area.[408] A horse will eat about 21 g of dry matter per kilogram of body weight per day. Thus, a minimal toxic dosage could be estimated at 1.7 mg/kg per day—a figure close to the previous estimate.

Although the evidence above suggests that horses might be more sensitive to lead than cattle are, a consideration of the grazing habits of horses precludes any firm conclusions. Horses occasionally pull forage out by the roots and eat the roots and attendant soil with the forage. Cattle rarely, if ever, do that, probably because their jaw structure makes it impossible. The soil near smelters usually contains far greater amounts of lead than does the forage. It is apparent that a horse showing a marked tendency toward this habit could ingest far greater quantities of lead than would be estimated from the analysis of forage alone.

Several workers have documented high concentrations of lead in grass along highways. Motto et al.[406] found in grass samples immediately adjacent to the roadside an average concentration of lead (dry weight) of 255 mg/kg; the concentration decreased with increasing distance from the highway (see Table 2–6). It is appropriate to consider whether concentrations in grass of this magnitude constitute a hazard to animals, such as cattle and horses.

Even if the entire diet of cattle were obtained from forage immediately adjacent to a major highway, overt clinical poisoning probably would not occur. Cattle eat approximately 22.5 g of dry matter per kilogram of body weight per day. Thus, the ingestion of grass immediately adjacent to the highway (255 mg/kg dry weight) would provide a daily intake of approximately 5.7 mg/kg. Horses, however, appear to succumb to lead poisoning at a lower daily intake than cattle. If their diet consisted exclusively of forage obtained 75 ft from a major highway (99 mg/kg dry weight, Table 2–6), overt lead poisoning conceivably could occur. If a horse eats approximately 21 g of dry matter per kilogram of body weight per day, the ingestion of forage containing 99 mg/kg (dry weight) would provide a daily intake of approximately 2.1 mg/kg. Exclusive consumption of forage 125 ft from the highway would provide a daily intake of approximately 1.4 mg/kg, somewhat below that associated with clinical lead poisoning in the horse.

It is emphasized, however, that it would be highly unlikely for animals to obtain their entire diet, the year around, from grazing within 125 ft of a major highway. Even in the absence of fences, animals usually prefer to graze in areas farther from major highways.

It is only natural for persons residing close to smelters near which animals are dying of lead poisoning to be concerned about their own health. In many cases, such persons eat produce from home gardens. Analyses of blood and urine of these persons by local public health officials have not revealed evidence of increased lead absorption. It is emphasized that horses and cattle are herbivores and, if raised in the vicinity of a lead industrial operation, may subsist entirely on contaminated vegetation. Probably only a small fraction of the total diet of human beings would consist of food grown in the vicinity of a lead operation. Furthermore, it is customary for people to wash garden produce (or to husk corn) before consuming it. This practice undoubtedly removes appreciable quantities of surface lead deposits. Inasmuch as the animal and human populations breathed the same air and human residents in the area did not show evidence of increased lead absorption, it may be concluded that the animals received nearly all their lead burden through oral ingestion.

All domestic species with lead poisoning exhibit various degrees of derangement of the central nervous system, gastrointestinal tract, muscular system, and hematopoietic system. Differences occur clinically, however, in the relative severity of signs referable to those organs and tissues. The most striking syndrome is presented by young calves. The calf may suddenly begin to bellow and stagger about with rolling eyes and frothing mouth, often blindly crashing into objects. This phase may last up to 2 hr, when there is sudden collapse. In less severe cases, depression, anorexia, and colic may be observed, and the animals may be blind and may grind their teeth, move in a circle, push against objects, and be ataxic. The less severe signs are more frequent in adult cattle, although the syndrome of maniacal excitement is not uncommon.

In sheep, the syndrome consists mainly of depression, anorexia, abdominal pain, and (usually) diarrhea. Excitatory phases have never been reported for sheep. Anemia is common during chronic ingestion of lead.

In horses, the syndrome consists mainly of depression, stupor, knuckling at the fetlocks, and laryngeal paralysis that produces an obstruction in the air passage and causes the horse to "roar." Anemia is commonly associated with lead poisoning in horses.[123]

Gastrointestinal or central nervous system signs are seen with equal frequency in lead poisoning in dogs. At some time during the course of poisoning, approximately 87% of dogs show gastrointestinal signs consisting of emesis, colic, diarrhea, and anorexia. Approximately 76% of dogs show central nervous system signs consisting of hysteria and convulsions. Anemia and basophilic stippling are commonly associated with lead poisoning in dogs and are considered to be of diagnostic significance.[155,599]

Abortions have been reported in ewes that graze in lead-mining areas. A high rate of abortions and of failures to conceive were noted in ewes fed finely divided metallic lead at a rate sufficient to induce signs of poisoning.[70] The lethal dose of lead appears to be considerably lower in pregnant than in nonpregnant ewes.[5] Cattle and horses have given birth to normal offspring after excessive lead exposure,[164,497] but the small number of animals reported (five) makes it impossible to state that lead has no effect on the fetus in these species.

A high concentration of lead in blood or tissues, associated with clinical signs, is considered to be the best criterion for a diagnosis of lead poisoning. The presence of basophilic stippling of red blood cells, immature (especially nucleated) red blood cells, and acid-fast inclusion bodies in the cells of the kidneys has been reported to be commonly associated with lead poisoning.[56,599] A discussion of the treatment and costs of lead poisoning in cattle is found in Appendix G.

BIRDS

Lead poisoning has been recognized in waterfowl and upland game bird species for at least 100 years. Lead poisoning was considered to be a serious problem in ducks and other waterfowl in the United States by 1919.[579] Recently it was estimated that a million ducks, geese, and swans die of lead poisoning each year in the United States.[12] This figure becomes even more impressive when it is considered that most of the birds die after the hunting season and thus represent a loss of breeding stock. The principal, and probably the only significant, source of lead is spent lead shot that is mistakenly ingested in the birds' search for gravel. Approximately 6,000 tons of lead shot are deposited on waterfowl habitats each year.[12] Cases of lead poisoning occur in upland game birds, as well as waterfowl.[27] As in the case of waterfowl, the primary source of lead appears to be spent lead shot, as evidenced by the recovery of the material from the gizzards of affected birds.

Efforts to develop a safer material than lead for shot began as early as 1936.[217] Copper and hard iron are safer materials, but ballistic considerations and damage to gun barrels and chokes make the materials unsuitable. The Sporting Arms and Ammunition Manufacturing Institute (SAAMI) recently supported a $100,000 study by the Illinois Institute of Technology to find a material more suitable than lead. Soft iron pellets were found to be the best substitute. Although soft iron pellets compared satisfactorily with lead for killing ducks in flight,[12] the cost of manufacturing them is at present prohibitive. Another problem with soft iron shot is that the material hardens with age. Two years after manufacture, shot has hardened by 25%, which will cause a scoring of gun barrels and chokes.[264]

As with mammals, the presence of lead in birds is a constant finding. A study including between one and 37 representatives of 28 different bird species with no known "excessive" lead exposure revealed concentrations in fresh liver ranging from 0.3 to 7.0 ppm.[26] Lead, as well as several other inorganic ions, was measured in pheasant populations in Illinois. Concentrations (wet weight) ranging from 0.22 to 0.27 $\mu g/g$ of blood, 0.09 to 0.84 $\mu g/g$ of liver, and 0.11 to 0.27 $\mu g/g$ of kidney were measured in apparently healthy pheasants.[11]

A lethal amount of lead for duck can be absorbed from one #6 lead shot. Variable mortality occurs after the ingestion of up to six #6 shot, which is nearly always lethal.[579] A daily dose of 6 mg/kg per day (as lead nitrate) for 137 days did not produce any observable ill effects, but when the dose was increased to 8 and 12 mg/kg per day, the survival periods averaged 28 and 25 days, respectively.[126] The deposition of lead in soft tissues was almost proportional to dosage, but no appreciable differences were measured for bone. When the dosage of lead for the two birds that received 6 mg/kg per day for 137 days was increased to 12 mg/kg per day, death occurred at about the time expected for the new dosage. The long period on the lower dosage seemed to have little effect on the rate at which clinical signs developed or on the deposition of lead in soft tissues. When excretion was expressed as a percentage of total dose, an average of only 3% was excreted in the first week, but the average increased to 67% and 63% for the second and third weeks, respectively.

Concentrations of lead in muscle are very low in mammals, but it has been reported that breast muscle and liver from a pheasant dying of lead poisoning contained 42 and 169 ppm, respectively.[267] A total of 29 shot were recovered from the gizzard. However, concentrations of lead in muscle of mallards dying of lead poisoning are considerably lower than 42 ppm (L. N. Locke, personal communication).

The usual picture of lead poisoning in waterfowl consists of lethargy, weakness, flaccid paralysis, emaciation, anemia, greenish diarrhea, impaction of the proventriculus, and distention of the gall bladder. The large pectoral muscles waste away, and in some cases the sternum is covered merely with a thin layer of fascia, muscle, and skin—the so-called "razor-keel" or "hatched" breast.[126,362,459,543] Acid-fast intranuclear inclusion bodies of the renal tubular cells are commonly but not always found in cases of lead poisoning.[361] A number of workers have stated that basophilic stippling of red blood cells does not occur.

It has been suggested that lead may be important in producing sterility among many birds that in other respects appear to have recovered completely from clinical lead poisoning.[579] This contention was not supported by a study designed to evaluate breeding performance of mallard drakes.[98] The data indicated that drakes recovering from lead poisoning did not exhibit a significant loss of fertility; similar studies with females, however, were not carried out. It has been reported that some green feeds, such as coontail (*Ceratophyllum demersum*), will prevent lead poisoning in mallards fed lead shot in amounts that will kill birds maintained only on cracked or whole corn.[282] In another study, ducks maintained on corn and on a diet of grain and duck pellets developed acid-fast intranuclear inclusions in renal tubular cells when given one or three #6 lead shot orally. No lesions developed in ducks maintained on a duck-pellet ration and fed the same number of shot.[360] It is not known whether these dietary factors affect the absorption or the biologic effects of the lead.

ZOO ANIMALS

Reports of lead poisoning in zoo animals are uncommon. Cases are reported in eleven nonhuman primates,[474] three Australian fruit bats,[600] one polar bear, and an unspecified number of lorikeets and ferrets.[385] These poisonings occurred in seven different zoos, and almost all cases were reportedly due to the ingestion of leaded paint. In addition to the documented poisonings, eosinophilic intranuclear inclusion bodies have been reported in the renal tubules of zoo-dwelling primates in a London zoo[255] and in parrots, primates, and other animals in a Philadelphia zoo.[129] A disease of unknown cause peculiar to zoo primates, acute amaurotic epilepsy, was described in 1935 (it appears to have occurred as early as 1915).[598] This disease has many clinical and pathologic features of lead poisoning.

Postmortem examinations at the National Zoological Park in Washington, D.C., have disclosed 41 lead poisonings in primates and parrots that were confimed by the finding of excess lead in the liver (3–500 ppm wet weight) coupled with typical lesions, including acid-fast intranuclear inclusions in all and brain lesions in most. In every instance, paint containing 3–66% lead was found peeling or partially removed from enclosures where the poisoned animals were kept; in several, the animals were observed removing and ingesting the leaded paint. Other significant sources of lead were largely ruled out (B. C. Zook, personal communication).

Preliminary work in regard to lead poisoning in New York City zoo animals and lead contamination of zoo animal environments has shown, in the great cats and primates tested, fecal lead as high as 4,000 ppm (ashed weight) and blood lead concentrations as high as 130 μg/100 ml. Sampling of the lead content of the outdoor zoo environments (soil, grass) revealed high lead contamination. The precise source of the lead is under investigation (Ralph Strebel, E. Garner, E. Dolensek, D. Craston, and T. J. Chow, personal communication).

AQUATIC ORGANISMS

Contamination of natural waters by effluent from lead mines has long been recognized in England. A report of the River Pollution Commission of 1874 (cited by Jones[279]) described the disappearance of fish from streams fouled by effluent from lead mines and deaths of waterfowl, horses, and cattle in the vicinity of streams. Lead also can be present in effluent associated with a number of industrial and manufacturing operations.

Probably the first definitive experiments on lead poisoning in fish were carried out by Carpenter.[85, 87, 88] An explanation was sought for the continued absence of fish in rivers passing through old mining areas. Minnows placed in a river in cages remained normal until heavy rains occurred. The concentration of lead in the river suddenly increased from an unmeasurable value to 0.3–0.4 mg/liter, and the minnows died. It was reasoned that the rain dissolved surface lead deposits and carried them into the river.

The effect of lead on lower forms of life is not well documented, but it appears to be less toxic than in higher forms. For example, insects were shown to be less sensitive than fish to the effects of lead.[568] Concentrations of lead in excess of 0.1 mg/liter appear to inhibit the self-purification of water by biologic means in water-storage reservoirs.[287, 593] Concentrations of lead in excess of 0.5 mg/liter have been reported to retard the growth of protozoa and to retard nitrification in sewage purification procedures.[287]

Acute Toxicity of Lead to Freshwater Fish

For purposes of this review, "acute toxicity" will be defined as including effects that occur within 2 weeks of exposure to lead.

Available evidence suggests that the principal biochemical lesion caused by lead in fish occurs outside the body. When fish were placed in a solution containing insufficient lead to cause death, a film of coagulated mucus formed over their bodies, with concomitant respiratory distress.[87] Recovery occurred when the film was shed. Analysis of the film for lead accounted for almost all the lead in the original solution. No lead could be found in the bodies of the fish, but it should be pointed out that the exposure was brief (hours) and that the method of lead analysis[19] was not as sensitive and accurate as methods in use today.

Observation of these effects led to formulation of the "coagulation film anoxia" theory.[167, 279, 578] The film of coagulated mucus that appears over the entire body is particularly prominent over the gills; the insoluble material interferes with the respiratory function of the gills, resulting in acute respiratory distress and death by suffocation. This effect is not peculiar to lead; it can be produced by toxic concentrations of other heavy metal ions, including zinc, iron, copper, cadmium, mercury, manganese, cobalt, nickel, silver, gold, and aluminum.[86, 157, 167, 279] The effect has been demonstrated for many species of freshwater fish, but apparently not for saltwater fish. Lead may precipitate in seawater before toxic concentrations are attained. Thomas[534] could not poison killiefish (which can live in both freshwater and seawater) with lead in seawater, because the material precipitated out of solution; in fresh water, lead nitrate (3 mg/liter) was fatal in 12 hr.

Some species of fish are considerably more susceptible than others to the toxic effects of inorganic lead. Carpenter[89] observed that the action of lead on goldfish was the same as on trout, sticklebacks, and minnows, but goldfish were more resistant. Jones[281] stated that goldfish appeared able to tolerate indefinitely 1 mg of lead per liter of soft tap water, whereas 0.1–0.2 mg/liter proved fatal to sticklebacks. The amount and nature of gill secretions may explain variations in species susceptibility to lead.[281] Goldfish produce a copious gill secretion. When exposed to 10 mg of lead per liter, goldfish produced so much precipitated mucus that the solution became milky and sediment collected on the bottom of the vessel. Ellis[167] suggested that, if the concentration of a pollutant, such as lead, were low enough or if the source were limited so that it acted on the fish for only a short time, the secretion of additional mucus might wash away the precipitated material before serious toxicity to the fish occurred.

It is difficult to define acutely toxic concentrations of lead for fish; experimental results from different laboratories vary considerably. Such variables as dissolved oxygen concentration, solution pH, volume and number of exchanges of experimental solution, and duration of exposure are not always controlled.[157] Water temperature is an important factor. A 10 C rise in temperature reduces survival time by 50%.[89] Probably one of the most important factors is the degree of water hardness. Lead is readily precipitated as the carbonate or hydroxide; thus, hard waters tend to decrease the effective concentration of lead. As water hardness (expressed as calcium carbonate) increased from 14 to 53 mg/liter, the concentration of lead in solution decreased from 8 to 1.6 mg/liter.[279] Another important point regarding the presence of calcium is that it appears to decrease the toxic effects of lead.[281] For example, in solutions containing 1 mg of lead (as lead nitrate) per liter with 0, 5, 10, 20, and 50 mg of calcium (as calcium nitrate or chloride) per liter, survival times averaged 1, 3, 6, 7, and 10.5 days, respectively. In this case, precipitation of lead could not account for the decreasing toxicity with increasing concentrations of calcium. It was concluded that calcium somehow prevents the precipitation of mucus by lead. Calcium was shown to have a similar protective effect on the toxicity of other metals.

Carpenter[87, 89] and Jones[281] have reported some of the lowest demonstrable concentrations of lead (0.1–0.4 mg/liter) toxic to fish. They used either distilled or soft tap water in their studies, which might be expected to provide optimal conditions for the toxic effects of lead. However, it has been pointed out[157] that other species of fish probably are more sensitive to lead than those studied by Carpenter and by Jones, and concentrations of 0.1 mg/liter therefore probably do not represent minimal concentrations of lead toxic to sensitive fish in the conditions most conducive to poisoning.

The behavioral effects of acute exposure to very low concentrations of lead in goldfish are discussed in Chapter 4.

Chronic Toxicity of Lead to Freshwater and Saltwater Fish and Other Aquatic Organisms

Few studies are available concerning the chronic toxicity of lead to fish. Anemia has been reported in catfish exposed to solutions of 50 mg/liter for periods of 16–183 days.[143] Somewhat similar findings were reported in guppies exposed to 1.24 and 3.12 mg/liter (total water hardness, 80 mg/liter) for periods of up to 129 days.[132] In addition to blood changes, histologic studies revealed renal changes consisting of expanded tubular lumina and a lack of lymphoid tissue, a lack of mesenteric fat, cellular elements in the myocardium suggestive of degenerative changes, and retarded gonadal development. There was no demonstrable consistent alteration of respiratory epithelium or evidence of an accumulation of coagulated mucus, but the possibility of some damage to the respiratory system was suggested by the frequent finding of granular debris in the branchial blood vessels. The histopathology, as well as growth inhibition and retardation of sexual maturity, suggested that the secondary effects of inanition or stress were the most prominent features of chronic lead poisoning in fish. Growth inhibition also was observed in saltwater plaice when exposed to solutions of 4 mg of lead per liter.[153]

There have apparently been no studies with freshwater fish in which concentrations of lead have been measured simultaneously in fish and water. Such information would be essential for evaluating the ability of fish to concentrate lead from a surrounding medium. Kehoe, Thamann, and Cholak[305] and Harley[239] have reported lead concentrations of 0.24 and 0.16 ppm in freshwater fish. Wetterberg[580] reported concentrations as high as 12 ppm in liver, 5.7 ppm in gills, and 1.4 ppm in muscle of fish taken from a lake near a rich lead mine. No analysis of the lake water for lead was reported.

Analyses of over 1,500 samples from natural water sources near water-treatment plants over a 5-year period throughout the United States revealed measurable quantities of lead in fewer than 20% of the samples analyzed, and 27 samples were over the U.S. acceptable limit for drinking water of 0.05 mg/liter.[314] The highest value recorded was 0.14 mg/liter in the Ohio River near Evansville, Indiana, a heavily industrialized area. The authors pointed out that the total concentration of lead in a body of water would be higher than that in flowing water because the presence of carbonate and hydroxyl ions in natural still waters tends to induce precipitation of lead as insoluble lead salts. This was borne out in a study measuring the concentration of lead in particles larger and smaller than 0.45 μm at various depths in Lake Hamilton, Arkansas.[422] The concentration of larger lead particles increased with increasing depth.

Information is not available to state with any degree of certainty whether the occurrence of lead in natural waters of the United States constitutes a serious threat to fish or to humans who eat the fish. There seem to be no reports of fish kills due to pollution of natural waters in the United States by lead. In addition to areas close to water-treatment plants, it would appear highly desirable to analyze both water and fish for lead downstream from industrial operations likely to emit lead. An evaluation of lead concentrations in the water and fish of lakes used heavily by motorboats would also be desirable. The amount of lead emitted into the water from an outboard motor burning leaded gasoline (0.7 g of lead per liter) appears to be related to the size of the motor and the speed of operation.[170] A 10-hp engine operated at one-half to three-fourths throttle was shown to emit into the water 0.229 g of lead per liter of fuel consumed, whereas a 5.6-hp engine operated at full throttle emitted 0.121 g/liter.

There is no question that some marine organisms can concentrate the lead present in seawater. The normal concentration of lead in seawater is stated to be around 0.00003 mg/liter.[571] Although concentrations of lead reported to occur in seafood are relatively low, they do indicate considerable concentration from the surrounding medium. For example, Schroeder et al.[480] reported a range of 0.17–2.5 ppm in seafood, with an average of 0.5 ppm and only one sample exceeding 0.87 ppm. Harley[239] reported a concentration of 0.31 ppm in shellfish. Pringle et al.[447] reported average wet-weight concentrations of 0.47, 0.70, and 0.52 ppm in eastern oysters, soft-shell clams, and northern quahogs, respectively. The remarkable ability of the eastern oyster to concentrate lead was demonstrated by exposing oysters to flowing seawater containing lead concentrations of 0.025, 0.05, 0.1, and 0.2 mg/liter. After 49 days, the total accumulations of lead amounted to 17, 35, 75, and 200 ppm (wet weight). The highest concentrations of lead in the oyster occurred in liver, and the lowest concentrations, in muscle tissue. Oysters exposed to the two lower experimental concentrations of lead appeared normal. Oysters exposed to the higher experimental lead concentrations (0.1 and 0.2 mg/liter), however, grossly showed considerable atrophy and diffusion of the gonadal tissue, edema, and less distinction of hepatopancreas and mantle edge.

In view of the insolubility of lead in seawater in usual conditions, it would be very interesting to know whether conditions could arise that would permit lead concentrations of 0.2 mg/liter to exist in seawater in a chemical state such that it could be absorbed by marine organisms to the extent shown in this experimental study.

SUMMARY

Lead poisoning is the most frequently diagnosed poisoning of domestic animals. The sources most commonly incriminated include lead-base paints, storage batteries, and used motor oil. Airborne lead from smelting and other lead-using industries has caused poisoning of cattle and horses in localized areas, by contaminating hay and pasture vegetation. Airborne lead from vehicular exhaust emissions has not been shown to cause poisoning of domestic animals.

Lead poisoning is an important health problem in waterfowl. The only source of lead ever reported to cause poisoning is spent lead shot from hunting.

There is no evidence that lead constitutes a health problem in fish in the United States, but there is very little information on which to base any firm conclusion. Very few analytic data have been reported on concentrations of lead in fish in natural or experimental conditions. The data that are available suggest that soluble lead is not present in natural waters of the United States in concentrations likely to be toxic to fish. There is no published evidence of any trend toward increased concentrations of soluble lead in natural waters. Much of the man-dispersed lead that is eventually washed into natural waters is probably precipitated, owing to the presence of carbonates, hydroxides, and organic ligands in the water, and settles to the bottom. There is no evidence that lead precipitated on the bottom of natural waterways is harmful to fish.

6

Airborne Lead
Alkyl Compounds

The atmosphere may contain gaseous lead alkyls, in addition to particulate inorganic lead. Lead alkyl vapors result from the production of lead antiknock compounds and their subsequent handling and use as gasoline additives. Precise information on the concentration of lead alkyl vapor in the ambient air is scanty, because until a few years ago the only available methods of analysis required the sampling of large volumes of air, and their precision and specificity were not as good as could be wished.

The analytic methods in use before 1962 were developed mainly to monitor the air in lead alkyl manufacturing plants.[339, 509, 510] Because the threshold limit value for tetraethyl lead (TEL) was 75 μg of lead per cubic meter of air, the analytic methods were designed to measure TEL concentrations close to this figure. That some of the analytic methods were inadequate even at this comparatively high lead alkyl concentration in the air is shown by the recovery of only 30–70% of the TEL in the air by the aqueous iodine method.[355] By 1967, a new method was developed, using an activated charcoal scrubber, that achieved an acceptable level of accuracy ($\pm$0.008 μg/m^3 of air) in the hands of well-trained personnel, and an effort was made to measure the much smaller quantities of lead alkyl compounds in suburban air.[508] However, the large volumes of air (100–200 m^3) that

192

had to be passed through the scrubber made the method suitable only for measuring average concentrations over periods of several days. Snyder carried out some limited sampling in Los Angeles with this method; at a time when the average concentration of inorganic lead in the air was 3.56 $\mu g/m^3$ of air over a 6-week period, the organic lead concentration averaged 0.078 $\mu g/m^3$ of air, with a range of 0.047–0.106 $\mu g/m^3$. The method of analysis used during the survey of atmospheric lead in three urban communities[554] was not accurate enough to allow more than the general comment that "at most the alkyl lead concentrations did not reach 10 percent of the inorganic lead values and probably were considerably less."

In 1970, A. Laveskog published a method that combined the use of gas chromatograph material to trap alkyl lead compounds, desorption, separation, and detection (carried out in a mass spectrometer). The method is sensitive to within 10 ng of tetramethyl lead (TML) or TEL per cubic meter of urban air.[335] This method made it possible, although by no means simple, to measure the TEL and TML in the urban air accurately with relatively short (15 min) periods of sampling.

LEAD ALKYLS IN THE AIR

Because lead alkyls are readily broken down by light and heat, their presence in the atmosphere is transient. In some conditions, however, sizable short-lived peak concentrations can be attained. For example, the combustion process within the engine coupled with the passage of the exhaust gases through the hot exhaust manifold and muffler system normally results in no more than 100 μg of lead alkyls per cubic meter of exhaust gas leaving the tailpipe. This gas is rapidly diluted by the surrounding air to give concentrations of 0.02–2 $\mu g/m^3$ of air. However, if measurements are made at the tailpipe of a poorly tuned car starting fully choked from cold, transient peak lead alkyl concentrations up to 5,000 μg of lead per cubic meter of air may occasionally be reached; such peaks last for a matter of seconds and fall below 1,000 $\mu g/m^3$ in 10 min. It must be remembered that these measurements are made in the exhaust gas stream before dilution with ambient air. If such a cold-started fully choked car were to pass a sampling station in the street where the average lead alkyl level might be 0.02–0.04 $\mu g/m^3$ of air, a peak of about 0.5 $\mu g/m^3$ might be measured as the car passed by.[335]

Other sources of lead alkyl vapor in the ambient air due to operation of a car are evaporation of gasoline from the fuel system, particularly from the carburetor after the hot engine is shut off, and crankcase "blow-by." The crankcase emissions contain a high percentage of unburned air–fuel mixture. Both these sources of lead alkyls have been or are being reduced or removed by antipollution devices built into new cars now being sold in the United States. The devices include the recycling of the blow-by gases and control systems designed to contain and recycle evaporative losses from the carburetor and fuel tank.

Sources that are more difficult to control involve the distribution and dispensing of gasoline containing lead alkyl and include displaced fuel-tank vapors, entrained fuel droplets in the displaced vapors, and liquid gasoline spillage.

Because of the much higher vapor pressure of gasoline than of TEL or TML and the small amount of lead alkyl in a gallon of gasoline, lead alkyl vapors are not present to a significant degree above liquid gasoline until almost all the gasoline has evaporated. When a gasoline spill occurs and the gasoline is allowed to evaporate completely, as may happen in filling a gasoline tank from a pump, a transient high concentration of lead alkyl in the ambient air can be found. Filling-station attendants, more than most persons, are exposed to the lead alkyls in the air around service stations, as well as to sources of inorganic lead, e.g., from cylinder head deposits, crankcase oil, and dust from mufflers and other parts of the exhaust system. In addition, some service-station attendants engage in the grinding of body solder. Such attendants have been studied and their urinary lead concentrations found to be within the range in the general public, although, as might be expected from the possibility of absorbing lead from more than one source, concentrations for individual attendants may be toward the high end of the normal range (up to 30 μg/liter).[303]

CLINICAL RAMIFICATIONS

Tetraethyl lead was discovered by Löwig in 1852,[365] but the first cases of occupational poisoning were reported in 1924, shortly after TEL began to be manufactured in the United States as a gasoline additive.

The main site of action in lead alkyl poisoning is the central nervous system. In severe cases in man, a toxic psychosis develops, with hallucinations, delusions, and excitement, which may end in delirium and death. If the mental symptoms disappear, recovery is very likely but may take 2–6 months. In contrast with poisoning with inorganic lead, lead alkyl intoxication seldom if ever is accompanied by abdominal colic, abnormalities of the red cells, or peripheral neuropathy. The earliest symptom of lead alkyl poisoning in man is insomnia; in cases of more severe exposure, it is followed by lack of appetite, nausea, vomiting, and diarrhea. Continuing exposure commonly leads to complaints of irritability, restlessness, nervousness, and anxiety, and these may be followed by the more serious mental symptoms mentioned earlier.

As with toxic effects of all chemicals, the relation of the amount of the chemical absorbed to the type and severity of the symptoms is very important in establishing whether a clinical picture is due to a particular chemical. Cassells and Dodds[90] and Kehoe[295] agree that, if the urinary excretion of lead is less than 0.1 mg/liter of urine at a time when symptoms like those described are present, the cause is probably not absorption of TEL. Mild symptoms may occur with a concentration of 0.15 mg/liter of urine, but TEL poisoning is generally associated with concentrations of about 0.3 mg/liter or greater. Stopps et al.[521] found no adverse effect of TEL exposure on health (as measured by history of important chronic diseases, height and weight, blood pressure, hematology, electrocardiographic abnormalities, or other findings on physical examination) when 348 TEL workers were compared with 348 matched controls not working in TEL production. Lead excretion in the TEL group was 0.064 ± 0.033 mg/liter of urine, and in the control group, 0.03 ± 0.016 mg/liter of urine. The health of those who had previously worked in TEL production but were no longer so engaged was also studied and compared with the health of the other two groups. No significant differences in health were found between any of the groups.

Although the acute toxicity of organic and inorganic lead differs considerably, it is possible that the chronic toxicity depends more heavily on the lead ion than on the chemical form of lead at the time of absorption. This is suggested by the fact that, if the lead concentrations in the urine of workers exposed to organic or inorganic lead are kept below 150 mg μg/liter and the concentrations in the blood are kept below 70 mg/100 g of whole blood, the workers' health is protected.[181, 327] It has not been found necessary to set lower biologic safety limits for exposure to organic lead than for exposure to inorganic lead; this suggests that the safety of long exposures to either inorganic or organic lead depends more heavily on the average amount of lead ion present in the soft tissues and less heavily on whether an inorganic or an organic form of lead enters the body.

Because TML is more volatile than TEL (TML boils at 110 C, TEL at 199 C), some concern was felt by manufacturing companies and public health authorities when TML was introduced as a component of gasoline antiknock mix around 1959. DeTreville *et al.*, however, reported in 1962[149] that in their experience there was less hazard associated with the manufacture of TML than of TEL. The smaller hazard associated with TML is explained partly by a slightly lower absorption of TML, as shown by the somewhat lower urinary lead concentration of workers in TML areas than of workers in TEL areas, at the same concentrations of TEL and TML vapor (measured as lead).[356]

EXPERIMENTAL STUDIES

In addition to observations in man, toxicity differences between TEL and TML have been found experimentally. Schepers[477] found that the approximate lethal oral dose of TEL in rats was 11 mg of lead per kilogram of body weight and that of TML was 83 mg/kg—about a sevenfold difference in acute toxicity. Similar differences have been found when the compounds were given by inhalation.[142] The metabolism of TEL suggests that it is a compound of very low toxicity, but that it is broken down in the body to triethyl lead, a water-soluble compound that causes the clinical picture typically associated with lead alkyl toxicity.[133] In experiments on liver and brain homogenates, Cremer[133] also showed that the enzyme system that converts TEL into triethyl lead is found only in the liver. Bolanowska[53] carried these studies a step further with rats and showed that 24 hr after the administration of TEL, 50% of the total lead in the soft organs was in the form of triethyl lead. The concentration of triethyl lead remained steady for several days. The other metabolite of TEL was inorganic lead, which was produced within the first 24 hr after a single exposure to TEL but was removed from the soft tissues within a week.

SUMMARY

Practical and precise methods of measurement of the concentration of lead alkyls in the ambient air have only recently become available.

Preliminary data based on these newer methods suggest that the broad generalization contained in the three-city survey,[554] that "at most the alkyl lead concentrations did not reach 10 percent of the inorganic lead values and probably were considerably less," remains true. It is now possible to demonstrate peak concentrations lasting from a fraction of a minute to several minutes during which the lead alkyl concentration may reach 50% of the inorganic lead concentration when the sampling point is close to a cold-started automobile or a spill of gasoline containing lead antiknock compounds. Offsetting this difference in ambient concentrations to some extent is the relatively greater acute toxicity of lead alkyls than of inorganic lead compounds. Judging from the few clinical cases, these differences do not appear in practice to apply to long human exposures extending over a working lifetime.

7

Nonbiologic Effects of Lead

The Panel has not looked exhaustively at the nonbiologic effects of airborne lead, but it has inquired specifically about possible effects on two important categories of material: natural and man-made textile fibers and glass. In addition, it offers some brief comments on automotive exhaust catalysts and microelectronic devices. The possible roles of lead aerosols in affecting atmospheric visibility and in serving as nuclei for water vapor condensation are also discussed.

NONBIOLOGIC EFFECTS ON MATERIALS

Organic fibrous materials used in clothing and in a large number of household and utilitarian items fall into two basic categories: the natural fibers, among which wool and cotton are economically the most significant, and man-made or synthetic fibers.

Normal values for lead content apply both to the cotton plant and to the cotton fiber grown in soils of normal lead content, and for plant ash they are between 0.008% and 0.18% (80–1,800 ppm).[265]

The lead content of wool has been reported to be 1–3 mg/100 g.[137] Data for human hair reported by Kraut and Weber[318] are consonant

198

with the overall lead content of 1.7 mg/100 g from normal persons not working in activities involving lead products. Data obtained during assessment of damage to wool fibers induced by the use of plumbite solutions in chemical treatments and photochemical degradation showed that the uptake of lead by wool is related to the formation of lead–sulfur complexes with sulfhydryl groups generated by the splitting of disulfide linkages in the wool structure (F. J. Rizzo, unpublished data). Thorsen[536] has more recently shown that staining of wool by lead occurs strongly in the paracortex of the fiber, and progressive levels of staining in this component may be taken as an indicator of increased damage to the fiber. By extrapolation from these facts, one may thus assume that the lead content of wool fibers is associated with free sulfhydryl groups. The distribution of lead in the tissues of animals in which lead salts are deliberately injected favors the bone structure,[472] which suggests that the concentration in the wool fiber will be limited even when feeds containing high concentrations of lead are ingested by the sheep.

In the modern fiber-producing facilities of the industry, lead as a structural element has been supplanted by other materials that greatly reduce the lead and other nonfibrous components that tend to interfere with the color of the fiber and its processing and chemical reactivity characteristics. The lead content of man-made fibers to which lead compounds have not been deliberately added is generally below that of natural fibers.

By far the most significant source of lead in textiles is its deliberate addition to achieve specific functional properties not inherent in the basic fiber of the fabric. In some instances, it is accidental—for example, in yarns that have been delustered by the use of titanium dioxide pigments in which lead is a natural impurity. Organolead compounds and lead compounds formed *in situ* with many organic acidic compounds of high molecular weight have been applied to textile materials to impart waterproofing or water-repellence, fungus-proofing, and occasionally delustering characteristics to textile materials.[127] Other compositions involving compounds with more favorable toxicologic and dermatologic characteristics are available today and are therefore more generally used both for clothing materials and for textiles that go into industrial and other nonclothing items. Where it is desirable to use lead compounds in processing clothing materials, it is obvious that preference is for nonabsorbable (not fat-soluble) forms that cannot enter the body through the skin (see Chapter 3).

The synthetic-fiber industry introduces small amounts of metal compounds into the polymer before its extrusion in fiber form to provide antioxidative properties,[390] heat stability, and photochemical stability and to depress some degradative tendencies. The degree and nature of chemical bonding of lead and other additives are not always clear, but the additives obviously are sufficiently bound to the polymer substrate by either physical or chemical processes to remain essentially undiminished during the active life of the textile materials. The protective qualities of lead against gamma and x rays are well known. Textile fabrics impregnated with lead salts[404, 492] and fabric composites with lead sheets are items of commerce for both laboratory and medical shielding purposes.

Deposits of airborne contaminants (including lead) are known to have deteriorative properties on textile materials, but it is not known how much, if any, of the deterioration may be due to lead itself. A significant factor that limits the impact of contaminants on clothing materials is laundering or dry cleaning, which reduces deposits to amounts that should be close to those in the fiber when it was produced.

Airborne lead has no effect on glass at low temperatures (25 C) and concentrations. Lead will react with glass at temperatures above about 400 C,[430] which precludes using glass where such high temperatures exist with lead.

The catalytic surface destruction by lead in automotive exhaust control devices appears to be of major importance. Such effects are not strictly from ambient atmospheric lead, but rather from lead that would otherwise have been distributed in the atmosphere. There appear to be some problems with respect to the effects of particulate matter in general on microelectronic devices, but it is not possible to assign any of these effects specifically to lead (J. R. McNesby, personal communication).

NONBIOLOGIC EFFECTS ON ATMOSPHERIC VISIBILITY

Charlson and Pierrard[96] estimated that automotive lead emissions could be responsible for one fourth or more of the visibility degradation noted at times near freeways. The magnitude of this estimate depends heavily on assumptions made because of lack of data on two important properties of the lead aerosol. These assumptions are that the lead aerosol always has a size distribution similar to that of the aged urban atmospheric aerosol and that short-term lead aerosol particle-mass concentrations in such areas exhibit large excursions about their longer-term mean values.

Since the appearance of that paper, further data have been published that suggest that the contribution of lead emissions to visibility reduction should be reconsidered. Daines *et al.*[135] reported a decrease of 50% in airborne lead mass concentration between 10 and 150 ft from a highway, with a similar reduction between 30 and 250 ft from the highway. The particle size distributions showed little change in the fraction of collected lead at the third impactor stage [mass median equivalent diameter (MMED) = 3.5 μm for ρ = 5.85 g/cm^3] as a function of distance from the highway, but they showed a decrease for larger particles and an increase for smaller ones. These observations support the approach of Mueller,[407] who estimated the size distribution of atmospheric suspendible lead (by assuming settling of all particles larger than 10 μm MMED) from Habibi's[223] size distributions of automotive emitted lead. Habibi *et al.*[224] have since reported that 57% of the mass of the lead emitted by the average car on the road is in particles larger than 9 μm MMED. However, atmospheric measurements by Robinson and co-workers[455, 456] and Lundgren[368] show MMED of 0.1–0.5 μm for lead-bearing particles.

These observations indicate that a rapid and significant change takes place in the size distribution of the lead aerosol in the time between its emission and its arrival at a point, even, say, 30 or 40 ft from the source. It appears that a suitable first approximation is that the air-suspendible fraction of the emitted aerosol (MMED more than about 10 μm) is conserved. The magnitude of the reduction in lead mass concentrations and the implicit change in size distribution over short distances suggest that an estimate of visibility reduction by lead particles cannot be soundly based on the assumption that the lead aerosol has, at the same time, a size distribution comparable with that of the atmospheric aerosol and a high mass concentration corresponding to proximity to the source.

In an effort to clarify the role of exhaust lead particles in visibility reduction, a sampling program was conducted in September and October 1970, at a site adjacent to the heavily traveled San Bernardino Freeway at El Monte, California, 15 miles west of downtown Los Angeles. Continuous records were made of (1) light-scattering coefficient, which is inversely proportional to visibility, (2) carbon monoxide concentration, (3) wind speed and direction, and (4) temperature and relative humidity. Although analysis of the data from this study is not yet complete, some useful points have already emerged (J. M. Pierrard, personal communication).

Visibilities encountered during the observing period varied over more than an order of magnitude. No deliberate bias was introduced in choosing periods for lead sampling runs, except that no samples were taken between midnight and 6 a.m. Ten-minute average values were formed from the records of the continuously recorded variables listed above, and these data analyzed statistically. Correlation coefficients between lead and carbon monoxide concentrations were slightly smaller than those (0.79–0.81) found at Los Angeles area sites during the three-city survey.[554] For visibility of less than 5 miles, the correlation coefficient between 10-min lead and carbon monoxide concentrations is 0.66 ($N = 156$); for visibility of greater than 5 miles, $r = 0.75$ ($N = 335$).

The statistical associations provide no information on the absolute magnitude of the contribution of lead particles to visibility reduction. The failure to find a significant association between visibility and the concentration of lead suggests that the effect of lead particles in visibility reduction is outweighed by other factors in the case of low visibility. The probable dominance of other elements, such as hygroscopic particles, is also suggested by the improved performance of complicated quadratic models in accounting for light scatter.

However, lead particles in the air must make some contribution to total light scatter. The size-fractionated aerosol collections mentioned earlier were made to provide estimates of this contribution. Unfortunately, analysis of these samples is incomplete, so no estimate is yet possible. It does appear that the large, easily settleable particles were already greatly depleted in the lead aerosol sampled at the site, in that the average of 18 lead size distributions analyzed to date yields an MMED of approximately 0.2 μm, in agreement with the results of others[455, 456] for the dispersed urban lead aerosol. The ratios of peak 10-min average lead concentrations to the averages over 1 and 2 hr were 1.20 and 1.28, respectively. Although peak: mean ratios of lead concentration may be larger than this closer to the source, large particles that would contribute strongly to mass concentration near the source would not make significant contributions to light scatter. It therefore appears unlikely that lead particles could contribute as much as 25% of visibility reduction.

Recent field tests in an idle traffic tunnel with late-model cars using leaded and unleaded fuel showed more severe visibility degradation with the latter.[443] This finding is in line with the facts that total volume of particles is more significant in visibility changes than is mass (MMED) and that unleaded fuel produces more particle volume than leaded fuel.[224]

WEATHER MODIFICATION BY AIRBORNE LEAD

The formation of large masses of ice crystals either increases or decreases precipitation and may be related to airborne lead insofar as lead contributes to the possibility of the formation of nuclei. Schaefer[475] observed the production of abundant freezing nuclei when iodine vapor was allowed to react with automotive exhaust; he interpreted the reaction as a lead–halide interaction. In a recent study in the Boulder–Denver area,[435] iodine vapor production of freezing nuclei was more than an order of magnitude above the background level, yielding concentrations of 10–300 nuclei/liter during both surface and airborne sampling. This concentration range is considered adequate for effective weather modification. Furthermore, the interaction with iodine vapor generated plentiful freezing nuclei even at 9,000 ft above sea level, which is frequently the level of summertime cumulus cloud bases in the Denver area. Sampling was conducted as high as 14,000 ft, where high concentrations of latent ice nuclei were found when conditions favored turbulent mixing. During periods of inversion, very low concentrations were observed at the higher levels.

A study by Hogan[256] of iodine-treated automotive exhaust indicated that 60% of the detected lead particles had a radius of 0.2–1.0 μm. The minimal detectable size was 0.2 μm, and therefore at least 60% of these particles will have low terminal fall velocities and long expected residence times in the atmosphere. Supportive evidence that lead contributes to nuclei formation is the fact that concentrations of lead and other particles are known to be effectively reduced by rainfall.[533] It should be noted that there is still little more than circumstantial evidence that lead particles, in the absence of artificial treatment, actually become ice nuclei, but the possibility of widespread effects should be kept in mind.[476]

SUMMARY

The reportedly low lead content in natural fibers is related to the relatively low solubility of most lead compounds found in the soil, the low natural concentration of lead in normal soils, and, in the case of wool, the metabolic balance in the tissues. Man-made textile fibers are produced today with very low lead content, except those to which lead is deliberately added for specific protective qualities. The low concentrations of lead in fibers encourage the conclusion that such concentrations may be within the tolerance limits of humans for lead compounds, even if the concentrations are labile to the point of complete transfer from the textile material to human skin. Given the knowledge that fiber producers subject their products to toxicologic and dermatologic testing for reasons of self-protection, the role of lead when it is deliberately added would not seem to achieve significance in terms of potential hazard to man, except where skin damage exists and lead is in a fat-soluble form. The secondary factor in this respect is the low level of addition that is effective in achieving the desired results.

Lead concentrations in the air are too small and usually not at a high enough temperature to affect glass. Lead-containing particles in automotive exhaust are destructive to metallic surfaces only when they are no longer airborne. It is not possible to assign a destructive role to lead in contamination of microelectronic devices.

Re-examination of the statistical association of concentrations of lead to carbon monoxide concentration, light-scattering coefficient, wind speed and direction, and temperature and relative humidity provided no information on the extent of lead's contribution to light scatter, especially at low visibility, where other ambient factors apparently come into play. There are few capable people working on these complicated problems, and there is much more work to be done before the problems can be treated adequately.

The modification of weather by interaction of lead with iodine vapor needs much more field research before conclusions can be drawn as to its usefulness.

8

General Summary
and Conclusions

EXTENT OF ENVIRONMENTAL POLLUTION
WITH AIRBORNE LEAD

The extensive information assembled in this document leaves little doubt as to whether man has substantially contaminated some parts of his environment with lead. It is also clear that one major source of general environmental contamination is the combustion and dispersion of lead alkyl compounds used as automotive fuel additives. The lead alkyls also are by far the most readily and completely dispersed of all the various substances generated by the lead-using industries, owing to their aerosol form. The air over the largest American cities has a concentration of lead 20 times greater than the air over sparsely populated areas of the country and 2,000 times greater than the air over the mid-Pacific Ocean. Although there is evidence that this concentration profile is due largely to gasoline-additive lead, the high degree of dispersion associated with the venting of burned lead alkyls into the air has minimized the effect of the rapid rise in consumption of leaded gasoline on the atmospheric concentration of lead, with the result that the average lead content of the air over most major cities apparently has not changed greatly over the last 15 years. The net result is that correspondingly little change in the character and magnitude of the effects of atmospheric lead on biologic systems will likely occur for some years to come. We are, in short, not dealing with a rapidly shifting scene in this respect. However, more recent information is not in complete agreement with this conclusion and might slightly modify it.

From the point of view of contamination of the total environment with lead, the lead-using industries have contributed more than has the single source of burned leaded fuel. Two to three times as much lead is added to the total environment in the form of paint pigments and metallic products as in the form of lead alkyls. Some undefined fraction of this nonrecycled lead finds its way into the ecosystem by surface weathering and leaching, dumping, and burning. The environmental fate of this lead is ill-defined, but it is probably chiefly returned to the soil without emission to the air. Any proposal for the removal of lead from automotive fuels to rid the environment of lead pollution must take into consideration the fact that the fate of other lead products, such as paints and manufactured items, is largely unknown. The Panel can do no more than call attention to the lack of information on this point.

The magnitude of transfer of lead from the atmosphere to the soil bears a direct relation to the density of automobile traffic. The surface soil of parks, the street dust in large cities, and narrow bands beside major roadways are heavily contaminated with lead. However, rural soils where crops are grown show little evidence of lead contamination attributable to burned lead alkyls. Similarly, the waters of streams and lakes have about the same concentration of lead today as in 1940, at which time the consumption of lead alkyls was considerably less than it is today.

There is no evidence that the amount of lead in the diets of people has changed substantially since 1940. This is consistent with the observed trends concerning lead in soil and water. Furthermore, the concentration of lead in edible plants is little affected by even large increases of lead in soil above rural concentrations. Surface deposition of lead on plants from the atmosphere occurs but seems to be small, except in the immediate vicinity of major roadways or of other sources of lead emission. The concentration of lead in animal food products also seems to have changed imperceptibly if at all over the last 30 years.

The general picture that emerges from consideration of lead in the environment is of a steep gradient of pollution emanating from the cities, in proportion to their size. The absence of significant upward trends in the concentration of lead in rural soils and water and in the food sources of man in the last 30 years indicates that the great increase in the combustion of lead alkyls has not had a large impact on the intake of lead by nonurban people and animals, except perhaps by direct inhalation. Air has not been monitored long enough or extensively enough to allow any firm conclusions on this point, although data from the urban centers since 1960 are inconclusive as to any general upward trend.

EFFECTS OF LEAD ON MAN

Toxic effects of lead on man and animals are numerous, are of variable severity, and have been studied extensively. The entity of severe clinical lead poisoning is manifested as a constellation of effects on the central nervous system, the gastrointestinal system, the hematopoietic system, and the kidneys. Other organs (such as the thyroid gland and the heart) may be involved to varying degrees. In the most severe form of poisoning, profound disturbances of the central nervous system are prominent, and permanent damage to the brain may occur. Damage to the kidneys also is prominent and may be permanent. The life-span of erythrocytes is shortened, with or without coexistent anemia. This form of lead poisoning is encountered today mainly among infants and heavy drinkers of illicitly distilled whiskey.

In its mildest forms, clinical lead poisoning is usually seen where close medical supervision (e.g., in industry) can facilitate early identification of toxic signs and symptoms. In such circumstances, mild anemia with shortened red-cell life-span is noted, often with headaches and generalized muscle aches. Constipation and diffuse abdominal pain generally follow. These effects can be readily reversed by removing the worker from the source of lead.

The concentration of lead in the blood has long been used as the major index of the biologically available concentration of lead in the body. This measurement has also been used extensively as an aid to the diagnosis of lead poisoning and in monitoring lead exposure in industry. The first clearly defined clinical signs of lead poisoning usually do not occur at blood lead concentrations lower than 80 μg/100 g of whole blood, except in cases where anemia prevails. In such cases, lower concentrations may be associated with signs or symptoms of poisoning, because the analysis of lead per unit volume of blood is performed on an abnormally low number of red blood cells, to which more than 90% of lead in blood is specifically associated.

At blood lead concentrations of 40–80 μg/100 g of whole blood, the excretion of the heme precursor ALA in urine is increased because of inhibition of the conversion of ALA to porphobilinogen (PBG) by the enzyme ALAD. With respect to hematopoiesis, this loss of heme precursor may be compensated completely, for there is no evidence at present of interference with the maintenance of normal hemoglobin concentrations in the blood of adults at this level of exposure. Implications for the synthesis of other heme pigments have not been adequately explored. Nonetheless, this action must be viewed as undesirable, in that it does represent an interference with the availability of an essential metabolite required for normal body function, which in some circumstances might prove deleterious.

At concentrations of blood lead below about 40 μg/100 g of whole blood, inhibition of ALAD in circulating red blood cells can be demonstrated *in vitro* and is in proportion to the concentration of lead found in the cells. This relation seems to apply even at the lowest concentrations of lead detectable *in vivo* in the peripheral blood of man, but its biologic significance is dubious, because it is unaccompanied by any detectable effects on the biologic function of intact man.

The suspicion has long been entertained that lead exposure of long duration at low concentrations might have some subtle effects on the health and behavior of people, apart from the classic syndrome of lead poisoning. Retrospective studies have been made of some health characteristics of populations that were exposed to abnormally high concentrations of lead but did not necessarily show classic lead poisoning. It has not been possible to link the incidence of human diseases other than lead poisoning to lead exposure unequivocally. Admittedly, the list of diseases to which such studies might be addressed is virtually inexhaustible, but the information gathered to date does not encourage the belief that lead at concentrations encountered in the general population increases the susceptibility of people to disease. However, people with iron-deficiency states and hemolytic anemia may be more susceptible than others.

The subtle effects on behavior of low lead exposure of long duration without prior acute exposure may be manifest in two types of disorders: the dulling of mentation and chronic hyperkinesis. No information is available regarding the possibility of cause and effect in what may be an extremely important problem.

SOURCES OF LEAD POISONING IN MAN

Poisoning clearly attributable to airborne lead exposure was at one time a serious and frequently encountered disease among workers in lead smelters and in the lead-using industries. Today, industrial lead poisoning is much less commonly encountered and is seldom seen in its more severe forms, because industrial hygiene programs and better diagnostic procedures have substantially reduced the hazard. However, in small shops with relatively little supervision, there are potentially dangerous conditions whose extent is at present unknown.

In addition to airborne lead in smelters and in lead-using industries, other sources of lead poisoning have been identified. The most serious and crippling current form of lead poisoning is encountered in infants and young children living in deteriorating housing in the cities; usually, the source of poisoning is leaded paint. This type of paint is no longer used for interior surfaces, but the prevalence of poorly maintained pre-1945 housing constitutes a special hazard to those who live in it.

Other miscellaneous sources of lead poisoning of both children and adults include illicitly distilled whiskey, improperly lead-glazed earthenware, old battery casings used as fuel, and an assortment of manufactured items, such as toys containing lead.

Only in the urban setting is man possibly exposed to hazardous circumstances relative to atmospheric lead pollution, occupational exposures in the lead-using industries excepted. The high concentrations of lead in urban air and on the surfaces of parks and streets constitute a source of intake additional to the usual dietary sources and in special circumstances may be a substantial source.

Although the concentration of lead in the air of cities poses no identifiable current threat to the general population, two special categories of people are exposed to lead of atmospheric origin to a degree that seems undesirable. The first category consists of men who are more or less continuously exposed to unusually high concentrations of lead in ambient air in the course of their work (e.g., garage workers, traffic policemen, workers in the lead trades), which may result in blood lead concentrations in excess of 40 $\mu g/100$ g of whole blood. Even within this small population, this level of blood lead concentration is probably attained by only a relatively small proportion of those exposed. To reach the very high blood lead concentration compatible with clinical lead poisoning would probably require in these special groups approximately a fivefold increase beyond current levels in lead assimilation for a long period.

The other special category of persons for whom the lead in ambient air poses a significant threat consists of infants and young children. Recent surveys of children in large cities indicate that many have blood lead concentrations in the range of 40–60 μg/100 g of whole blood. These high blood lead concentrations cannot be ascribed specifically to the inhalation of lead, although that is a possibility. It is also possible that these infants and children eat leaded paint in quantities too small to produce acute poisoning and that at least some of their lead burden comes from the ingestion of lead-bearing street dust and soil, which often attains lead concentrations in excess of 2,000 μg/g. Assuming the validity of the relation between daily lead intake and blood lead content, the daily ingestion by a child weighing 10 kg of 0.41 g of street dust with a lead content of 2,000 μg/g would result ultimately in a blood lead concentration compatible with clinical lead poisoning, even without allowing for additional lead acquired by inhalation, from normal dietary sources, or from coincident ingestion of leaded paint. Likewise, approximately 44 mg of street dust daily would suffice to increase the daily lead assimilation from that associated with a blood lead content of 20 μg/100 g of whole blood to that associated with 40 μg/100 g of whole blood. This is an undesirable level of exposure. These estimates of the amount of street dust or soil that ultimately would increase the concentration of lead in the blood to dangerous levels may be too low, because they assume continued intake for prolonged periods. Unfortunately, the amount of street dust or city soil swallowed or inhaled by young children is totally unknown.

There is no doubt that the general population also assimilates lead from air, food, and beverages and that the magnitude of assimilation is greatest in the cities. The contribution of atmospheric sources of lead to the total body burden of city dwellers varies considerably and depends on the particular urban complex and on the place of residence and of work within that complex. An extensive survey of men in three large urban complexes has suggested but not shown with definitive evidence a strong association between the concentration of lead in the blood and time spent in areas of high automobile traffic density. Although this evidence of the impact of lead inhalation is inferential, limited experimental data are consistent with the conclusion that the amount of inhaled lead is about one half (and in special circumstances twice) the amount that comes from diet, depending on the particular urban microclimates encountered in the course of daily activities. However, it is not possible, on the basis of available epidemiologic evidence, to attribute any increase in blood lead concentration to exposure to ambient air below a mean lead concentration of about 2 or 3 $\mu g/m^3$; only special small groups of people in large cities have been identified as being exposed to higher mean atmospheric concentrations.

Autopsy data strongly suggest that the body burden of lead in the general population increases with age. Most of the increase is attributed to an increase in the amount of lead in bone, but it seems likely that some other tissues also are involved. The concentration of lead in the blood does not increase with age. This suggests that the readily exchangeable pool of lead in the body generally reaches a steady state early in life and that the increases in body burden with age probably involve a relatively inert, slowly exchangeable pool of lead whose toxicologic significance has not been evaluated.

SIGNIFICANCE TO OTHER FORMS OF LIFE

Most livestock and wildlife are far removed from the high ambient air concentrations of lead that have been shown to warrant some concern with respect to the health of man. It is conceivable that the grasses along heavily traveled roadways (more than 50,000 vehicles/day) would in some cases acquire enough surface deposition of lead to constitute a hazard to grazing animals. However, for a hazard to exist, animals would have to confine their grazing to a band of 125 ft or less on either side of the heavily traveled roadways, which is extremely unlikely. The actual atmospheric hazard is to livestock grazing in the vicinity of lead smelters when stack emissions are not well controlled. There is no evidence that clinical lead poisoning of household pets can be attributed to atmospheric sources of lead. The etiology of lead poisoning in pets is similar to the etiology in infants, in that it is most common in very young animals, which share with human infants the tendency to eat or chew on foreign objects, including many that contain lead. It is not known, however, whether household pets eat lead-contaminated street dust and soil any more than it is known whether infants do.

Lead does not appear to be a hazard to aquatic animals, such as fish. This is no doubt related to the fact that only very low concentrations exist in solution, most of the lead in natural waters being insoluble and apparently nonavailable.

Lead poisoning is an important health problem in waterfowl. The only source of lead reported to cause poisoning is spent lead shot from hunting.

As in the case of animals, there is no evidence that atmospheric sources of lead are injurious to plants. Although some plants may be susceptible to lead in the natural environment, lead in soil and water is generally in a form that is largely nonavailable to them.

9

Recommendations for Research

EXTENT OF ENVIRONMENTAL POLLUTION WITH AIRBORNE LEAD

Recommendation 1
Improved Aerometric Data Gathering and Sampling near Populations at Risk

Currently, after 26 years of being concerned with air pollution, our meteorologic broadcasts are limited to announcements of the local air pollution index in a relatively few cities of this country. Much effort should be expended in the field of meteorology, coupled with the use of tracer techniques, to use this important branch of science for a more complete understanding of the factors that bear on dissipation of air pollutants. Specifically, most meteorologic data are now collected at airports near the fringes of urban centers and do not necessarily describe the conditions in the city, where the industrial, municipal, traffic, and other emission sources are, or in the surrounding rural environs. Also, some polluting elements (such as lead) are

213

difficult to measure in a built-up area. A network of aerometric stations should be established in each urban area to obtain meteorologic and pollutant data that are representative of the area and can be used to provide overall values for the city as a whole. Furthermore, this network should be extended to cover the natural air movements from one district or region to others, to form a national meteorologic program that is air-pollution-oriented. The continued and orderly development of the Storage and Retrieval of Aerometric Data (SAROAD) system by the Environmental Protection Agency is a step in this direction, whose usefulness will be determined by the quality of the data that enter the system. For individual air sampling sites, the Panel believes it important to point out that the site should be related to the community at risk. If air samples are for analysis of pollutants potentially hazardous to man, for example, they should be taken where the population is greatest—near the street, rather than on the roof of a tall building. If young children constitute the population at risk, then the sampling intake should be closer to the surface than if adults are the only concern. This principle also applies to testing of natural waters subject to industrial contamination. In this case, it would be desirable to collect representative samples from sites removed from water treatment facilities to obtain complete data on the concentrations of lead (and other trace elements) resulting from discharge by lead-using or lead-producing industries along the waterways. The importance of these measurements is apparent when it is realized that the lead may be concentrated by different species of fish or other aquatic organisms.

Recommendation 2
Expanded Study of Lead Chemistry in Nature

The Panel encourages the study of the chemistry of lead in the environment—in emitted particulate matter, in soil, and in water. A prerequisite to research on the chemistry of lead in the environment is the training of atmospheric chemists competent to undertake it or the reorienting of trained chemists in this direction. The physics of particles and aerosols in general is comparatively well known, but the chemical forms of lead need elucidation before its movement in the environment can be fully understood. Similarly, knowledge of the complex chemistry of biotransformation of lead by lower organisms is of considerable importance.

Recommendation 3
Monitoring Food and Drink for Lead Content

It is recommended that an extensive monitoring program of lead in common items of food, drinking water, and miscellaneous beverages be instituted now, to provide reliable bench marks for the future. The protocol for securing this information should be standardized and should be detailed as to description of sampling technique, analytic procedure, specification of water content, and geographic and other environmental characteristics of the sampling site. The lack of firm evidence that concentrations of lead in food and drinking water are increasing is not very reassuring. Past studies of lead in foods have been so poorly described and so deficient in sample size as to make the data of very questionable value as bench marks for measuring changes over the years. In assessing the dietary sources of lead, the possible contamination during preparation and storage of food and drink must be taken into account. Periodic publication of updated figures in a useful form would enhance the value of such studies to nutritionists and public health officials.

EFFECTS OF LEAD ON MAN

Recommendation 4
Additional Information on Dose-Response Relations of Lead

A fuller understanding of the biologic significance of the *in vitro* inhibition of ALAD in blood is needed. Because it is likely that heme synthesis will be inhibited in other tissues, as well as in blood, it seems likely that the assay in blood may be a model of the effects of increasing lead content in other organs. Dose-response relations with respect to heme synthesis need studying in other tissues and particularly in the central nervous system. Relations between ALAD, ALA, and the "mobile" or "chelatable" fraction of the total body lead burden require further careful clinical study, especially in the range of 5–80 μg/100 g of whole blood, to determine more accurately the apparent "threshold" for this effect. All age groups, as well as subgroups of the population that may be less able to compensate for impairment in heme synthesis, should be studied. Such studies not only should have sound epidemiologic design, but should use timed, quantitative urine collections, standardized mobilization techniques, and more specific methods for measuring A L A than have been used in the past. Dose-response relations that can be worked out in intact experimental animals should be evaluated in correlative studies in man, in whom careful control of dosage is not altogether possible. A clear understanding of the dose-response relations with respect to lead in this area of metabolism can serve as a basis of reference in the study of other, less well understood adverse metabolic and functional effects that have been attributed to lead.

More precise studies are needed of the relation between atmospheric lead exposure in the urban environment and the concentration of lead in the blood, perhaps by the use of personal monitors. Only by balance studies of individual subjects can the proportion of body burden due to atmospheric intake be precisely determined.

Because dosages can be only approximated in human populations, carefully controlled studies in intact animals are needed to buttress apparent dose-response relations that are now estimated for man. Particular attention should be given to central and peripheral nervous function and to renal function at dosages that produce subclinical effects. Assays of endocrinologic functions may also offer a readily available avenue of approach, as may studies of rates of catabolism of various drugs, both in intact animals and in isolated systems. Investigations of interactions between lead and other metals may also be productive, and a thorough understanding of the binding and transport of lead in the tissues is urgently needed.

There is need to carry out animal studies to determine the threshold at which metabolic abnormalities begin to occur in such fundamental processes as oxidative phosphorylation and electron transport, as well as the threshold for effects on dithiol enzymes. Studies should be done in a large population of animals (e.g., rats) raised on a hydroponically grown diet extremely low in lead, measuring the length of exposure, the concentrations of lead in blood and other tissues, and effects on heme synthesis. Comparison of these results should be made with animals on a "normal" diet and a diet with a moderate lead content—e.g., 100 $\mu g/g$ dry weight.

With suitable guidelines from studies in animals, prospective correlative investigations in man may be undertaken. Some of the questions obviously in need of answers are: (1) At what low but chronic degree of overexposure are behavior and performance compromised? (2) Does aging, particularly as it may affect renal and vascular function, modify man's response to minimal increases in soft tissue lead content? (3) Are fetuses, infants, and young children more sensitive to lead than adults? Answers to these questions are needed most to permit proper medical supervision of children and industrial workers, in whom subclinical adverse effects are most likely to be found.

More lead balance studies of the type pioneered by Kehoe are needed, but they should be designed to include atmospheric lead intake along with intake from food and beverages. Fortunately, this type of study is under way and is expected to yield significant information. Comparable studies pertinent to the metabolism of lead in human fetuses, infants, and children should also be done. Owing to ethical considerations, much of this type of experimentation will have to be carried out in appropriate experimental models. Nonhuman primates may be particularly valuable in the study of effects related to nervous system function.

Recommendation 5
Further Search for Possible Subtle Effects of
Prolonged Low-Level Exposure to Lead

There is need for further study of the possible relations between disease and lead exposure. The particular population studied should be relatively stable, and whole family groups should be studied. The study should include several health indices and other aspects of health besides those related to environmental pollution.

The importance of determining whether insidious poisoning due to low-level exposure to lead occurs is apparent. Current information does not afford an adequate basis for the evaluation of this critical area of concern. The only studies available on the effects of long-term inhalation of lead on animal behavior are those of the Russian investigators. It is important for research in this area to confirm or deny the development of behavioral toxicity at comparably low, chronic exposures to lead. Although frank encephalopathy produced by early exposure to lead seems to result in mental retardation, the evidence on the late effects of less severe early poisoning is still unclear.

Recommendation 6
Study of the Ingestion Patterns of Children

The Panel recommends that research be intensified on the broad subject of pica. This behavioral activity has implications for social problems far beyond those associated with lead poisoning in children.

SOURCES OF LEAD POISONING IN MAN

Recommendation 7
*Establishment of Comprehensive Medical and Environmental
Control Programs to Eliminate Clinical Lead Poisoning in
Special Groups*

Occupationally exposed workers and young children are in urgent
need of sustained medical supervision and effective environmental
control programs. Prospective epidemiologic programs are needed to
evaluate the extent of the risk to these groups and to assess the effectiveness of measures designed to minimize such risks. In such programs, consideration should be given to total exposure derived from
all environmental sources. There is urgent need for evaluation of the
importance of city street dust and soil as a source of lead for young
children. It is hoped that implementation of the Occupational Safety
and Health Act of 1970 and the Lead-Based Paint Poisoning Prevention Act of 1970 will provide much of the needed epidemiologic data
and facilitate the realization of these goals.

Analysis of confiscated samples of illicitly distilled whiskey indicates that this may also be a significant cause of lead poisoning.
Sampling of populations known to be at risk is needed to evaluate
the extent of this problem. Potential sources of hazard, such as improperly lead-glazed earthenware, should be controlled by systematic
sampling before distribution to the general public.

There is no substitute for astute clinical observation and case-
finding. These techniques provide clues concerning incompletely understood aspects of lead poisoning, which should be studied experimentally. The obvious adverse effects of excessive lead on the
nervous system, kidneys, and hematopoiesis are well recognized at
the clinical level, but they are not adequately understood at the subclinical level. Furthermore, dose-response relations need to be established with regard to these effects. Case studies suggest that neuropathy and myopathy may be significant but inadequately recognized
aspects of lead poisoning both clinically and subclinically. These pos-
sibilities are in need of careful study. Even less well understood are
the apparent effects of lead on various endocrine organs. Experimental and clinical investigative efforts are appropriate to elucidate
the clinical significance and mechanism of these effects.

Wider availability of adequate laboratory diagnostic services is essential if progress is to be made toward these recommended clinical and epidemiologic goals. Analytic problems inherent in the determination of lead in biologic samples suggest that reliable data may be obtainable only in larger laboratories with adequate quality-control procedures and experience in lead determinations. In addition to estimates of the level of exposure and of the mobile fraction of the total body lead burden, adequate medical supervision also requires measurement of some metabolic response, such as ALAD or ALA.

Recommendation 8

Research on Body Burden and Distribution of Lead as Related to Age and Its Biologic Significance

More age-related studies are needed to evaluate further the concept that the "mobile" fraction of the total body lead burden remains constant throughout life; this hypothesis is presently based on very limited data. Age-related studies should also include some measure of biologic response to increasing concentrations of lead in soft tissues (e.g., ALAD in blood and excretion of ALA in urine). The concept that the nondiffusible fraction is tightly bound in bone and therefore biologically inert requires more detailed examination. In mammalian systems, the relations between parathyroid hormone, thyrocalcitonin, bone, and kidney are intimate and important in the metabolism of bone mineral. Research concerning the effects of these relations on lead metabolism and clearance from the body should therefore be carried out. Data obtained from such studies will provide a better understanding of the significance of the "nondiffusible" fraction of body lead to health.

Recommendation 9

Standardization of Diagnostic Tests and Study of Therapy

In relation to estimates of the mobile fraction of the body burden of lead, there is a need to develop a standardized CaEDTA mobilization test for use in asymptomatic adults and children. The dose of CaEDTA is related to the size of the person (preferably estimated by height or surface area), and CaEDTA is given parenterally over a defined period. Urine should also be collected over a carefully defined interval. Modification of the test for use in renal disease needs exposition. Also, data should be accumulated on the efficacy and safety of repetitive chelation therapy with CaEDTA and D-penicillamine.

SIGNIFICANCE TO OTHER FORMS OF LIFE

Recommendation 10
Additional Study of Susceptibility of Animals and Plants to Lead

Long-term studies are needed to define more precisely the level of
lead intake that can be tolerated by the major species of domestic
animals likely to be exposed to environmental lead hazards. The
newer methods for the assessment of the body burden of lead and its
biologic effects in man should also be investigated and applied to
these animals.

The assimilation of and susceptibility to lead of a wide range of in-
digenous plant species should be studied, especially those that are
consumed by man and domestic animals. These studies are important
to determine the possibility that some plants have an unusual capacity
to assimilate lead from the biosphere or a high susceptibility to lead.

Plant studies should also be made on a wide range of exposures to
lead, but especially at the lower concentrations that the plant might
be expected to encounter, rather than at very high experimental concentrations. The importance of such studies lies in acquiring information on and detecting a possible threshold for mutagenesis in plants.

APPENDIXES

Appendix A

Particle Size

Many disciplines are involved in the study of particles. Each appears to have devised its own system of nomenclature to classify particles with respect to size, physical state, origin, etc.[558]

In terms of particle size, the main reason for this confusion is that an irregularly shaped particle has no unique dimension. Its size can be expressed only in terms of the diameter of a sphere that is equivalent to the particle with regard to some stated property.[250] Such "equivalent" spheres are those with the same volume as the particle, the same surface area as the particle, the same free-falling velocity in a fluid as the particle, and the same projected area as the particle when viewed in a direction perpendicular to the plane of greatest stability.

It is evident that different methods of particle-size determination measure different equivalent diameters. For example, microscopes measure equivalent diameter based on projected area, whereas sedimentation techniques measure equivalent diameter based on free-falling velocity. It is also evident that the numerical values for the various equivalent diameters can be the same only for spherical particles and that the divergence of the values will increase with particle irregularity.

In dealing with atmospheric particles, size is usually presented as the diameter of a sphere of unit density that has the same terminal fall velocity in still air as the particle in question. For spherical particles larger than approximately 1 μm, the terminal fall velocity in still air can be calculated by Stokes's law:

$$v = \frac{gd^2 (\rho_1 - \rho_2)}{18n},$$

in which

    v = terminal velocity, cm/sec
    g = acceleration of gravity, cm/sec^2
    d = particle diameter, cm
    ρ_1 = density of particle, g/cm^3
    ρ_2 = density of air, g/cm^3
    n = viscosity of air, poises

The expression has an upper limit of applicability, because, when some terminal fall velocity is reached, the particle generates a significant "wake." A lower limit of applicability is reached when the particles become small enough that air resistance is no longer continuous but is the result of individual collisions with air molecules.

For most purposes, the terminal velocity of particles smaller than about 1 μm can be determined with the Stokes-Cunningham equation:

$$v = \frac{gd^2 (\rho_1 - \rho_2)}{18n} \left(1 + \frac{2A\lambda}{d}\right),$$

in which A is a constant close to unity (0.9 is often used) and λ is the mean free path of the fluid.

When comparing the geometric and equivalent diameters of a particle with a density greater than 1 g/cm^3, it is evident from Stokes's law that the geometric diameter will be smaller. Consider, for example, a spherical particle of lead sesquioxide with a geometric diameter of 0.9 μm and an assumed density of 10 g/cm^3. The equivalent diameter, d, in micrometers, as calculated from Stokes's law, is

$$d^2 (1 - \rho_2) = (0.9)^2 (10 - \rho_2).$$

Assuming that the density of air is negligible, compared with the lead particle,

$$d^2 = (0.9)^2 \times 10 = 8.1$$
$$d = 2.84 \ \mu m.$$

Similarly, the equivalent diameter of a lead sesquioxide spherical particle of 0.05 μm with an assumed density of 10 g/cm^3 can be calculated by using the Stokes-Cunningham equation:

$$d^2 \ (1 + \frac{2A\lambda}{d}) = \left(\frac{0.05}{10^4}\right)^2 \ 10 \ (1 + \frac{2A\lambda}{0.05} \times 10^4).$$

Taking a value of 0.9 for constant A and 10^{-5} cm for the mean free path of air, the equivalent diameter is

$$d = 2.61 \times 10^{-5} \ cm$$
$$d = 0.26 \ \mu m.$$

In the case of polydispersed aerosols, the size distribution of the particles can be presented in a number of ways. Because atmospheric particles usually follow a log-normal distribution, the accepted method is to plot a cumulative distribution on special graph paper with log-probability scales. Thus, the equivalent diameter is plotted on a log scale on the Y axis, and the total fraction of particles that are larger than that diameter is plotted on a probability scale on the X axis. The equivalent diameter is determined by size-measuring instruments, such as impactors calibrated in terms of spherical particles of unit density. The particulate fractions are conveniently calculated as the cumulative weight percent oversize. For a truly log-normal distribution, this type of size-distribution plot will provide a straight line. The equivalent diameter corresponding to the 50% oversize value is known as the "mass median equivalent diameter" (MMED) of the aerosol.

A number of workers have determined the MMED's for lead in the atmosphere and report values in the range of 0.15–0.3 μm.[340,454]

Appendix B

Sampling and Analytic Methods for Lead

The methods presented in this appendix are reliable, sensitive, and essentially free from interference.

LEAD IN THE ATMOSPHERE

Dithizone Method

The Tentative Method of Test for Lead in the Atmosphere, ASTM Designation D 2681–68T,* is recommended for the sampling and analysis of particulate and nonparticulate (organic) lead.

1. Scope

1.1 This method covers the determination of lead in the atmosphere. It involves separate measurements of particulate lead and nonparticulate lead. For the purpose of this method, nonparticulate lead is that which will pass a 0.45-μm membrane filter and includes

*Reproduced with permission of the American Society for Testing and Materials, 1916 Race Street, Philadelphia, Pennsylvania 19103. This method is currently being evaluated for accuracy and precision by the ASTM, "Project Threshold," which is conducted with cooperating laboratories under actual field conditions.

the organic lead. This procedure is designed to measure ambient lead concentrations above 0.2 μg of lead/m^3. The method employs a special short-term sampling procedure using an iodine absorber for the nonparticulate lead, and a membrane filter to collect particulate lead. It is satisfactory for measuring lead with an accuracy of ±0.2 μg of lead/m^3.

2. Summary of Method

2.1 *Sample*—The sample of air is drawn through a sampling train consisting of the 0.45-μm pore membrane filter and then through a special sampling tube containing crystalline iodine (1,2,3,5).[2] A sample of 2 m^3 is collected.

2.2 *Particulate Lead*—The membrane filter is digested with nitric, sulfuric, and perchloric acids to remove all organic matter and to dissolve the lead. The lead is determined by the colorimetric dithizone procedure (4).

2.3 *Nonparticulate Lead*—The iodine crystals are dissolved in acidified potassium iodide solution and the excess iodine is reduced with sodium sulfite. The lead is determined by the colorimetric dithizone procedure.

2.4 *Dithizone Method*—The dilute acid solution containing the lead is treated with citric acid and is made alkaline with an ammoniacal buffer solution. The lead is extracted with successive portions of a chloroform solution of dithizone. The lead is then transferred into the aqueous phase by extraction with an acidic buffer. This acidic buffer is treated with an ammoniacal buffer solution and the lead is re-extracted into chloroform as lead dithizonate. The lead dithizonate is measured spectrophotometrically at 510 mμ (4).

[1] Under the standardization procedure of the Society, this method is under the jurisdiction of the ASTM Committee D-22 on Methods of Atmospheric Sampling and Analysis. A list of members may be found in the ASTM Year Book. Accepted Feb. 14, 1968.
[2] The boldface numbers in parentheses refer to the list of references appended to this method.

3. Significance

3.1 This method is sensitive and relatively free from interferences. While it is intended primarily for measuring ambient atmospheric lead concentrations above 0.2 μg of lead/m^3 for atmospheric survey, careful attention to details and effective control of contamination will allow lower concentrations to be determined.

3.2 The procedure is based on the removal of particulate lead by a membrane filter and the reaction of nonparticulate lead with crystalline iodine.

4. Definitions

4.1 *particulate lead*—the lead collected on a membrane filter with a nominal pore size of 0.45 μm.

4.2 *nonparticulate lead*—that lead which passes an 0.45-μm membrane filter and is collected on crystallized iodine in accordance with the described sampling procedure.

4.3 For definitions of other terms used in this method, refer to ASTM Definitions D 1356, Terms Relating to Atmospheric Sampling and Analysis.[3]

5. Interferences

5.1 Dithizone gives colored complexes with bismuth, cadmium, cobalt, copper, gold, lead, mercury, nickel, palladium, platinum, silver, stannous, thallous, and zinc ions. Stannous and thallous ions are oxidized in the wet-ashing technique to prevent interference. Aluminum and iron are complexed with citric acid. Cadmium and zinc are complexed with cyanide in ammoniacal solutions. Bismuth is removed in the double extraction procedure which leaves the lead in solution free from interference from other metals.

6. Precautions

. 6.1 Dithizone is insoluble in water, but is soluble in ammonium hydroxide, and many organic solvents. Mild oxidizing

[3] Appears in this publication.

agents convert it to diphenylcarbadiazone which is yellow and does not react with metals. The presence of hydroxylamine hydrochloride in the solution prevents the oxidation. If the reagent contains some yellow oxidation product, it must be removed by recrystallization.

6.2 The determination of lead in small quantities by this method requires meticulous attention to technique. Good precision is not usually obtained without some experience with a dithizone procedure. Precision may be improved by knowledge of, and close adherence to, the suggestions that follow.

6.2.1 All glassware used in the method must be borosilicate glass. It is also imperative that contamination be prevented by rinsing with nitric acid (1+1) and completing the cleaning with several distilled water rinses.

6.2.2 For the dithizone extraction, always use separatory funnels that have not been used in the other parts of the procedure. After use for the dithizone extraction, the separatory funnel is lead-free if rinsed only once with distilled water. Washing with a mixture of dithizone solution and buffer solution is one of the most effective ways of deleading and of testing for the absence of lead.

6.2.3 Use the same reagents and solutions in the same quantities for a group of determinations and the corresponding blank. When a new reagent is prepared or a new stock of membrane filters is taken or new stock of chemicals is required, a new blank *must* be prepared.

7. Apparatus

7.1 *Absorption Cells*, matched, chemically strengthened aluminosilicate glass, covered or stoppered, 50 mm long.

7.2 *Iodine Crystal Scrubber*—See Fig. 1.

7.3 *Carbon Trap*—Pack a glass tube 18 in. long by 2.5 in. in diameter with activated carbon 10 to 30 mesh with 3 in. of glass wool between the activated carbon and the one-hole rubber stopper located at each end of the tube.

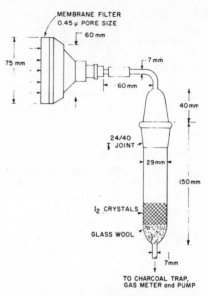

Fɪɢ. 1—Sampling Train.

7.4 *Borosilicate Glassware* shall be used in this method.

7.5 *Erlenmeyer Flask*, wide-mouth, 500-ml capacity.

7.6 *Filter Holder*,[4] for a membrane filter with a diameter of 2 in. or 47 mm (see Fig. 1).

7.7 *Gas Meter*—An integrating gas meter capable of measuring from 10 liters of air/min.

7.8 *Membrane Filter*,[5] of 0.45 μm pore size. Blanks must be performed for each lot of filters (see Fig. 1).

7.9 *Separatory Funnels*, Squibb-type, 125-ml and 250-ml capacity.

7.10 *Spectrophotometer*.[6]

7.11 *Vacuum Pump*, capable of drawing 10 liters of air/min.

---

[4] Gelman No. 1200A Open Filter Holder 2 in., or No. 4273 Dispoz-It 2 in. with filter; Millipore Aerosol Open-type Filter Holder (47 mm) XX50 047 10 or MAWP 0 37 AO Aerosol Gravimetric Analysis Monitor with Filter, have been found satisfactory.

[5] Millipore membrane filter Type HA, 0.45-μm pore size; Gelman AM-6, 0.45-μm pore size; or Schleicher and Schuell, Type B, 0.45-μm pore size may be acceptable.

[6] Beckman Model DU or equivalent, equipped with 50-mm cells, has been found satisfactory.

8. Reagents and Materials

8.1 *Purity of Reagents*—Reagent grade chemicals shall be used in all tests. Unless otherwise indicated, it is intended that all reagents shall conform to the specifications of the Committee on Analytical Reagents of the American Chemical Society, where such specifications are available.[7] Other grades may be used, provided it is first ascertained that the reagent is of sufficiently high purity to permit its use without decreasing the accuracy of the determination.

8.2 *Purity of Water*—Unless otherwise indicated, references to water shall be understood to mean distilled water or referee reagent water conforming to ASTM Specification D 1193, for Reagent Water.[3]

8.3 *Ammonium Hydroxide (sp gr 0.90)*—Concentrated ammonium hydroxide (NH₄OH).

NOTE 1—Low-lead ammonium hydroxide and hydrochloric acid manufactured for the electronics industry are available and are satisfactory.

8.4 *Buffer Solution*—Dissolve 400 g of citric acid in water, add 6 drops of phenol red indicator solution, then add NH₄OH until the solution turns pink, then add 50 g of potassium cyanide. To another beaker add 13.5 g of hydroxylamine hydrochloride and sufficient water to dissolve the salt. Add 6 drops of phenol red indicator solution, and add NH₄OH until the solution turns pink. Mix the two solutions and dilute to 1570 ml with water.

8.5 *Clark and Lubs Buffer Solution pH 3.4*—Dissolve 17.0 g of potassium acid phthalate in water. Add 1.4 ml of HCl and dilute to 1000 ml with water.

8.6 *Chloroform*—Place 1000 ml of chloroform in a 2000-ml separatory funnel. Dissolve approximately 10.0 g of hydroxylamine hydrochloride in 50.0 ml of water and make the solution ammoniacal to phenol red indicator solution with NH₄OH. Add this solution to the chloroform in the separatory funnel. Shake well. Allow the aqueous layer to separate and filter the chloroform through a fluted filter. To stabilize, add 10 ml of absolute alcohol to the filtered chloroform.

8.7 *Dithizone*—An especially pure grade is required.[8]

8.8 *Dithizone Solution*—Dissolve 40 mg of dithizone in 1000 ml of chloroform. This solution is stable for only 4 weeks and should be kept in a refrigerator. Allow the solution to warm to room temperature before use.

8.9 *Hydrochloric Acid (sp gr 1.19)*—Concentrated hydrochloric acid (HCl) (Note 1).

8.10 *Iodine Crystals*—Sieve crystals through a 16-mesh stainless steel sieve, and use only the portion that passes the sieve. Store crystals in the dark in lead-free brown glass bottle (Note 2). Purify the sieved crystals by washing with dilute nitric acid (Note 3).

NOTE 2—Iodine crystals tend to segregate in a storage bottle. When weighing 20.0 g for an analysis, invert the bottle and mix the fine particles with some of the larger ones to obtain a representative portion of the sieved particles. About 30 percent of particles finer than 30 mesh are necessary for complete lead recovery at high sampling rates.

NOTE 3 —Delead the surface of the iodine crystals by adding 30 to 50 ml of HNO₃ (1+1) to the iodine scrubber. Rinse with 25 to 30 ml of water. Add 25 ml of methanol solution and with a rubber bulb force all extraneous alcoholic solution from the scrubber. Care must be exercised to prevent the solution of the fine particles in the alcoholic water wash solution.

8.11 *Indicator Solutions*—Phenol red and methyl orange. Dissolve 0.1 g of the indicator in water and dilute to 100 ml.

---

[7] "Reagent Chemicals, American Chemical Society Specifications," Am. Chemical Soc., Washington, D. C. For suggestions on the testing of reagents not listed by the American Chemical Society, see "Reagent Chemicals and Standards," by Joseph Rosin, D. Van Nostrand Co., Inc., New York, N. Y., and the "United States Pharmacopeia."

[8] Eastman Kodak white label requires no purification and has been found satisfactory.

8.12 *Methanol Solution*—Add 600 ml of methanol to 300 ml of water.

8.13 *Nitric Acid (1+1)*—Prepare by adding 1 part of nitric acid (HNO_3, sp gr 1.42) to 1 part of water.

8.14 *Nitric Acid (1+4)*—Prepare by adding 1 part of HNO_3 (sp gr 1.42) to 4 parts of water.

8.15 *Potassium Cyanide Solution*—Dissolve 15 g of potassium cyanide (KCN) in 1000 ml of NH_4OH (sp gr 0.90). **Caution,** see Note 4.

NOTE 4: **Caution**—Handle potassium cyanide with rubber gloves in a vented hood and wash hands and gloves frequently. Drain excess and waste solutions in a hooded sink that is not used for the disposal of acids, and flush with water.

8.16 *Perchloric Acid (72 percent)*.

8.17 *Potassium Iodide, Acidified*—Prepare just before each analysis by mixing 5 parts of potassium iodide solution with 1 part of HNO_3 (1+4).

8.18 *Potassium Iodide Solution*—Dissolve 500 g of potassium iodide (KI) in water and dilute to 1000 ml with water.

8.19 *Sodium Sulfite Solution*—Dissolve 200 g of sodium sulfite in 1000 ml of water.

8.20 *Standard Solution I*—Dissolve 0.1600 g of lead nitrate in 200 ml of water in a 1000-ml volumetric flask. Add 8 ml of HNO_3 (sp gr 1.42) and dilute to 1000 ml with water (lead concentration = 0.10 mg/ml).

8.21 *Standard Solution II*—Add 10 ml of Standard Solution I to a 1000-ml volumetric flask and dilute to 1000 ml with Clark and Lubs pH 3.4 buffer (8.5) (lead concentration = 1 μg/ml).

8.22 *Sulfuric Acid (sp gr 1.84)*—Concentrated sulfuric acid (H_2SO_4).

9. Sampling

9.1 Draw air at the rate of at least 10.0 liters/min through the sampling train (Fig. 1). The components of the sampling train are: (*1*) 0.45-μm membrane filter to collect the particulate matter and particulate lead, (*2*) a tube containing 20 g of crystalline iodine to collect the nonparticulate lead. (Note 3), (*3*) an activated carbon trap to protect the pump from volatilized iodine, (*4*) a gas meter to measure the air, and (*5*) a pump to draw the air sample.

9.2 Collect approximately 2 cm^3 of air (*V*) per sample. Do not take an air sample so large that it would reduce the iodine below 10 g, the minimum amount that should remain after each test (see Note 6).

9.3 Tap the sides of the iodine scrubber every 5 to 10 min with a pencil or rod to ensure an even bed (cross section) of iodine crystals.

9.4 Treat the membrane filter for particulate lead as described in 11.1. Treat the iodine scrubber for nonparticulate lead as described 11.2.

9.5 *Blank*—Prepare a reagent blank of all reagents. Use the same portions of each reagent used in the analysis. Treat the reagent blank similarly as the sample in all steps; (*1*) for the membrane filter as described in 11.1 and 11.3; and (*2*) for the iodine scrubber as described in 11.2 and 11.3. Read the micrograms of lead from the calibration curve and subtract the appropriate blank from the amount of lead found in the sample.

9.5.1 A blank is not required for each determination once an average blank has been established. A new blank must be prepared when the supply of any reagent including distilled water or of membrane filters is changed.

10. Calibration Curve

10.1 *Lead from Particulate Filter*—Pipet 0.0, 2.0, 5.0, 10.0, 15.0, and 20.0 ml of Standard Solution II respectively into each of six Squibb-type 125-ml separatory funnels and dilute each solution to 50 ml with Clark and Lubs buffer. Add 2 drops of methyl orange indicator solution and treat the solutions as described in 11.1.2. Subtract the absorbance of the 0.0-ml sample from the absorbances of the other solutions.

10.1.1 Construct a calibration curve by plotting the absorbances of the solutions against micrograms of lead.

10.2 *Lead from Absorption on Iodine Crystals*—The amount of iodine in the scrubber at the end of the sampling procedure may influence the zero reading of the curve. Separate calibration curves must, therefore, be prepared for 10 and 20 g of iodine remaining in the scrubber.

NOTE 5—The influence of iodine on the results is in dispute. The calibration of lead with varying amounts of iodine present is offered so that a check can be made. If the amount of residual iodine has no effect on the results, the curve prepared in 10.1 will suffice. If the iodine has an effect on the results, the calibration curves prepared as described in 10.2.1 will be required.

10.2.1 Pipet 0.0, 2.0, 5.0, 10.0, 15.0, and 20.0 ml of Standard Solution II respectively into each of six beakers containing 10 g of iodine crystals. Prepare a similar series of samples using 20 g of iodine in each beaker. Treat the samples as described in 11.2.1, 11.2.2, and 11.2.3. Subtract the absorbance of the 0.0-ml sample from the absorbances of the other solutions.

10.2.2 Construct a calibration curve by plotting the absorbances of the solutions against micrograms of lead.

11. Procedure

11.1 *Particulate Lead:*

11.1.1 Remove the membrane filter from the holder. Place it in a 100-ml beaker and add 5 ml of water, 5 ml of HNO_3 (sp gr 1.42), 3 ml of H_2SO_4 (sp gr 1.84), and 0.5 ml of perchloric acid (72 percent). Digest on the hot plate until the solution is white or pale yellow. Finally, remove the last of the carbonaceous material by heating the sample until dense white fumes appear. Allow the solution to cool. Add 10 ml of HNO_3 (1+4) and boil the solution to dissolve any lead sulfate. Dilute the mixture to 25 ml and filter into a 250-ml Squibb-type separatory funnel. Use another 25 ml of water to wash and transfer the sample.

11.1.2 Add phenol red indicator solution. Add NH_4OH (sp gr 0.90) until

the solution turns yellow. Add 25 ml of buffer solution and 10.0 ml of the dithizone solution, shake for 1 min, allow to separate, and run the dithizone-chloroform layer into a 125-ml Squibb-type separatory funnel. Repeat the treatment with 5-ml portions of dithizone solution until the last addition retains its original green color. Discard the aqueous layer.

11.1.3 Treat the combined chloroform-dithizone layers as described in 11.3.

11.2 *Nonparticulate Lead:*

11.2.1 Set the iodine scrubber in a beaker of suitable size and dissolve the iodine crystals in the scrubber by adding acidified KI in small quantities until all of the crystals are dissolved. Rinse the scrubber with water and collect all washings in the beaker.

11.2.2 Add sodium sulfite solution until the iodine color disappears (2.6 ml of sulfite solution is equivalent to 1.0 g of iodine). Use 3-ml portions, adding each portion with stirring until all the iodine color is gone (Note 6). Transfer the mixture to a 250-ml Squibb-type separatory funnel. Add phenol red indicator solution. Add NH_4OH (sp gr 0.90) until the solution is ammoniacal. Add 25 ml of buffer solution and 10.0 ml of the dithizone solution, shake for 1 min, allow to separate, and run the dithizone-chloroform layer into a second 125-ml Squibb-type separatory funnel. Repeat the treatment with 5.0-ml portions of dithizone solution until the last addition retains its original green color. Discard the aqueous layer.

NOTE 6—The volume of reducing solution required is a measure of the amount of iodine that has remained in the tube following the period of sampling. At least 10 g of iodine should remain in the tube after sampling. If less than 10 g remain, discard the test. Practice has shown that the air scrubbing for nonparticulate lead becomes inefficient and erratic if the iodine level drops below 10 g.

11.2.3 Treat the combined chloroform-dithizone extracts as described in 11.3.

11.3 Lead Determination-Dithizone Extract:

11.3.1 Add to the chloroform-dithizone extracts (obtained in 11.1.3 and 11.2.3) 50.0 ml of the Clark and Lubs pH 3.4 buffer, 2 drops of methyl orange indicator solution, and shake. Adjust the pH of this solution to 3.4 by matching the color against 50 ml of pH 3.4 buffer solution to which 2 drops of methyl orange indicator solution have been added. Use HCl or NH4OH to make the match. Shake for 1 min. Compare colors. Match again if necessary. Shake for 1 min and let stand to allow the layers to separate. Discard the chloroform layer. Add 5 ml of chloroform to the solution in the funnel. Shake, let stand to separate layers, and discard the chloroform layer. If the lead concentration is 10 μg or less per sample, treat the aqueous layer as described 11.3.3. For concentrations above 10 μg per sample, treat the aqueous solution as described in 11.3.2 *and* 11.3.3. Usually the particulate lead level will be above 10 μg and 11.3.2 and 11.3.3 should be followed. For the nonparticulate lead sample, proceed as in 11.3.3.

11.3.2 Drain the aqueous layer into a 100-ml volumetric flask. Dilute to volume with Clark and Lubs buffer solution. Place a 10-ml aliquot in a 125-ml Squibb-type separatory funnel and dilute to approximately 50 ml with Clark and Lubs buffer solution.

11.3.3 Add ammonium hydroxide to the aqueous solution until ammoniacal. Add 20 ml of the KCN solution. Add 20 ml (buret or pipet) of dithizone solution and shake for 1 min (Note 7). Drain and discard the first 2.0 ml of dithizone solution and then fill a 50-mm absorption cell with the chloroform-dithizone solution. Read the absorbance compared to chloroform with the spectrophotometer set at 510 mμ.

Note 7—Usually a 1-min shaking period is specified for shaking the solution with dithizone-chloroform to extract the lead. If shaking is done by hand, care must be exercised to prevent warming the container by the hand since the solubility of lead dithizonate in aqueous phase or in the chloroform phase will vary depending on the temperature of the mixture. The extraction of the lead dithizonate at this step must be done exactly in the same manner each time to reduce errors or variations in the results.

11.3.4 Determine the micrograms of lead by comparison with the previously prepared calibration curve and correct for blank.

12. Calculation

12.1 Particulate Lead:

12.1.1 Calculate the concentration of particulate lead, C_p, in micrograms per cubic meter of air sample as follows:

$$C_p = \frac{W_p \times 1000 \times 10}{V}$$

where:
W_p = micrograms of particulate lead from calibration curve,
V = liters of sample volume,
1000 = factor to convert to cubic meters, and
10 = factor for aliquot (11.3.2).

12.2 Nonparticulate Lead:

12.2.1 Calculate the concentration of nonparticulate lead, C_{np}, in micrograms per cubic meter of air sample as follows:

$$C_{np} = \frac{W_{np} \times 1000}{V}$$

where:
W_{np} = micrograms of nonparticulate lead from calibration curve,
V = liters of sample volume, and
1000 = factor to convert to cubic meters.

References

(1) Cholak, J., "Analytical Methods for Determination of Lead," Archives Environmental Health, AEHLA, Vol 8, 1964, p. 222.
(2) Snyder, L. J. and Henderson, S. R., "A New Field Method for the Determination of Organic Lead Compounds in Air," Analytical Chemistry, ANCHA, Vol 33, 1961, pp. 1175–1180.

(3) MacPhee, R. D., Eye, M. G., and Parkinson, E. E., "A Method for Monitoring Organic Lead in the Atmosphere," Air Pollution Control District, County of Los Angeles, APCPA, September, 1962.

(4) "Methods for Determining Lead in Air and Biological Material," American Public Health Association Inc., APHYA, 1790 Broadway, New York, N. Y., 1955.

(5) Snyder, L. J., "Determination of Trace Amounts of Organic Lead in Air," Analytical Chemistry, ANCHA, Vol 39, 1967, pp. 591–595.

COMMENT

The Millipore type H A filter, with a 0.45-μm pore size, is reported to have a 99.9% efficiency for collecting particles as small as 0.03 μm.[516] Blank filters from each new batch should be analyzed by the selected procedure, and the appropriate averaged correction value must be applied to the results of sample analyses.

Crystalline iodine, used in this method to collect organic lead, is not 100% efficient for this purpose, according to L. J. Snyder and H. R. Henderson.[510] Snyder has since used 30- to 50-mesh activated charcoal to sample organic lead in 100- to 200-m^3 air samples near a Los Angeles freeway at a rate of 0.7 cfm. The lead was converted to inorganic lead and analyzed by the dithizone method[508] with a precision of ± 0.008 μg/m^3, based on laboratory experimentation with tetramethyl lead.

Alternate Method for the Determination of Lead by Atomic Absorption Spectrophotometry

During the last 6 years, atomic absorption spectrophotometry has emerged in the United States as a very rapid, specific, and sensitive method for the analysis of metallic elements, including lead, in any type of sample that can be put into solution. Using an air–acetylene flame to produce the "atomic cloud" of sample constituents, a sensitivity of 15 μg/100 g of whole blood is now being achieved routinely with dilute acid solutions of ashed blood samples. The accuracy and precision of this method are extremely high; results obtained by this method compare very favorably with those provided on duplicate samples with a spectrographic procedure applied in other laboratories. Thus, the reliability and rapidity of atomic absorption analyses for lead are making this technique attractive to many laboratories.

The coefficient of variation of the atomic absorption method, as determined by repetitive measurements of a set of blood lead standard samples over a period of 6 months, was found to be 8%. However, by the preparation of a separate standard curve for each group of samples, the true coefficient of variation can be reduced to 1.5%.*

APPARATUS

All glassware must be borosilicate and must be freed of lead by rinsing with warm 1 : 1 nitric acid and distilled water before use.

1. Atomic absorption spectrophotometer. Numerous instruments, available commercially, are being used for the analysis of lead in sample solutions. The Techtron models AA4, AA5, and AA120, or equivalent, have been found satisfactory.
2. Volumetric flasks, glass-stoppered, 50 ml.
3. Pipets, volumetric, assorted sizes.
4. Beakers, Phillips, conical, 125 and 250 ml.

REAGENTS AND MATERIALS

1. Acid, hydrochloric (sp gr 1.19), A.C.S. grade. Prepare dilute reagent as needed.
2. Acid, nitric (sp gr 1.42), A.C.S. grade.
3. Acid, sulfuric (sp gr 1.84), A.C.S. grade.
4. Distilled water, shown to be lead-free by atomic absorption spectrophotometric analysis. Used throughout the method where water is mentioned.

PROCEDURE

To the cooled acid digest of the sample resulting from the treatment described in Sec. 11.1.1 of ASTM Method D 2681, add 10 ml of HNO_3 (1 : 4) and boil the solution, as stipulated, to dissolve any lead sulfate. Transfer the solution to a 50-ml volumetric flask, dilute to volume with water, and mix. Analyze the solution, or a diluted aliquot if the lead content is high, by atomic absorption spectrophotometry. The following characteristics apply to the Techtron instruments:

Current	6 ma
Slit	300 nm

*Unpublished data of R. I. Grunder and R. G. Keenan from "An atomic absorption method for the analysis of lead in particles," in preparation.

Burner height setting	3.0
Support pressure (air) setting	15
Fuel flow (acetylene) setting	3
Analysis line	2170 Å

Obtain the absorbance of the sample solution. Correct this value by subtracting from it the absorbance of an unused membrane filter carried through the entire procedure.

CALCULATIONS

Estimate the micrograms of lead per milliliter of sample solution from the standard curve prepared daily at the *same time* each group of unknown samples is analyzed. Multiply by 50 (and by any additional aliquot reciprocal if further dilution of the prepared sample solution was required for a high-lead sample) to obtain the total number of micrograms of particulate lead in the total air sample. The concentration of lead per cubic meter of air is calculated as follows:

$$\mu g/m^3 = \frac{\mu g/ml \times 1{,}000 \times 50 \times \text{any additional aliquot reciprocal}}{\text{liters of air sampled}}.$$

COMMENT

The atomic absorption method may be used for the analysis of lead in any prepared dilute acid solution ($<3\,N$) of a sample following the wet oxidation of organic material and the solubilization of lead with mineral acids. By standardization with a set of lead solutions of known concentrations with each group of samples, it is possible to minimize the effect of varied gas-flow regulator settings and to reduce the relative standard deviation to less than 1.5%. The acidity of the sample solutions should be less than $3\,N$ to prevent corrosion of the burner. Modification of this method for continuously measuring lead is currently being field-tested by the Environmental Protection Agency.[400]

LEAD IN BIOLOGIC MATERIALS

Lead in blood, urine, feces, and body tissues may be analyzed by the "USPHS" method for determining lead in air and in biologic materials[293] or by the APHA methods for determining lead in air and in biologic materials[10] (the latter provides for the separation of bismuth dithizonate at pH 3.4). Methods and precautions for the collection, preservation, and storage of biologic samples are described in Appendix D.

"USPHS" Method for Determining Lead in Air and in Biologic Materials*

THE USPHS method for the determination of lead is a double-extraction, mixed-color dithizone procedure which is especially convenient for lead analysis in the absence of bismuth. Although this method has evolved from the early experimentation conducted with dithizone procedures in this Division starting in 1937, it has never been published in complete detail but only in an abbreviated form as part of a committee report.[1] Many chemists have suggested that the complete procedure along with its supporting data should be published.

During the past 26 years, the method has been refined through the efforts of the chemists who have used it in this Division. Consequently, these improvements have been incorporated on a gradual basis in the separate series of mimeographed copies of the method distributed to those requesting them. Hence, it is appropriate now to publish the complete details of the fully refined method along with the associated information on sample collecting, ashing and other preparative procedures.

Of equal importance, however, is the need to report on the results of the repetitive testing of the method of which the accuracy and precision have been evaluated periodically by the analysis of replicate samples of blood and urine. For these evaluations, pooled biological samples have been used. In each series of test samples, one set of replicates contained lead only in its physiologic form whereas the remaining sets contained this lead plus known incremental quantities of an inorganic lead

compound. Statistical analyses of the resulting lead recovery data have been made. The results of the analyses of the latest series of test samples of blood are reported in this paper.

Reagents

Analytical grade reagents are used. Purification is essential when analyzing biological tissues and fluids because of the very low levels of lead in these materials; purification of reagents may not be required for air samples containing quantities of lead sufficiently greater than that present in the reagent blank. A reagent blank sample is carried through the entire procedure with each set of unknown samples (air, biological, or other type) and its analyzed lead content is subtracted from each analytical result to calculate the net quantity of lead in each unknown sample.

A boiling rod is used to prevent bumping in the flasks when distilling reagents. This is prepared by cutting 3 or 4 mm O.D. glass tubing to a length which is one cm greater than the height of the flask. The tubing is sealed at a spot about one cm above the bottom end which is firepolished but left open. Before each use, the liquid is shaken out of the bottom section and the rod inserted in the flask. As the flask is heated a steady stream of air and vapor bubbles issues from the open space, thus providing nuclei for smooth boiling.

Double-distilled Water.—To distilled water in an all borosilicate-glass still add a crystal each of potassium permanganate and barium

The use of trade names in this paper does not constitute an endorsement by the Public Health Service.

*Reproduced with permission of the American Industrial Hygiene Association, 25711 Southfield Road, Southfield, Michigan 48075.

hydroxide and redistill. Use for reagent and biological sample solutions unless tests indicate that single-distilled water is satisfactory; single-distilled water is usually adequate for determinations or air samples.

Nitric Acid, Concentrated.—Redistill in an all borosilicate-glass still the ACS reagent grade acid, 69.0% minimum, specific gravity 1.42. Use an electric heating jacket on the boiling flask to minimize danger of its breakage, and a boiling rod to prevent bumping, which otherwise would be severe. Discard the first 50 ml of distillate; this may be combined with the acid allowed to remain in the flask at the end of the distillation and used for washing glassware. The reagent is conveniently dispensed from a small automatic burette. No grease should be used on the stopcock.

Nitric Acid, 1:99.—Dilute 10 ml of the redistilled, concentrated acid to one liter with double-distilled water.

Ammonium Hydroxide, Concentrated.—Distill in an all borosilicate-glass still 3 liters of the ACS reagent grade, 28.0% minimum, specific gravity 0.8957 at 60°F, into 1.5 liters of double-distilled water, contained in a 2-liter reagent bottle which is chilled in an ice bath. Continue the distillation until the bottle is filled up to the previously marked 2-liter level. Submerge the condenser tube deeply in the water in the receiver, but withdraw it before discontinuing the heat to avoid siphoning back of distillate. This reagent may be prepared more conveniently from tank ammonia, using a small wash bottle to scrub the gas and a sintered glass delivery tube which extends to the bottom of the reagent bottle. The ammonia gas is absorbed in double-distilled water until the solution reaches the desired specific gravity.

Chloroform.—Use a brand with a statement on the label that the chloroform passes the American Chemical Society test for suitability for use in dithizone procedures. In addition, each batch of chloroform should be purchased in glass containers only and should be tested as follows in the laboratory to make sure that it is satisfactory for preparing the dithizone solutions: add a minute quantity of dithizone to a portion of the chloroform in a test tube, shake gently, then stopper with a cork. The faint green color should be stable for one day. Our experience has indicated that the procedures for reclaiming used chloroform are tedious, time-consuming, sometimes unsuccessful, and no longer warranted in view of the commercial availability of acceptable reagent grades.

Extraction Dithizone.—Dissolve 16 mg of diphenylthiocarbazone (dithizone), Eastman Kodak Co. No. 3092, or equivalent, in one liter of chloroform. Store in a brown bottle in the refrigerator.

Standard Dithizone.—Dissolve 8 mg of diphenylthiocarbazone in one liter of chloroform. Store in a brown bottle in the refrigerator *but allow to warm to room temperature before using.* Age for at least one day, then standardize as described in the procedure. Restandardize every few months.

Sodium Citrate.—Dissolve 125 gm of the $2 Na_3C_6H_5O_7 \cdot 11 H_2O$ salt in sufficient distilled water to provide a solution nearly 500 ml in volume. Adjust the pH to 9-10, using a very small quantity of phenol red indicator solution (strong red color) and *fresh,* pHydrion test paper to check the pH. Extract in a large separatory funnel with a 100 mg per liter solution of dithizone and finally with the extraction dithizone reagent until a green extract is obtained with the latter reagent. Add a small volume of lead-free citric acid until an orange color (pH 7) appears. Extract the excess dithizone repeatedly with chloroform until a colorless extract is obtained. Remove the last traces of chloroform.

Hydroxylamine Hydrochloride.—Dissolve 20 gm of the salt in distilled water to provide a volume of 65 ml. Add a few drops of m-cresol purple indicator, then add ammonia until the indicator turns yellow (pH 3). Add a sufficient quantity of a 4% solution of sodium diethyldithiocarbamate to combine with metallic impurities, then mix. After a few minutes extract repeatedly with chloroform until the excess carbamate reagent has been removed, as indicated by the absence of a yellow color in the final chloroform extract tested with a dilute copper solution. To the aqueous solution of the hydroxylamine hydrochloride add redistilled, 6N hydrochloric acid until the indicator turns pink, and adjust the volume to 100 ml with double-distilled water.

Potassium Cyanide.—(Danger! Highly poisonous!!) To 50 gm of potassium cyanide in a beaker, add sufficient distilled water to make a sludge. Transfer the sludge to a separatory funnel previously marked to show 100-ml volume. Add a small amount of distilled water to the beaker and warm. (Potassium cyanide cools the solution as it dissolves, thus retarding the solution process.) Add this warm water to the separatory funnel but do not permit contents to exceed the 100-ml mark. Shake, then let stand until the contents come to room temperature. A practically saturated solution results.

Extract the lead by shaking repeatedly with portions of the extraction dithizone solution until the lead has been removed. Part of the dithizone dissolves in the aqueous phase but enough remains in the chloroform to color it. A green extract indicates that all the lead has been completely extracted. Most of the dithizone in the aqueous phase is then removed by repeated extractions with pure chloroform. Dilute the concentrated solution of potassium cyanide with double-distilled water to 500 ml. It should not be necessary to filter the solution, if the directions are followed precisely. Extraction is carried out before dilution because the higher pH of the dilute solution is less favorable.

(NOTE: A colorless solution usually results if above directions are followed. Occasionally aging results in a brown color or precipitate due to polymerization of hydrogen cyanide. This does not interfere with use of the reagent if it is carefully decanted. Old potassium cyanide reagent may lose enough strength to cause insufficient complexing of large amounts of zinc.)

Ammonia-cyanide Mixture.—Mix 200 ml of the purified 10% potassium cyanide reagent with 150 ml of distilled ammonium hydroxide (specific gravity 0.9, corresponding to 28.4% NH_3) and dilute to one liter with double-distilled water. If the measured specific gravity of the ammonia is not 0.9, use the equivalent volume as calculated from a table of specific gravity vs. percentage ammonia.

Standard Lead Solution.—Dissolve 1.5984 gm of pure lead nitrate in one liter of 1:99 nitric acid to provide a strong stock solution containing one mg Pb per ml. Pipet exactly 20 ml into a 500-ml volumetric flask and make to mark with 1:99 nitric acid to give a dilute stock solution containing 40 μg Pb per ml. (A standard lead solution, 10 μg Pb/ml, was stable in 1:99 nitric acid for three years.) Prepare a working solution, containing 2 μg Pb per ml, just before it is needed by pipetting 5 ml of the dilute stock solution

into a 100-ml volumetric flask and making to mark with 1:99 nitric acid.

Phenol Red.—0.1% aqueous solution.

Ashing Aid Acid.—Dissolve 25 gm potassium sulfate in sufficient redistilled concentrated nitric acid to make 100 ml.

White Petrolatum.—Supplied in a glass jar, for greasing stopcocks. To check on the purity, put a pinch of this petrolatum in a beaker, add a few milliliters of the standard dithizone and swirl. If the dithizone is no longer green after a few minutes, the material is unsatisfactory for greasing stopcocks.

Apparatus

A Beckman Model DU Spectrophotometer has been used in this laboratory since this instrument became available in the 1940s. However, the Beckman Model B and the Bausch and Lomb Spectronic 20 have been shown to give comparable results for blood lead determinations, provided that appropriate standardizations are conducted with each instrument. Other laboratories, whose results are reported in this paper, have presumably used a diversity of available photometers and spectrophotometers. In our laboratory, 22 x 175 mm matched test tubes are used in most spectrophotometric procedures employing the Model DU, which is fitted with a tube holder which does not interfere with the use of the instrument with regular cells.[2] These same tubes are used in the Model B fitted with a test tube adaptor. A ¾-inch tube, supplied by the manufacturer, is used in the Bausch and Lomb Spectronic 20.

Borosilicate glassware is used throughout the procedures (except for vacutainers used for blood sampling). Ashing is performed in 125- or 250-ml Phillips beakers. Automatic burettes are used for the addition of most reagents. The extractions are conducted in Squibb-type, 125-ml separatory funnels supported in electrically operated shakers provided with timer switches. The stopcocks of the separatory funnels are greased with white petrolatum (purchased in a glass jar rather than in a metal can or tube) unless Teflon stopcocks, which require no grease, are used. All glassware should be reserved for trace analysis only, to avoid possible gross contamination.

Soak all ashing beakers in a detergent solution (Alconox or Duponol is suitable) immediately after each usage to prevent any material from drying on the surfaces. Rinse 8-10 times with hot water and store in a dust-proof drawer or cabinet until needed. Use the following acid cleaning, lead-freeing techniques *immediately before* the next use of the glassware: Rinse the ashing beakers with a saturated solution of sodium dichromate in concentrated sulfuric acid. Leave a 1-2 ml portion in the beaker or flask (proportionally less in a small volumetric flask!). Add about 5-10 ml of warm tap water and allow the hot solution to flow over all inner surfaces to remove the last traces of grease. Rinse with three or four portions of cold tap water. Rinse with one portion of either concentrated or 1:1 nitric acid, as preferred. (This wash nitric acid may be used repeatedly until it loses its strength.) Then rinse successively with three or four portions each of tap water, distilled and double-distilled water. Set the beakers upright on the bench and cover with a clean dust-case or a large piece of filter paper (or otherwise protect from dust). *Under no circumstances is glassware turned upside down to drain on a towel or cheesecloth placed on a laboratory bench.* Use an oven operating at 105°C if dry glassware is required.

Separatory funnels are rinsed with tap water immediately after use. If a high lead sample was present or if a visible precipitate remains on the inside, it is rinsed with a small portion of 1:1 wash nitric acid (which is discarded), followed by tap water. The stoppered funnels are stored in double-deck racks. Immediately before use, stopcocks are regreased if necessary. Then the funnels are rinsed with wash acid, four times with tap water, and four times with distilled water. Each rinse is accomplished by shaking with the stopper, then draining through the stopcock with two or three turns.

Spectrophotometer tubes are rinsed four times each with tap and distilled water immediately after use. They are placed upright in a large beaker and dried in an oven at 105°C, then stored under a dust-cover. Occasionally they are cleaned with dichromate-sulfuric acid and nitric acid as described above.

(NOTE: With this method of cleaning glassware we have never encountered cross-contamination from chromium, lead, or from any other trace element being determined routinely in this laboratory.)

Analytical Procedure

1. Warm the sample ash (prepared as described in the following sections) with 2 ml of concentrated nitric acid for a few minutes, then add 25 ml of distilled water, heating on the hotplate until a clear solution is obtained.

2. Cool to room temperaure. Add to the solution in the beaker one ml of hydroxylamine hydrochloride, 4 ml of sodium citrate (10 ml is required for a urine sample), one drop of phenol red indicator, and titrate to a strong red color with concentrated ammonia reagent. Add a few drops excess of ammonia to make sure that the pH is between 9 and 10, using *fresh* pHydrion test paper to check the pH.

(NOTE: Phenol red has a weak orange-red color in strong acid, yellow in weak acid, and a red color in alkaline solution. Do not mistake the first color for that produced in alkaline medium!)

3. Transfer the sample quantitatively with double-distilled water rinsings to a 125-ml Squibb separatory funnel containing 5 ml of the potassium cyanide reagent.

4. Add 5 ml of the extraction dithizone and shake two minutes, after releasing the initial pressure by momentarily opening the stopcock of the inverted separatory funnel. Allow the chloroform layer to settle.

5. Draw off most of the extraction dithizone into a second funnel containing exactly 30 ml of 1:99 nitric acid.

6. Add a second 5-ml portion of extraction dithizone to the first funnel and shake as before. Allow the layers to separate and combine the extracts in the second funnel. Continue this process with fresh portions of extraction dithizone until the reagent remains green. A rough estimate of the lead present in the sample may be made on the basis of 20 μg for each cherry-red 5-ml extract portion.

7. Shake the second funnel for two minutes to transfer the lead to the 1:99 nitric acid layer. Allow the layers to separate. Discard the chloroform layer.

8. Shake the nitric acid solution with approximately 5 ml of reagent chloroform and let settle. Drain the settled chloroform through the stopcock bore as completely as possible without loss of the aqueous layer. Evaporate the last drop of chloroform clinging to the upper surface of the liquid.

(NOTE 1: Start a zero lead standard at the beginning of this step by placing 30 ml of 1:99 nitric acid in a separatory funnel. This zero lead standard will be used to set the spectrophotometer at zero absorbance for each series of samples being analyzed.)

(NOTE 2: If the quantity of lead estimated for any sample exceeds the 25 μg range of the colorimetric determination, pipet an appropriate aliquot of the nitric acid solution at the end of step 7 into a clean separatory funnel containing 5 ml 1:99 nitric acid to minimize errors caused by possible leakage of the stopcock, add sufficient additional 1:99 nitric acid to make 30 ml total volume, and continue with step 8.)

(NOTE 3: Start lead standards at this point if required. Add 5-ml portions of 1:99 nitric acid to each of four separatory funnels, then 2.5, 5.0, 7.5, and 12.5 ml of dilute standard lead solution (2 μg Pb/ml) from a burette, respectively to the separatory funnels, finally add the proper quantity of 1:99 nitric acid to make total volume 30 ml in each. Continue with step 8.)

9. Add 6.0 ml of the ammonia-cyanide mixture, *exactly* 15.0 ml of the standard dithizone, and shake two minutes. Allow the layers to separate. Drain the chloroform layer containing the lead dithizonate into a clean, dry test tube, and cork the tube immediately.

10. Decant this solution carefully into a dry photometer tube leaving the water behind. If any water spots are visible in the optical light path, transfer again to another photometer tube.

11. Set the spectrophotometer at a wavelength of 510 mμ.

12. Set the instrument at zero absorbance using the zero lead standard solution.

13. Read the absorbances of the samples and of the reagent blank.

14. Calculate the lead content of each by multiplying its absorbance by the standardization factor (which is the slope of the stanardization plot in micrograms of lead per unit of absorbance.) Subtract the blank value from the gross lead content of each sample to obtain the net amount of lead expressed in micrograms.

Special Materials for Blood Sampling

1. Vacutainers, Becton-Dickinson, No. 3208, 20-ml or 10-ml, complete with stoppers are used for blood sampling. The vacutainers are used repeatedly and are lead-freed by the technique described previously. Blood is removed from the vacutainers and the stoppers, after each use, by soaking in cold tap water. When no further visible trace of blood remains on these items, they are soaked overnight in the detergent solution. They are then rinsed repeatedly with hot tap water to remove alkaline materials. The vacutainers are then subjected to the chromic and nitric acid cleaning procedures. The stoppers are soaked for 20- to 30-minute periods, three times, with single distilled water and finally three times with double distilled water. The

lead-freed vacutainers are dried at 105°C, fitted with clean stoppers, and stored in a drawer reserved for them. Layers of cheesecloth are placed between the separate layers of vacutainers and the drawer is sealed with masking tape to prevent the admittance of any dust. They are evacuated just before shipment to the field. A vacuum tester is used both in the laboratory and field to test for loss of vacuum, which usually will not occur until stoppers have been used several times.

2. Vacuum Tester, High Frequency, Fisher Cat. No. 1-179, or equivalent.

3. Needles, Becton-Dickinson, Gauge 20, one and one-half inches in length, *stainless steel,* B-D No. 3200 N. As these needles are used repeatedly, check the tips for burrs by drawing them across the thumb nail. When burrs develop either discard the needles or file off the burrs. After filing, they must be recleaned. Vacutainer needles are soaked in a dilute detergent solution. A Becton-Dickinson Needle Cleaner, No. 3200 C, is used to force detergent solution and subsequent rinse water through the needles. Needles are subjected to thorough rinsing with distilled water. They are then placed in steritubes and either autoclaved or heated for two hours in a drying oven operating at 180°C. The steritubes are then fitted with rubber caps.

4. Steritubes, Becton-Dickinson, No. 3200 D, with rubber caps.

5. Stillets for No. 3200 N needles, 20 Gauge, two and seven-eighths inches long.

(These BD items are available from the Becton-Dickinson Company, Rutherford, New Jersey.)

Collecting and Ashing Blood Samples

Collect a 10-ml sample of whole blood using a lead-free vacutainer and a sterilized, stainless steel needle. In the laboratory, transfer the sample to a weighed, lead-free, 125-ml borosilicate Phillips beaker. No aliquoting of the blood is permissible, as most of the lead is present in the clot. Determine the weight of the blood sample to the nearest 0.01 gram, weighing rapidly to minimize evaporation. Add 2 ml of ashing aid acid reagent. Add 7 ml of concentrated nitric acid. (This ashing system permits the analyst to handle a large number of samples at a time as the blood clot breaks up readily and smoothly without bumping and without requiring the constant attention of the analyst.) Place the samples on a hotplate operating about 130°C and evaporate just to dryness. After the water is driven off in the initial evaporation to dryness, keep the beaker covered with a lead-free watchglass to increase the reflux action of the concentrated acid. This serves to wash solids down from the sides to the hotter zone at the bottom, and also reduces the amount of acid needed. Cool the beaker briefly and then add successive portions of the nitric acid ranging from 2 ml down to 0.5 ml as the ashing proceeds. Do not remove the watchglass at any time but merely slide it back sufficiently to facilitate each new addition of the acid. Each time, as soon as the residue becomes light colored, heat on a 400°C hotplate *just long enough to blacken the residue*, then remove and cool the sample. Throughout the remainder of the ashing procedure, alternately heat the sample with a few drops of nitric acid on the 130°C hotplate and bake the residue for the few minutes required to darken it on the 400°C hotplate. Finally, the residue will remain pale yellow or light brown (due to iron content) after heating for 5-10 minutes at the high temperature. *Avoid excess baking at this stage as the ash will become decomposed to a difficultly soluble form.* It is now ready for solution and analysis. Report results as milligrams of lead per 100 grams of whole blood.

Collecting and Ashing Urine Samples

Use lead-free, narrow-mouthed, reagent-type, borosilicate, 250-ml bottles provided with standard taper glass stoppers to collect grab samples of urine. Add 2.0 ml of a 37% formalin solution as a preservative, shaking the bottle 10-12 times after the contribution of the urine to mix the specimen with the formalin thoroughly.

Alternatively, urine specimens may be collected in 125-ml polyethylene bottles containing as a preservative 100-200 mg of EDTA (acid form) per bottle.[3] This is convenient and economical for shipping samples considerable distances.

If the urine sample is clear and only one or two days old, measure a 50 ml portion into a graduated cylinder. However, if the sample is older, much of the lead may be in a sediment or on the walls of the bottle and must be dissolved before aliquoting. Transfer the entire specimen to a glass-stoppered graduated cylinder, record the volume, rinse the sample bottle with three small portions of concentrated nitric acid and add these rinsings to the cylinder. Mix thoroughly (Caution! Old samples may foam over.) Note the total volume and remove an aliquot equivalent to 50 ml of urine for analysis. Transfer the aliquot portion to a lead-free, 250-ml borosilicate Phillips beaker and add 5 ml of redistilled concentrated nitric acid. Evaporate just to dryness on a hotplate operating at about 130°C. Cool, add sufficient nitric acid to moisten the residue and cover the beaker with a lead-free watchglass. Heat on the 130°C hotplate and then alternately bake for a few minutes and digest with minimal amounts of nitric acid (as described in the ashing method for blood) until a white residue remains after the final heating for 5-10 minutes at the high temperature. The sample is now ready for solution and analysis. Report results as milligrams of lead per liter of urine.

Procedure for Air Samples

It is convenient to wash out samples in electrostatic precipitator tubes with redistilled ethanol, using a special policeman made with a rubber disc cut to fit the tube like a piston, and transferring the sample through a short stem funnel into a 250-ml Phillips beaker; gently evaporate just to dryness. (Ethanol is helpful in removing greasy deposits on the walls of the precipitator tube. Some chemists may prefer hot 1 to 5% nitric acid to transfer the sample.) Transfer impinger samples or membrane filter samples to Phillips beakers. If little ash is expected (usually for impinger or membrane filter samples), add 2 ml of ashing aid acid reagent. (The presence of this salt will prevent loss of lead by glazing onto the surface of the beaker during ashing.) Otherwise add 1-2 ml nitric acid. Evaporate to dryness. Continue ashing with nitric acid at a moderate heat until organics are destroyed.

Dissolve the ash in 2 ml of concentrated nitric acid and distilled water and then transfer quantitatively to a 100-ml volumetric flask and make to mark. Pipet a suitable aliquot into a separatory funnel, containing about 5 ml of double-distilled water, add sufficient additional double-distilled water to make the total volume about 25 ml, and apply the Analytical Procedure, starting with step 2. In step 3, as the sample is already in a separatory funnel, merely add the cyanide. The amount of lead present in the aliquot may be estimated as described in step 6. If it is less than a few micrograms, an additional aliquot may be added to the same funnel, and the pH readjusted with ammonia. The extraction is then continued, and extracts combined with those collected previously in the second funnel. If the estimated amount of lead exceeds the range of the method (25 micrograms), take an aliquot as described in Note 2, step 8.

When calculating the results, make allowance for the total number of aliquots. If convenient, aliquot the reagent blank in the same manner so that the correction represents the same amounts of ashing and extraction reagents as are present in the sample. However, the blank correction is usually small for air samples. Report results as milligrams of lead per cubic meter of air.

Lead in Paint on Sheet Metal

Cut a small disc of known area from the sheet without dislodging the paint. A 7/32-inch shearing type metal punch is convenient. Weigh the disc to the nearest 0.01 milligram. Transfer the disc to a 125-ml Phillips beaker and add 3.0 ml of methylene chloride. Swirl the beaker for several minutes. If necessary, use a fresh, clean wooden stick to help dislodge the paint completely from the metal surface. Remove the stripped metal disc with clean forceps, blot with filter paper, and air-dry. Reweigh. Calculate the loss in weight as the amount of paint film removed by the methylene chloride treatment.

Transfer the beaker to a steam bath and evaporate off the methylene chloride. Add 3.0 ml of concentrated nitric acid and heat until a clear solution results. Apply the procedure for air samples, beginning with the second paragraph. Results obtained with this method may be expressed both as milligrams of lead per square inch of surface and as percentage lead in the paint film.

Comments on Analysis of Biological Materials

This method may be regarded as essentially specific for lead in biological materials. Any tin which may be present is oxidized during the ashing procedure to the stannic state, which is not extracted by the dithizone. Although bismuth is an interference with the procedure it is very rarely found in biological samples. The bismuth present in oral medications generally appears in the feces and does not enter the blood or urine unless taken over a prolonged period.[4] The intravenous injection of bismuth medication for treatment of such diseases as syphilis is now seldom practiced as it has been supplanted by penicillin. Thallium would be measured

as lead but, as it is rarely encountered in biological materials, it does not constitute an interference from the practical viewpoint.

Studies were made of the losses of lead in blood samples shipped in vacutainers fitted with rubber stoppers. There was no loss of lead present in its normal physiologic form, although lead in the inorganic form added to whole blood was shown by analysis to be lost on the rubber stoppers. In the latter case shipment must be made using sealed glass ampoules. Experimentally it was shown that inorganic lead, in the form of either the chloride or nitrate, was not lost when samples were stored so that there was no contact between the blood and the rubber stoppers.

Experimental studies also were made of losses of lead during the ashing of blood samples. If the samples were overheated deliberately so that carbonized material flashed into flames, up to one-third of the lead was lost.

By adding 0.5 gram of potassium sulfate (in the ashing aid acid) good results were obtained; even in the absence of flashing, 5% more recovery was obtained for inorganic lead added to blood samples. The final color of the ashed residue depends upon the degree of heating but does not affect the recovery of lead. Overheated samples have a brownish residue due to presence of iron oxides and may require prolonged heating before a clear solution of the ash is obtained at the start of the analysis. No loss of lead was found to occur upon standing of the dissolved sample for 20 hours prior to completion of analysis.

Evaluation of Method for Lead in Blood

A supply of citrated human blood from expired stock in a blood bank was mixed in a lead-free, borosilicate glass carboy. Approximately 2,000-gram portions of this pooled specimen were transferred to each of four previously weighed, lead-free, glass-stoppered, borosilicate glass bottles. The weight of the blood in each bottle was then determined to the nearest gram. Appropriate quantities of lead, as a solution containing one mg Pb per ml, were added from a burette to provide *inorganic lead* concentrations of 0, 0.050, 0.125, and 0.271 mg Pb per 100 gm of whole blood in the bottles, which were labelled P, S, T, and W, respectively. These concentrations of added lead, plus the mean normal value of 0.020 mg Pb per 100 gm blood determined by analysis of 12 replicate portions of sample "P" using the described method, provided total lead concentrations of

TABLE I

Replicate Analyses by USPHS Laboratory

(All values expressed as mg Pb per 100 gm whole blood
or per 100 ml of 1% HNO₃ solution)

Sample	Pa	Sb	Tb	Wb	Xc	Yc
Calcd. Lead Content	0.020	0.070	0.145	0.291	0.075	0.150
Replicate Analyses	0.0186	0.0693	0.1469	0.2876	0.0717	0.1485
	0.0237	0.0700	0.1424	0.2819	0.0753	0.1510
	0.0212	0.0714	0.1434	0.2809	0.0722	0.1456
	0.0195	0.0700	0.1433	0.2791	0.0753	0.1524
	0.0179	0.0708	0.1406	0.2916	0.0703	0.1426
	0.0204	0.0689	0.1376	0.2721	0.0734	0.1451
	0.0200	0.0697	0.1349	0.2741	0.0706	0.1448
	0.0192	0.0680	0.1339	0.2853	0.0737	0.1511
	0.0203	0.0670	0.1590	0.2890	0.0731	0.1543
	0.0236	0.0620	0.1360	0.2780	0.0740	0.1451
	0.0187					
	0.0182					
Sum	0.2413	0.6871	1.4180	2.8196	0.7296	1.4805
Mean	0.0201	0.0687	0.1418	0.2820	0.0730	0.1481
Percent Recovery of Total Pb	95.7d	98.1	97.8	96.9	97.3	98.7
Standard Deviation from Calcd. Value	0.0019	0.0030	0.0081	0.0115	0.0028	0.0045
Coefficient of Variation, %	9.5	4.3	5.6	4.0	3.7	3.0

(a) Unspiked blood sample containing 0.020 mg Pb per 100 grams of blood, as determined from analyses reported in table.
(b) Blood sample containing calculated 0.020 mg Pb per 100 grams spiked with 0.050, 0.125, or 0.271 mg inorganic Pb/100 grams blood.
(c) 1% nitric acid solutions spiked with indicated amounts of inorganic lead.
d) From intercept of line in Figure 1.

0.020, 0.070, 0.145, and 0.291 mg Pb per 100 gm of whole blood for the series of four samples. The blood was kept under refrigeration except during laboratory handling prior to shipment to the collaborating laboratories.

Replicate sets of samples, of approximately 10-ml volume, were removed periodically from the bottles during the initial 10-day period, weighed, and analyzed. This procedure was repeated for five sets of samples to make sure that the calculated lead content of each sample was correct. Upon obtaining this assurance, sets of lead-free vacutainer tubes were loaded with approximately 10 ml of the blood samples and the tubes were flame-sealed. During the next two months five sets of these vacutainer samples which had been retained in our laboratory under refrigeration were analyzed. These latter analyses were spread out over this period while the remainder of the samples were being analyzed by the collaborating laboratories. The results of all of the analyses conducted in this laboratory on the blood samples are presented in Table I. In addition to the blood lead values, this table also lists the results of our analyses of standard samples X and Y which contained respectively 0.075 and 0.150 mg Pb per 100 ml in 1% nitric acid.

The data presented in Table I (excluding sample P) showing the mean lead recoveries ranging from 96.9 to 98.7%, demonstrate the accuracy to be expected of the method. The lower portion of Table I shows the standard deviations and the coefficients of variation. The coefficients of variations in the 3% to 5% region indicate the highly satisfactory precision possible with this method.

The same data are reproduced graphically in Figure 1. The quantity of lead added is plotted as the abscissa and the total amount of lead found is plotted as the ordinate. Extrapolation of the linear curve to zero ordinate has provided a value of 0.021 mg Pb per 100 grams of whole blood as the probable true initial concentration of lead in the supply of pooled blood. The slope of this curve is 0.971, which represents a mean recovery of 97.1%. Furthermore, the 0.0201 mg Pb per 100 gm of blood obtained as the mean of the 12 replicate analyses of the pooled blood supply is in close agreement with the 0.0204 analytical value from the graphical computation (0.021 x 0.971).

The analytical data reported for this same series of samples by the 10 collaborating laboratories of State and local occupational health agencies using the USPHS method, are presented in Table II and plotted in Figure 1. These data show satisfactory lead recoveries except for sample P which yielded mostly high results. It should be noted that each value is the mean of two analyses in contradistinction to the individual analyses reported in Table I. With the diversity of analysts, reagents, and instrumentation employed in this collaborative effort, one might expect larger coefficients of variation than those obtained by a single analyst. These

TABLE II

Replicate Analyses by Ten Collaborating Laboratories

(All values are the mean of two analyses and are expressed as mg Pb per 100 gm of whole blood or per 100 ml of 1% HNO₃ solution)

Sample		Pa	Sb	Tb	Wb	U₁c	U₂c
Laboratory	Calcd. Value of Total Pb	0.020	0.070	0.145	0.291	0.075	0.150
A		0.032	0.078	0.150	0.270	0.068	0.149
B		0.022	0.067	0.134	0.277	0.081	0.148
C		(0.008)d	0.060	0.150	0.260	0.080	0.160
D		0.026	0.067	0.130	0.255	0.068	0.133
E		0.028	0.088	0.137	0.290	. . . .	. . . .
F		0.030	0.070	0.135	0.280	0.080	0.160
G		0.023	0.066	0.128	0.256	0.073	0.147
H		0.028	0.071	0.142	0.303	0.078	0.158
K		0.025	0.068	0.145	0.307	0.071	0.140
L		0.024	0.065	0.130	0.288	0.080	0.160
Sum		0.238	0.700	1.381	2.786	0.679	1.355
Mean		0.0264	0.0700	0.1381	0.2786	0.0754	0.1505
Percent Recovery of Total Pb		125.7	100.0	95.2	95.7	100.5	100.3
Standard Deviation from Calcd. Value		0.0082	0.0078	0.0110	0.0227	0.0055	0.0098
Coefficient of Variation, %		41.0	11.1	7.6	7.8	7.3	6.5

(a) Unspiked blood sample containing 0.020 mg Pb per 100 grams of blood, as determined from analyses reported in table.
(b) Blood sample containing calculated 0.020 mg Pb per 100 grams spiked with 0.050, 0.125, or 0.271 mg inorganic Pb/100 gm.
(c) 1% nitric acid solutions spiked with indicated amounts of inorganic lead.
(d) Discarded.

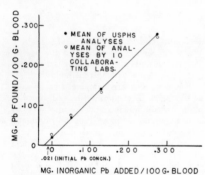

FIGURE 1. Evaluation of the method for lead in blood.

coefficients for the collaborators' results are about double those obtained by one chemist in our laboratory for the corresponding samples. However, it is pertinent to mention that the majority of these collaborating laboratories do not perform blood lead determinations on the routine basis that has been our practice for many years. Therefore, we believe that these data also demonstrate a remarkably good performance of this method for blood lead analyses.

Summary

The complete details of the USPHS method for the determination of lead in air and in biological materials have been presented. Also included is a rapid procedure for the removal of a known area of paint film from a sheet metal surface and the determination of its lead content in terms of percentage or of milligrams of lead per square inch of surface.

Complete information has been provided on the successful associated procedures for the cleaning of glassware, the collection of blood and urine samples, the transfer of atmospheric particulate samples for the ashing treatment after collection by the common sampling techniques, the wet ashing procedure using nitric acid, and the purification of reagents.

The method has been tested periodically with resulting minor procedural changes during the past quarter-century. The results of the most recent evaluation of the final method in this laboratory provided a mean lead recovery of 97.1% for lead in whole blood samples. The coefficient of variation was 9.5% for twelve replicate analyses of the pooled blood supply and it ranged from 4.0% to 5.6% for ten replicate sets of the other three blood samples which contained total lead ranging up to 0.291 milligram of lead per 100 grams of whole blood.

References

1. COMMITTEE ON CHEMICAL PROCEDURES OF THE OCCUPATIONAL HEALTH SECTION, AMERICAN PUBLIC HEALTH ASSOCIATION, INC.: *Methods for Determining Lead in Air and in Biological Materials.* American Public Health Association, Inc., 1790 Broadway, New York 19, N. Y. (1955).
2. SALTZMAN, B. E.: Matched Test Tubes in the Beckman DU Spectrophotometer. *Anal. Chem. 27:* 1207 (1955).
3. NELSON, KENNETH W.: Personal communication.
4. ELKINS, H. B., and B. P. W. RUOTOLO: Notes on Determination of Lead by Dithizone Method. Part II. Interference from Bismuth and Tin. *Amer. Ind. Hyg. Assoc. Quart. 14:* 111 (1953).

COMMENT

The "USPHS" method is free from interference except bismuth, thallium, and stannous tin. Tin, however, is oxidized to the noninterfering stannic form during ashing. Thallium and bismuth are currently seldom encountered in biologic samples. If bismuth is expected to be present, the APHA dithizone method or the atomic absorption or spectrographic methods described previously should be used.

LEAD IN FOODS

The standard methods of the Association of Analytical Chemists (formerly the Association of Official Agricultural Chemists), 1965[17] or 1970 Edition, should be consulted for the analysis of lead in foods. Procedures are given for the separation of lead from some metallic interference—notably, from tin present in canned foods, alkaline earth phosphates, bismuth, and iron in some food products—before analysis by the dithizone method.

Many food products contain substances that precipitate in the ammoniacal solution of the sample from which lead must be extracted as the dithizonate. These precipitates include the phosphates of calcium and magnesium, iron and aluminum hydroxides, and silicates. Lead is occluded in the precipitates and thus may be lost during the analysis. Substances containing more of these substances than can be kept in alkaline solution with the citric acid reagent must be subjected to a removal of lead as the sulfide after ashing. This may be accomplished by the following procedure.

Dissolve the ashed sample in hydrochloric acid. Add 20 ml of a 50% solution of lead-free citric acid, and adjust the pH to 3.0–3.4 with ammonium hydroxide, using bromophenol-blue indicator. If the iron content colors the solution strongly, a spot plate may be used to assist in adjusting the pH. If the anticipated lead content of the sample is small (less than 0.1 mg), 5–10 mg of lead-free copper sulfate ($CuSO_4 \cdot 5H_2O$) must be added to serve as a coprecipitant and "collector" of lead sulfide. Precipitate the sulfides by passing hydrogen sulfide into the solution for 3–5 min to achieve saturation. Then filter the solution immediately through a fine-fritted filter disk, using suction.

Dissolve the sulfides (without previous washing) with 5 ml of hot nitric acid, drawing solution through the filter disk into the original flask in which the samples had been gassed. Wash the filter with hot distilled water. Stopper the flask and shake to dissolve any sulfides adhering to the walls. Boil to expel residual hydrogen sulfide. The sample is now ready for analysis by the dithizone or other analytic procedure.

LEAD IN DUST AND SOILS

Lead in street or factory dusts[10, 51] should be dissolved by digesting and leaching with nitric acid (1 : 4) and hot 20% ammonium acetate. The extracts are filtered and analyzed, after appropriate dilution with distilled water, using one of the recommended dithizone, atomic absorption, or spectrographic methods. The selected dithizone method must be applied after proper provisions for the elimination of interfering substances. The atomic absorption and spectrographic methods are highly specific and may be used successfully. Care must always be taken to avoid molecular absorption errors with atomic absorption (the salt effect); this is accomplished by lowering the sample concentration in the solution as required for lead (or other elements) being analyzed.

The emission spectrograph, with its unparalleled degree of specificity, has been used to great advantage since 1933 for the determination of lead in biologic and environmental samples.[113, 115] This method offers the advantage of detecting and measuring simultaneously other elements that are in the sample and constitute possible interference with the dithizone method. Although its precision is not as great as that of the dithizone method, its error of measurement of lead may be reduced to about ±10% by the use of wisely selected internal standard and spectroscopic buffer conditions plus the analysis of biologic samples in triplicate. Industrial laboratories are using direct-reading spectrographs for routine, rapid analysis of many thousands of biologic samples of blood each year.[320] Under rigorously controlled conditions, this method has proved to be extremely reliable for the periodic blood lead analyses required for monitoring workers' exposures—an excellent example of a biologic monitoring technique. However, its expense puts the spectrograph beyond the budget of many hospitals and health departments.

Other methods that have been popular for lead analyses include electrolysis and polarography. However, these methods are capable of handling relatively few samples per day and still require extensive preliminary treatment of the samples to avoid spurious results.

Personal samplers are available from several manufacturers. These samplers are battery-operated; are complete with a rotameter, which should be calibrated with the sampling device attached in-line; and are used in monitoring individual worker exposure to dusts and fumes in mines and factories. A low cyclone attachment separates the collected particles into respirable and nonrespirable portions, the respirable portion being collected on a preweighed membrane filter. The sampling device is usually worn on the lapel in the approximate breathing zone; the pump is clipped to the belt. The use of this sampler permits the evaluation of a person's inhalation exposure to a dust or fume.

GENERAL COMMENTS ON METHODS FOR LEAD

The several published dithizone methods for lead will provide reliable data if the analyst is alert to the requirements of a high degree of purity of reagents, lead-free sample containers and laboratory glassware, lead-free Vacutainers and needles without a soldered joint, a thoroughly clean laboratory, and the isolation of glassware likely to have become contaminated with a "high-lead" sample until it has been deleaded. The last requirement is frequently overlooked and can cause spurious lead values in samples analyzed later in the same glassware. Extreme care must be taken to ensure the complete removal of traces of lead from such glassware, using hot nitric acid and rinsing; this glassware must be tested analytically to confirm that it has been completely freed of lead before permitting its reuse for any types of samples.

In wet-ashing biologic materials, care must be taken to avoid the "flashing" of samples, which always results in a loss of lead.

Molecular membrane filters are recommended, whenever feasible, for collecting particulate lead from the atmosphere. They are easily mounted for microscopic analysis, and they are readily digested with oxidizing acids, thus permitting rapid preparation of a sample for analysis. Airborne lead should be sampled at a height of 5–10 ft above ground level to keep the sampler above most of the coarser particles stirred up at ground level. In some studies conducted close to highways, it is necessary to use an elutriator to remove the coarse particles (greater than $10 \mu m$) before they reach the filter.

Several other methods for the quantitative determination of lead in biologic samples are being developed or are now in use. Further evaluation of these methods may be necessary to assess their value as analytic–diagnostic tools, but it is appropriate to mention them here.

The use of an ion-selective electrode consisting of a lead sulfide–silver sulfide crystal membrane has been used to determine lead in urine samples; a sensitivity down to the parts-per-billion level is claimed.[421] The method requires no sample preparation and is relatively rapid and inexpensive. The ion-selective electrode can measure only free ions; therefore, the method does not readily lend itself to the analysis of lead in blood, in which lead is usually bound to red cell constituents to a significant degree. Other blood proteins also may interfere with the electrodes. The method may prove applicable to hydrolyzed blood samples.

A method that requires relatively small amounts of sample, as well as very little sample preparation, is anodic stripping voltammetry (ASV). This method, as described by Matson,[374] relies on the concentration of an electroactive ion, such as lead, on a negative electrode during a relative long plating time (5–60 min). After plating, the polarity of the electrode is reversed and increased over a relatively short period (2–30 sec), resulting in a sharp current peak proportional to concentration. Sample treatment involves digestion of the sample in perchloric acid and dilution with water before ASV. Because different forms of the metals, as well as different organic complexes, will affect the plating kinetics of ASV, this method, in conjunction with other qualitative or quantitative methods, may lend itself to the study of the nature and kinetics of metallo-organic complexes in biologic and nonbiologic systems.

Hammer et al.[230] have recently used atomic absorption spectroscopy to analyze hair lead content and have demonstrated a correlation of hair lead content with environmental exposure to lead. Although the study did not attempt to relate hair lead content to clinical or subclinical illness, the use of hair samples to estimate subacute or chronic exposure to heavy metals is clearly feasible.

Appendix C

Data and Calculations for Figure 3-3

Blood Lead Content, $\mu g/100$ g Whole Blood	Air Lead Content, $\mu g/m^3$ Air	Total Daily Lead Assimilation, μg^a	
		At 30% Lung Retention	At 37% Lung Retention
12	0.12	30.83	31.02
16	0.5	33.45	34.26
13	1.0	36.90	38.51
21	1.0	36.90	38.51
19	1.9	43.11	46.17
19	2.2	45.18	48.72
24	2.4	46.56	50.42
25	2.2	45.18	48.72
30	3.8	56.22	62.34
31	4.2	58.98	65.74
21	5.2	65.88	74.25
31	5.5	67.95	76.81
30	6.3	73.47	83.61
48^b	2.0	148.80^c	152.02^c
63^d	2.0	221.30^c	224.52^c

^{a}Assumptions: 23 m^3/day inhaled air; 30 μg/day lead assimilated from food and water; data from California Department of Public Health.[80]
^{b}Subject M.R.[298]
^{c}Daily oral lead intake: of M.R., 1.350 mg; of E.B., 2.075 mg;[298] 10% absorption assumed.
^{d}Subject E.B.[298]

Appendix D

Collection and Storage of Biologic Samples

Valid analytic data require not only reproducible and accurate analytic techniques, but also great care to prevent either contamination or losses of lead and metabolites during collection, transport, and storage of biologic samples. A number of reports refer to the collection of blood and urine in "plastic" containers and the use of "plastic" syringes and "disposable" needles. With the introduction of newer microtechniques of analysis, specimen collection will require even greater care than in the past.

Polypropylene and Teflon are the preferred plastic materials for trace metals analysis, so blood and urine are best collected with polypropylene syringes and sample containers. Similarly, needles should be of stainless steel with a polypropylene hub. Vacuum tubes of silica glass designated as "lead-free" are also in wide use and are suitable. Anticoagulants (such as heparin or citrate) added to blood-collection outfits and acids or other preservatives added to urine must be shown on analysis to be "lead-free" (i.e., maximal permissible quantity of lead should be insignificant in relation to the quantity of lead in the sample). In general, collection equipment must be washed in mineral acids and then rinsed in copious amounts of water that has been "deionized" by passage through mixed ion-exchange resin beds; such water (resistance, 2–3 $\times 10^6$ ohms) may contain up to 200 ppb of lead.[445] In general, specimen collectors should be obtained either from an experienced laboratory performing the analyses or with their advice regarding the use of commercially available special lead-free equipment. In general, for urine containing CaEDTA (from patients receiving the drug), addition of hydrochloric acid to the collection bottle permits analysis for both lead and ALA and storage of urine for up to several weeks before analysis.

The stability of ALA[226] and coproporphyrin[226, 486] in urine has been studied and reported. The data may be summarized as follows: Samples are preferably collected and stored in the dark at 4 C. Repeated thawing and freezing can result in serious losses, so freezing should be avoided. ALA is stable in acid urine (pH, 1–5), so an acid preservative, such as hydrochloric or, possibly, glacial acetic acid, is needed, unless the analysis is carried out within a few hours. For 24-hr collections, enough acid must be added to yield a final concentration of 0.001–0.1 N.[106] The ALA content of acidified and refrigerated urine specimens remains constant for several months. Schwartz et al.[486] noted that unpreserved urine samples should be analyzed for coproporphyrin within 30 min because of the instability of this substance at the usual acid pH of urine. Samples collected and preserved with sufficient sodium carbonate to yield a final pH of 6.5–8.5 are suitable for analysis for up to 10 days if kept refrigerated in dark bottles. For 24-hr collections, sulfanilamide may be added to sodium carbonate in the collection bottle to suppress bacterial growth (J. J. Chisolm, Jr., unpublished data).

The most widely used method of determining ALA in serum is that of Haeger-Aronsen,[226] who analyzed her samples within 5 hr. Hernberg et al.[247] found that ALAD activity, as measured by the technique of Bonsignore et al.,[57] was stable up to 5 hr at 3, 25, and 30 C, but all analyses in their laboratory were done within 3 hr of sampling. Millar et al.,[391] who used a somewhat different technique for measuring ALAD activity in red blood cells, carried out the analysis within 1 hr of sampling. The available reports do not include data on the stability of protoporphyrin and coproporphyrin in blood; in view of the known difficulties in handling these substances in the laboratory, it is suggested that protoporphyrin and coproporphyrin determinations in blood be carried out as soon as possible.

Measurement of lead in blood and urine provides at once indices of exposure and absorption. Lead in these fluids may be measured by spectral analysis, the colorimetric dithizone technique, atomic ab-

sorption spectrophotometry (AAS), polarography, and anodic stripping voltammetry (ASV); these methods are discussed in Appendix B.
Each technique requires suitable preparation of the sample before
final determination. Spectral analysis is considered the most accurate,
but its use is limited by economic considerations. Polarography is
widely used in Europe but not in the United States. In the United
States, the dithizone technique and AAS find the widest use for lead
determinations in clinical laboratories. Long experience with and re-
finement of the dithizone technique make it the standard of reference. A minimum of 0.5 µg (preferably 1 µg) of lead in the final
sample volume is needed for accurate results. For blood, this requires
a sample of 5–15 ml. In recent years, because of the time-consuming
and exacting requirements of the dithizone method, AAS has been
explored in the hope of speeding and simplifying the analytic procedure and reducing the sample volume needed for accurate analysis
in blood and urine. Methods have sometimes been hastily introduced
without reference to comparability with older methods. Selander and
Cramér have published an AAS method for measuring lead in urine[489]
that shows excellent agreement with a dithizone technique. Their
AAS methods[488] for lead in blood give results that, even at low concentrations, are comparable with the results of spectral analysis.
These and other reports make it clear that important interference
does exist and must be corrected in AAS techniques: (1) In sample-
preparation techniques that omit the ashing or wet-digestion step,
blood and urine must be totally free of clots and particulate matter,
to avoid low recoveries. (2) With single-beam AAS instruments, the
sample must be read not only at an absorbing lead line (2170 or
2833 Å), but also at an adjacent nonabsorbing lead line, to correct for nonspecific light-scattering and light-absorbing effects.
(3) Double-beam AAS instruments with provisions for background
correction presumably accomplish the same correction, but the published data are inadequate to evaluate this point. (4) An ultraviolet-
sensitive photomultiplier is essential when the 2170 Å line is used for
analysis. Micro-AAS techniques[148] and ASV techniques[374] have the
potential for measuring lead in nanogram and subnanogram quantities
and hence may reduce the sample requirement for blood to less than
0.2 ml, which is readily obtainable by capillary sampling; these techniques are currently being developed.

Regardless of the method used, it is clear that the analyzing laboratory should be experienced in the technique, have experienced personnel, be performing lead analyses regularly, and incorporate ade-

quate quality and specificity control measures into its procedures. These factors are especially important when low concentrations of lead in blood and urine are being measured. It is unlikely that a laboratory that performs such analysis only occasionally will produce consistent and reliable results. A recent report[307] showing wide discrepancy between different laboratories points up the further need for interlaboratory studies when new techniques are introduced and at other times to ensure maintenance of adequate standards of quality with established techniques.

APPENDIX E Summary of Toxicologic Data on Experimental Lead Poisoning

Ref. No.	Type of Study	No. Animals Used[a]	Material Given	Dosage[b]	Route of Administration[c]	Result
63	Acute	150	Lead acetate	?	IP	MLD_{50}: 15 mg Pb/100 g body wt
			Lead monoxide	?	IP	MLD_{50}: 40 mg Pb/100 g body wt
			Lead orthoplumbate	?	IP	MLD_{50}: 45 mg Pb/100 g body wt
			Lead tartrate	?	IP	MLD_{50}: 70 mg Pb/100 g body wt
			Lead sulfide	?	IP	MLD_{50}: 160 mg Pb/100 g body wt
			Metallic lead (325 mesh)	>100 mg Pb/100 g body wt	IP	No deaths to 40 days
69	Acute	?	Lead acetate in H_2O	130 mg/kg	IP	Died in 2 days; kidney, liver, spleen, and tissue damage
	Acute	?	Lead thiocyanate in H_2O	70–100 mg/kg	IP	Lived several weeks; acute tubular nephritis; blood changes; appearance of normoblasts, anisocytosis, poikilocytosis, achromia, polychromatophilia, Hb reading
	Acute	?	Lead thiocyanate	150 mg/kg	SC	Survived; blood changes; local necrosis; kidney, liver, spleen, and tissue damage
	Acute	?	Lead potassium thiocyanate	42 mg/kg	IP	All animals dead in 3 days[d]
	Acute	?	Lead nitrate	120–330 mg/kg	IP, SC	Some animals died within 2.5 hr; others survived with nephritis and inflamed liver; others lived several weeks with kidney, liver, spleen, and tissue damage
	Acute	?	Loeser's colloidal lead	?	IP	[e]
	Acute	?	Glyceroplumbonitrate in glycol	50 mg/kg	IP	"Killed rapidly"
	Acute	?	Lead diphenyl propionate in olive oil	55 mg/kg	IP	"Is lethal"
	Acute	?	Lead diphenyl nitrate in H_2O	?	IP	MLD, "about" 20 mg/kg; marked blood changes absent

Ref	Duration	No.	Compound	Dose	Route	Effects
	Acute	5	Triethyl lead phosphate in H_2O	5–21 mg/kg	IP, SC	1 survived, others lived up to 2 days; MLD, 5–8.5 mg/kg
	Acute	5	Triethyl lead chloride	5–8 mg/kg	IP, SC	1 survived, others lived 3–8 days; MLD, 5 mg/kg; CNS signs and low body temperature
	Acute	8	Trimethyl lead chloride in H_2O	9–20 mg/kg	IP	5 survived, 2 with CNS signs at 1–5 weeks; 3 lived 8–9 days, with CNS signs at 3–4 days; MLD, approx. 17.0 mg/kg
	Acute	11	Tripropyl lead chloride in ethanol	3–14 mg/kg	IP, SC	1 survived, others lived 1 hr–7 days; MLD, <3 mg/kg; abdominal irritation; fluid
	Acute	8	Tributyl lead chloride in ethanol	2–7 mg/kg	IP	1 survived; others lived 2 min–4 days; MLD, 2 mg/kg; prostration; Cheyne-Stokes respiration[f]
	Acute	10	Tetraethyl lead in olive oil	11–46 mg/kg	IP	Lived 2–8 days; MLD, approx. 10 mg/kg; 8 had CNS signs at 2–6 days; some weakness and nose discharge
	Acute	5[g]	Tetraethyl lead in 20% gum arabic	14–38 mg/kg	IV	Died within 1 day; MLD, 15–30 mg/kg
	Acute	17	Tetramethyl lead in olive oil	23–101 mg/kg	IP	15 survived with mild reversible CNS signs; 2 lived 6–7 days, with CNS signs at 4 days; watery eye and nose discharge; MLD, 70–100 mg/kg
	Acute	13[g]	Tetramethyl lead in 20% gum arabic	62–159 mg/kg	IV	3 survived with no CNS signs; 2 survived, with CNS signs at 3–8 days; 8 lived 3–7 days, some with CNS signs; MLD, 70–100 mg/kg; little blood picture change
566	Acute	50[h]	Lead arsenate	300–1,000 mg/kg	PO	LD_{50}: 450 mg/kg
	Acute	60	Lead arsenate	500–1,000 mg/kg	PO	LD_{50}: 825 mg/kg
	Acute	63[g]	Lead arsenate	20–200 mg/kg	PO	LD_{50}: 125 mg/kg
434	Chronic	?	Lead acetate	3.3 mEq/kg 3 × per wk for 63 days	PO	Oral lead acetate delayed intestinal H_2O, IV lead did not; wt increase of stomach, small intestine, liver, kidneys, and adrenals
	Chronic	?	Lead acetate	13.3 mEq/kg 3 × per wk or less for 98 days	PO	
	Acute	?	Lead acetate	0.67 mEq/kg	IV	

APPENDIX E (Continued)

Ref. No.	Type of Study	No. Animals Used[a]	Material Given	Dosage[b]	Route of Administration[c]	Result
434	Acute	5	Lead acetate	6.7 mEq/kg (PO) and 0.33 mEq/kg (IV)	PO, IV	Antidiuretic effect of nicotine increased with large dose of lead acetate
13	Chronic	12	Lead acetate	1% of diet for 24 weeks	PO	Inclusion bodies found in kidneys after 2 months on diet
353	Chronic	7	Lead acetate	512 mg/kg diet for about 70–90 days	PO	Fasted (7–8 days) rats with lead had lower rate of protein catabolism measured by liver arginase concentrations
	Acute, fed	8	Lead acetate	21–22.5 mg total in 10–11 days	IP	
	Acute, fasted	8	Lead acetate	4.5 mg total in last 3 days of fast	IP	
563	Chronic	32	Basic lead acetate	0.1% of diet for 29 months	PO	Decreased rate of growth; normal blood; kidney tumors after 1½ yr; chronic interstitial nephritis; calcium deposits
	Chronic	24	Basic lead acetate	1.0% of diet for 24 months	PO	Anemia; kidney tumors after 1 yr; inclusion bodies in convoluted tubules after 1 month
151	Chronic	30	Lead acetate	90 mg/day for 50 days; every 7th day omitted	T	Hypertension; no significant blood vessel alteration; basophilic cytoplasmic inclusions in kidney and liver
100	Chronic	?	Lead acetate	2 cc of 4.5% daily for 9–365 days	T	No blood pressure change; increased kidney weight; degenerative lesions in cells of Henle's loop
99	Chronic	9	Lead acetate	2 cc of 4.5% daily	T	With 40% fat diet, death in 6–19 days, stomach dilatation, liver hypertrophy, fatty infiltration, and necrosis; without excess fat, no hepatic damage or death during experiment
412	Chronic	17	Lead acetate	2% in drinking H_2O 4 to 12 months	PO	Cystic changes in kidney; renal tumors; enlarged kidneys; decreased renal radio-

No.	Exposure	Ref.	Compound	Dose	Route	Effects
						active Hg uptake; decreased urinary osmolality
219	Chronic	15	Lead acetate	90 mg/day for 80 days; every 7th day omitted	T	All rats that survived 40 days were hypertensive
162	Chronic	20	Lead acetate	1% of diet for 1 year	PO	Kidney tumors in 15; adenomas; some carcinomas
403	Chronic	18	Lead acetate.	64 mg/kg diet for 1 year	PO	No change in fertility or fecundity; maternal transfer of lead to fetus: newborn had 8 times lead of controls
18	Chronic	18	Lead acetate	512 mg/kg diet for 1 year	PO	No change in fertility or fecundity; newborn had 40 times lead of controls
37	Chronic	20	Basic lead acetate	0.05%, 0.1%, 1.0% in H_2O; 1% in H_2O + 10 g% in food; for 7 months	PO	Intranuclear inclusions in proximal convoluted tubules of kidneys at 0.1% or higher
481	Chronic	104[i]	Lead acetate	5 ppm in H_2O for 36 months	PO	Not carcinogenic; incidence of tumors in males decreased; male longevity decreased; no lead accumulation noted
467	Chronic	3[j]	Lead acetate	289 mg Pb in 113 days; 9.5 g Pb in 143 days; 10.4 g Pb in 160 days	PO	1 died; all had increased coproporphyrin excretion and porphyrinuria
184	Chronic	1[j]	Lead acetate	32.5 g Pb over 3 years	T	No blood pressure change; 5 acute attacks of lead poisoning
	Chronic	1[j]	Lead acetate	1.9 g Pb	T	No blood pressure change; died at unspecified time of 2nd acute attack
298	Chronic	4[k]	Lead acetate or lead chloride	0.3, 1, 2, 3 mg Pb per day for 16 weeks–4 yr	PO	No clinical symptoms; increased lead content in urine and blood
	Chronic	1[k]	Lead sesquioxide	0.075, 0.15 mg Pb/m^3 per 37.5-hr week for 40 weeks	H	No systemic changes or progressive hematologic or urinary changes
332	Acute	6	Lead acetate in H_2O	77 mg Pb for 24 hr	A	1.8 µg Pb/g of kidney (wet wt)
	Acute	8	Lead orthoarsenate paste	102 mg Pb for 24 hr	A	0.85 µg Pb/g of kidney (wet wt)
63	Acute	12	Lead oleate ointment	148 mg Pb for 24 hr	A	1.3 µg Pb/g of kidney (wet wt)
	Acute	5	Tetraethyl lead	106 mg Pb for 24 hr	A	64.2 µg Pb/g of kidney (wet wt)

Ref. No.	Type of Study	No. Animals Used[a]	Material Given	Dosage[b]	Route of Administration[c]	Result
333	Chronic	14	Lead arsenate	3.53 mg Pb in 63–101 days	PO	Males had decreased growth rate, but not females; lead storage in femora, liver, kidneys, brain, and hair
	Chronic	32	Lead arsenate	1,320 mg Pb in 6–7 weeks (213 mg/kg body wt daily)	PO	Males and females had decreased growth rate; kidney and spleen hypertrophy and lead storage
81	Chronic	20[j]	Lead acetate or lead arsenate	12.8, 38.4, 64.0 mg Pb/kg diet or 0.32–2.56 mg Pb/kg average body wt daily for 15–356 days	PO	No difference in toxicity between acetate and arsenate; high retention in bone, kidney, liver; newborn pup of dam on lead had high lead content; 15 died of severe lead poisoning in 15–229 days; all had behavioral and CNS changes
63	Chronic	10[g]	Lead acetate	30 mg Pb/kg, 5 × in 16 days	PO	Killed 40–90 days later; basophilic cells rose sharply; "typical lead poisoning"
			Lead carbonate	200 mg Pb/kg, 5 × in 16 days	PO	
			Lead monoxide	200 mg Pb/kg, 5 × in 16 days	PO	
384	Chronic	3[l]	Lead arsenate	2 g/day	PO	2 died after 3½ days, 1 after 7 days; hemorrhagic erosions of lumen wall; severe enteritis; pneumonia
	Chronic	6	Lead arsenate	1.0, 0.5, 0.25 g/day, 3½–35 days	PO	5 died within 35 days; black bone marrow; temporary polycythemia
317	Chronic	16[m]	Lead carbonate	150 mg/day for 3 days; followed for 30 days	PO	Early punctiphilia, polychromatophilia, reticulocytosis, and normoblastic output; temporary marrow block; no tolerance by hemolytic and hematopoietic systems with repeated leading; no correlation between fatalities and blood crises

175	Chronic	53	Lead carbonate	15 mg $PbCO_3$/day for 6 weeks	PO	Lead deposited in softer tissues, diminished after 2 weeks on normal diet; lead in bone increased; reversible severe kidney damage and spleen changes
564	Chronic	11[n]	Lead chloride	10 mg/week for 1 month, then 20 mg/week for 7 months	IV	Anemia; basophilic stippling of red blood cells; increased urinary lead excretion; albuminuria; reversible depression of estrogenic activity; microscopic damage to primordial oöcytes
597	Chronic	?	Lead phosphate	20 mg/week (total dose, 40–760 mg)	SC	Adenoma, papilloma, and cystadenoma of renal cortex in 16 months
136	Chronic	78 pairs	Metallic lead in lubricating-grease–contaminated diet	3.5 mg/100 g diet (0.5–12 mg) for 9 months	PO	High incidence of death at birth of second generation; stunted growth; anemia of survivors in second generation
391	Chronic	?	Lead acetate	4% Pb in maternal diet, 30–40 days	PO	Suckling rats had significant increase in lead in kidneys, liver, spleen, and blood; decreased ALAD in liver, brain, and blood
54	Acute	34	210Pb-labeled lead acetate	1 mg Pb/kg	IV	8 animals' excretion 50% injected Pb in 1 week, observed 98 days after single dose; 100% "immediately" in blood, heart, lungs, liver, kidneys, spleen, gastrointestinal tract, 7% in 1 week; muscles, skin, 11% after 1 day to 8% after 1 week; bones, tail, 40% after 1 week

[a]Rats unless specified otherwise.
[b]mg/kg = milligrams of "material given" per kilogram of body weight, unless otherwise specified.
[c]IP = intraperitoneal, SC = subcutaneous, IV = intravenous, PO = per os, T = intubation, H = inhalation, A = skin application.
[d]Authors do not think this result is correct.
[e]Author's comment: same effect as of inorganic lead salts.
[f]Author's comment: results similar to those with propyl lead.
[g]Rabbits.   [k]Men.
[h]Chickens.   [l]Sheep.
[i]Mice.   [m]Guinea pigs.
[j]Dogs.   [n]Rhesus monkeys.

Appendix F

Treatment and Costs of Lead Poisoning in Man

TREATMENT OF LEAD POISONING

The management of asymptomatic increased lead absorption (arbitrarily defined as a blood lead concentration greater than 50 μg/100 g of whole blood in the presence of a normal hematocrit) and symptomatic acute lead poisoning in man consists of two interdependent components: separation from nonoccupational sources of exposure to lead and selective use of chelating agents as an important adjunct for the rapid safe reduction of high lead content in the soft tissues. Control of environmental exposure is the *sine qua non* of any treatment program. The adjunctive use of chelating agents should be instituted at the asymptomatic stage of illness. The need for this approach is supported by the evidence that single episodes of acute encephalopathy and recurrent episodes of less severe acute lead poisoning may be associated with irreversible injury to the nervous system and kidneys.[78, 106, 110, 168, 169, 354, 402, 442, 452] Chelating agents have been used almost exclusively for the treatment of acute lead intoxication; brief courses of chelation therapy have not been shown to mobilize the entire body lead burden, as estimated by the CaEDTA mobilization test.[106] In the case of occupational exposures, separation from the source is readily achieved by a variety of means known to industrial physicians and plant sanitarians. Selander and Cramér[490] have presented evidence that rotation of workers may, in some conditions, minimize exposure. In cases of lead poisoning associated with the burning of battery casings, improperly lead-glazed culinary ware, and other unusual sources of lead, the patient can be quickly and permanently separated from the source once it is identified. If undue exposure can be quickly controlled, asymptomatic patients with blood lead concentrations less than about 70 or 80 $\mu g/100$ g of whole blood may be treated on an ambulatory basis, and patients with higher blood lead content, with or without symptoms, may require only brief periods of hospitalization for parenteral injection of chelating agents and supportive care. However, when the environmental exposure and other social and behavioral factors cannot be controlled quickly, prolonged hospitalization is necessary if the patient is to be separated effectively from such environmental exposures as leaded paint in deteriorating housing or lead-contaminated whiskey. The medical literature contains one report of the treatment of children with pica for lead paint on an ambulatory basis, including some cases of encephalopathy;[465] the authors deemed the ambulatory-treatment program a success, in the sense that there were no fatalities; but the adequacy of the environmental control measures cannot be judged from this report, and no evaluation of residual effects is given. The treatment of children with blood lead concentrations greater than 80 $\mu g/100$ g of whole blood on an ambulatory basis may involve considerable risk to the patients in view of the very high levels of absorption associated with this type of exposure (Figure 4–2 and Table 4–6).

There is considerable clinical experience with three chelating agents that are effective in lead poisoning: calcium disodium ethylenediaminetetraacetic acid (CaEDTA), 2,3-dimercaptopropanol (BAL), and D-penicillamine. Diethylenetriaminepentaacetic acid (DTPA) and dimercaptosuccinic acid (DMS) have received only brief clinical investigative trials. CaEDTA and BAL are effective only when administered by injection.[106] Both parenteral and oral preparations of D-penicillamine are available in Europe. Few comparative studies have been reported, but one report indicated that D-penicillamine is almost as effective as CaEDTA when given parenterally, but less effective when given orally.[491] In the United States, parenteral preparations of D-penicillamine are not available, and the single oral preparation (205-mg capsules) for adults is currently classified as an investigational drug by the Food and Drug Administration (FDA) when used for the treatment of lead poisoning. (Its use for the treatment of Wilson's disease and cystinuria is not restricted.)

Chisolm[106] has proposed that the choice in dosage of chelating agents should be based on the physician's estimate of the mobile fraction of the body lead burden in patients with current and recent increased lead absorption. Thus, the highest doses consistent with safety would be indicated in the patients estimated to have the highest lead content in the soft tissues. Limited clinical experience indicated that the simultaneous administration of BAL and CaEDTA is more effective in terms of survival, reversal of metabolic toxicity, and rate of reduction of soft-tissue lead content than is CaEDTA alone in patients with acute symptomatic lead poisoning and in patients with blood lead concentrations greater than 80 μg/100 g of whole blood without symptoms but with known gross exposure. Although they are more efficacious in some situations, the intramuscular use of CaEDTA and the higher doses of BAL used in this regimen are not currently approved by the FDA. In patients with lower blood lead content, either parenteral CaEDTA or oral D-penicillamine provides adequate therapy.[106, 198, 491] The rationale for this approach, critical aspects of supportive therapy, and adverse drug reactions are reviewed elsewhere.[106, 198] Limited clinical data suggest that the use of D-penicillamine in patients with renal insufficiency must be approached with great caution; further experience may prove that it is contraindicated in such patients. The incidence of adverse drug reactions cannot be estimated from the available clinical data, although experimental studies indicate that adverse reactions are dose-related.[182]

It has been reported that the excretion of heme precursors in urine, as quantitatively measured in 24-hr samples, provides the best index of the quantity of lead that will be excreted under the influence of chelating agents and a better index of the "chelatable lead" in subjects with current and recent abnormal exposure to lead than blood and urine lead content.[109, 131] This is particularly useful in asymptomatic subjects with blood lead content of 50–80 μg/100 g of whole blood and acute or intermittent abnormal exposure to lead. In such patients, there may be considerable variation in the adverse metabolic responses to lead and the need for chelation therapy.

Alternatively, the response to chelating agents can be measured directly by determining urinary lead output during therapy. Therapy should be terminated when the diuresis of lead diminishes toward normal. However, only oral D-penicillamine can be given practically and safely on a continuous basis for more than a few days.[106, 198] Although the above statements are based entirely on the limited clinical reports of a few authors, it should be noted that chelation therapy without careful clinical supervision may be dangerous. Facilities for determination of lead in urine or blood and for repeated evaluation of a patient are essential for the proper use of chelating agents.

The lack of wider clinical experience and a more systematic approach to chelation therapy can be traced largely to the general unavailability of the necessary laboratory techniques in the general community (especially blood and urine lead analyses). Even accurate analyses are of little clinical use in the day-to-day management of patients if the results are not immediately available. At present, the use of chelating agents varies widely from clinic to clinic and is based largely on clinical evaluation and whatever laboratory techniques happen to be available in a particular clinic.

In patients with asymptomatic increased lead absorption, chelation therapy promptly suppresses the adverse metabolic effects of lead on heme synthesis. Because the subclinical effects of lead on the nervous system are not well defined, no evaluation can be made in this regard. Limited data with respect to kidney function indicate that the Fanconi syndrome[106] and the altered renin–aldosterone response to sodium deprivation are reversible and respond quickly to chelation therapy.[101, 106, 378] In patients with chronic nephropathy, CaEDTA has been used largely for diagnostic purposes only.[168, 169, 402, 442] The scarring and other permanent tissue damage reported in such patients make it unlikely that they would be responsive to chelation therapy. The spectrum of renal injury suggests, however, that subclinical functional renal injury may be reversible at some point before the late and apparently irreversible form in which it is now recognized clinically. No evaluation of the efficacy of chelation therapy in this type of patient has been found in the literature. With respect to encephalopathy, it is clear that at least 25% of childhood survivors sustain permanent and often profound brain damage, regardless of the form of therapy used. The efficacy of chelation therapy as it may relate to minimal cerebral injury is unknown.

In summary, the available but limited data suggest that chelation therapy should be instituted in patients with increased absorption and storage of lead. Soft-tissue concentrations of lead definitely should be maintained well below those associated with clear-cut clinical symptoms and functional injury. Chelation therapy is effective for this purpose, provided that subsequent exposure is controlled. There are insufficient data to judge the extent to which an excessive body burden of lead, once accumulated, can be safely and effectively mobilized. Control of hazardous exposure offers the most effective means of preventing the accumulation of an increased body lead burden. Chelation therapy is of limited efficacy in persons with acute encephalopathy, in terms of the occurrence of central nervous system sequelae in survivors, despite therapy.

DIRECT MEDICAL COSTS OF LEAD POISONING

No comprehensive estimate of total medical and related expenses attributable to lead poisoning can be made at this time because of the many medical and environmental factors involved. In general, the type of exposure, the age of the patient, and the severity, recurrence, and sequelae of the illness are the important variables that influence total direct medical costs in cases of human lead poisoning. In cases associated with circumscribed types of exposure (e.g., occupational exposures) or such sources as unsafe earthenware culinary items, direct medical costs may be limited to the costs of brief hospitalization and professional care. Provided that treatment is instituted before the occurrence of irreversible tissue injury and that hazardous exposure is promptly terminated, no further direct medical expenses would be anticipated. In cases associated with late diagnosis, "high-dose" types of exposure, and the initiation of medical treatment after the occurrence of irreversible tissue injury, even a single episode of acute encephalopathy without re-exposure will entail long-term medical expense for the sequelae of severe acute lead poisoning. In cases associated with uncontrolled types of environmental exposure, the likelihood of recurrence of acute illness, recurrent hospitalization, and expenses related to permanent injury is increased. Recurrent exposure and illness are major considerations in children with pica, in unsupervised small-shop occupational situations, and in the use of moonshine whiskey.

In young children, separation from exposure is the essential component of therapy; therefore, hospitalization is frequently indicated. Outpatient treatment with daily injections of chelating agents in children with persistent pica and continued intense environmental exposure is neither effective nor humane. Outpatient treatment may reduce public medical expense, but it increases costs to the parents of the affected children in the form of transportation costs, loss of time from work, and neglect of other members of the family. The epidemiology of childhood lead poisoning is such that these costs fall most heavily and directly on the poor, who are least able to pay.

Treatment costs may be divided into six general categories: (1) direct medical costs for acute and convalescent care, (2) after-care and excess school costs for the partially brain-damaged, (3) custodial care for the permanently and severely injured, (4) correction of hazards in housing, (5) preventive health supervision, and (6) supporting municipal and state health-department activities.

No broad generalizations concerning the economic impact of childhood lead poisoning can be made at this time. Diagnostic and treatment facilities vary widely among communities, few of which have programs that can be considered either comprehensive or wholly adequate. However, limited experience in one community with regard to direct medical expenses in a group of 45 children may be illuminating. These children were treated under the general medical policy that no child, when found to have increased lead absorption, with or without symptoms, is returned to a "leaded" home. Under this medical policy, the child is first treated in a general hospital for a brief period and then placed in a convalescent facility until a safe dwelling* is found for the family. (At present, Baltimore, Maryland, is the only U.S. city known to have such an "extended pediatric care" or convalescent facility for young children.)

Table F–1 lists actual direct medical costs incurred in 1965–1970 by a group of 45 children with increased lead absorption. The group of 45 included 10 survivors of acute encephalopathy. The average total time of acute and convalescent hospitalization was 100 days, and the average direct hospital cost for 34 patients was $2,746. Almost all these children were hospitalized at public expense in hospitals that at the time of hospitalization had a blanket basic charge and did not charge for such extras as special nursing and intensive care. Not represented in Table F–1 are the two highest hospital bills, which were over $8,000 each. In one instance, the high cost resulted from repeated hospitalization for complications of encephalopathy, and in the other, from an excessively long wait for admission to public housing. This experience is not unique, and the cost would be greater in other cities where children are retained in general hospitals for periods of 1–3 months while informal quests for safe housing go on. In view of the rapid rise in hospital costs during the last 5 years, it can

---

*"Safe dwelling" in this sense is defined as modern public housing or adequately repaired old housing.

TABLE F-1 Total Days of Hospitalization and Estimated Direct Medical Costs for 45 Children with Initial Blood Lead Content Greater Than 80 $\mu g/100$ g of Whole Blood (Including 10 Children with Acute Encephalopathy) Who Are Not Discharged to Home until Removal of Old Lead-Pigment Paints from Home Environment—Baltimore, Maryland, 1965–1970

	Duration of Hospitalization, Days		
	Acute Care (General Hospital)	Convalescent Care (Happy Hills Hospital)	Total
Total	1,108	3,402	4,510
Mean per patient	24.7	75.7	100.4
Median per patient	21	50	71
Range (80% of patients)	4–70	20–203	25–253

	Actual Costs for 34 Patients, $[a]
Total	93,377
Mean per patient	2,746
Median per patient	2,175
Range (90% of patients)	1,068–4,814

[a]Basic hospital rates roughly doubled between 1965 and 1970. Most of the 34 children for whom complete hospital charges could be verified were hospitalized during 1965, 1966, and 1967 at public expense.

be estimated that direct hospital costs for the 45 children shown in Table F-1 would average $5,486 in 1970 (Table F-2). Chelation therapy with BAL and CaEDTA followed by oral administration of D-penicillamine requires an average of only 10 days of hospitalization. Asymptomatic children do not require treatment in a general hospital; they can be handled in a convalescent facility at a lower cost. Under

TABLE F-2 Estimated Current Average Direct Medical Costs to 45 Children, Based on 1970 Basic Hospital Rates in Baltimore, Maryland[a]

	Estimated Costs, $		
	Acute Care	Convalescent Care	Total
Unit	100/day	40/day	—
Total	110,800 (1,108 days)	136,080 (3,402 days)	246,880 (4,510 days)
Mean per patient	2,462 (24.6 days)	3,024 (75.6 days)	5,486 (100.2 days)

[a]Children were handled under the general policy that no child is discharged until home is "deleaded" or family moves into safe modern housing; length of hospitalization is determined by this factor, rather than by severity of acute illness.

these circumstances, hospital costs beyond 10 days are attributable directly to delays in the completion of necessary housing repairs. Baltimore allows up to 6 weeks for completion of housing repairs before legal action is taken. New York and Philadelphia now limit the time allowed for compliance, repair an apartment at municipal expense, and take out a lien on the property to recover the costs.

Sustained medical follow-up for children with pica who live in substandard old housing is indicated for preventive purposes throughout the years of pica or for an average period of 3 years. The current costs for this are estimated at $120, on the basis of a fee of $15 per outpatient clinic visit. For those with lead poisoning, the follow-up period ranges from 2 to 10 years, or $225–675 per patient. The salary of a medical social worker or comparable paramedical personnel at one worker per 50 cases should be added to this figure. For children with moderately severe permanent brain damage who require special schooling, excess school costs related to transportation costs and smaller classes are currently estimated at $1,200 per pupil per year, or $14,400 for 12 years of school through high school for each damaged child. For children who require institutionalization for custodial care, current costs at the Rosewood State Hospital in Maryland are approximately $4,000 per year per patient. Data for other institutions in Maryland where such patients have been hospitalized in the past are not available, and comparable data from other parts of the country are not immediately available to the Panel. During the last 13 years, 19 children have been admitted to the Rosewood State Hospital as a result of lead encephalopathy during early childhood (J. J. Chisolm, Jr., personal communication); one has died and two have recently been given leave of absence, leaving 16 children in residence at a current cost of $64,000 per annum. These patients have been hospitalized for a total of 148 patient-years, or 7.7 years per patient. None of the 16 remaining in residence is considered suitable for discharge. If they survive to the age of 65, the expenditure for 60 years of institutional care at $4,000 per annum would be about $240,000 per severely damaged child. The total direct medical cost can therefore be roughly estimated, according to the final clinical outcome, as follows: (1) asymptomatic increased lead absorption without obvious residual permanent injury, $1,500–2,000 per patient; (2) moderate permanent brain damage (special schooling required), $18,000 per patient; and (3) severe permanent brain damage (institutional care required), $245,000 per patient at current medical costs.

These direct treatment costs may be contrasted with the cost of the repairs to substandard housing to eliminate the paint hazard. In Baltimore, estimated costs range from $150 to $1,200 per apartment, depending on the extent of repairs needed. New York City estimates costs at $1,263 per apartment.[514] Because New York City repairs many apartments itself through the municipal emergency repair program, actual figures may be available soon; the program was instituted in April 1970. Adequate housing repair is therefore comparable in dollars with the direct medical costs of treatment of a single asymptomatic child with increased body lead burden. Also, repairs to substandard housing can prevent lead poisoning in all the children who may live in a given house during the remainder of the house's useful existence. If houses were inspected and repaired before the onset of pica, direct medical costs could be totally eliminated.

Preventive health care costs for children cannot be precisely estimated. The program in New York City is the only comprehensive program in the United States. New York City estimates such costs at $12.50 per child for initial case finding and $6.51 per child for each follow-up visit, including blood lead tests. Current research is aimed at reducing the cost of screening both children and housing through improved techniques with a potential for automation and portability for field testing.

Appendix G

Treatment and Costs of Lead Poisoning in Cattle

Lead poisoning of domestic animals is generally considered to be a disease of low morbidity and high mortality. In general, it is felt by clinicians that, if an animal lives, the prognosis for recovery is good. For example, many calves are blind during acute manifestations of the disease. If a calf lives, sight usually returns within a week, at least enough for the animal to move about with no difficulty.

TREATMENT OF LEAD POISONING

The chelating agent calcium disodium ethylenediaminetetraacetate (CaEDTA), used as a successful treatment for lead poisoning in man, has also been used successfully as an antidote for lead poisoning in cattle.[235, 257, 348, 349, 540]

The dosage of administration of CaEDTA to lead-poisoned cattle in the reports cited was based largely on toxicity and metabolic studies in laboratory animals.[183]

To establish a more definitive basis for the use of CaEDTA in the

269

treatment of lead poisoning, a study was made in which CaEDTA was administered at various dosages to calves previously given lead.[16] Previous studies had established that the amount of lead mobilized by a single rapid intravenous injection into calves of 110 mg of CaEDTA per kilogram of body weight was proportional to the concentration of lead in their erythrocytes at the time of treatment.[233] This dosage probably produced the maximal amount of lead that could be mobilized in calves by a single rapid intravenous injection; a range of doses of 11–165 mg/kg did not produce significantly greater urinary excretion. This relation served as the standard base of reference for evaluating other dosages of CaEDTA administration. The study indicated that optimal conditions of lead mobilization were provided by concentrations of approximately 135 μm of CaEDTA per liter of plasma and higher, maintained for 10–12 hr.[16] These concentrations could be achieved by the constant intravenous infusion of CaEDTA at 110–220 mg/kg over 12 hr or approximated by two rapid intravenous injections of 6 mg/kg 6 hr apart. More than twice as much lead could be mobilized by these procedures as with a comparable dose given as a single rapid intravenous injection. The administration of CaEDTA as a 12-hr infusion for 3 consecutive days proved to be no more effective in mobilizing lead than a single 12-hr infusion.

Because these experiments were carried out with calves that did not have clinical signs of lead poisoning, it might be argued that the conclusions would not necessarily apply to clinical cases of bovine lead poisoning. It cannot be stated unequivocally that higher concentrations of lead in the body would not require higher concentrations of CaEDTA for maximal lead mobilization. However, the concentrations of lead measured in liver (2.3–3.2 μg/g wet wt), kidney cortex (2.8–15.0 μg/g wet wt), and blood (0.27–0.58 μg/ml) of untreated animals given lead were about half the concentrations commonly encountered in clinical cases of lead poisoning.[236] Furthermore, there was no significant difference in lead mobilization when CaEDTA was infused for 12 hr with a fourfold variation in the rate of administration (110–440 mg/kg). This suggests a ready capacity to cope with the greater amounts of lead that would be involved in actual poisoning.

With regard to the lack of additional benefit attained by repeating 12-hr infusions beyond the first infusion, a clinical situation might yield different results, because there might be a much larger reservoir of unabsorbed lead in the gastrointestinal tract, which would provide a greater continuing absorption of metal by the circulation. However, multiple daily infusions at 220 mg/kg over 12 hr would be hazardous because of the toxicity of CaEDTA.[16] It would therefore seem that, even in the presence of tissue concentrations of lead greater than those produced experimentally, 12-hr infusions of CaEDTA should not exceed 220 mg/kg and probably should not be instituted more than once every other day. Probably no more than three treatments should be given. A rational basis for an intermittent schedule of therapy also is provided by evidence that CaEDTA acts to remove some lead from bone and that additional time is required for redistribution of lead from soft tissues to the CaEDTA-sensitive sites in bone.[234]

ESTIMATES OF COSTS OF LEAD POISONING

A very crude estimate of what the economic cost of lead poisoning might be in cattle affected with clinical lead poisoning in the United States is based on an extrapolation of the estimated incidence of lead poisoning in Tompkins County, New York, an area served by the Ambulatory Clinic of the New York State Veterinary College. No estimate is being made for the cost of lead poisoning in other species of animals or for the cost of a pasture or crops contaminated by lead fallout from a smelting or mining operation. This probably conservative estimate indicates the difficulty of trying to assess the cost of a disease in domestic animals for which no reporting system exists. A survey of a knackery[539] (an establishment that receives and processes animal carcasses) in Northern Ireland estimated that lead poisoning accounted for 1.7% of the deaths of adult cattle and 4.5% of the deaths of young calves.[540] This incidence was considerably greater than the number of clinical diagnoses and suggested that cases of lead poisoning were not being diagnosed, for a variety of reasons.

The cost estimate of lead poisoning in cattle is based on the following facts, estimates, and assumptions. The total cattle population of the United States in 1969 was 123,784,000 head.[551] In Tompkins County, New York, the cattle population was 24,410.[548] From this county, the Ambulatory Clinic of the New York State Veterinary College treats approximately four cases of lead poisoning per year, or approximately one case of lead poisoning per 6,000 cattle per year. If this rate holds throughout the United States, it is estimated that 20,000 cases of lead poisoning occur in the United States per year. At an assumed cost of treatment per animal (based on two calls plus drugs) of $25, an assumed mortality of 50% (probably higher), and an assumed average value of an animal of $150, the cost of treatment is $500,000, and the loss is $1,500,000—or a total cost per year of $2,000,000 for lead poisoning in cattle.

Glossary

This glossary consists of terms not explained in the text, and they are defined in the sense in which they are used. Specialists and Panel members in the several disciplines have been consulted, in addition to the usual dictionary sources.

AAS: Atomic absorption spectrophotometry.

Abdominal colic: See *Colic*.

Absorption (of lead): Transfer of lead into an organism via intestinal wall, alveolar surface, or skin.

Accumulation (of lead): The net positive difference between intake and output of lead over an extended period.

Acid-fast: Describes a cell or bacterium that retains a dye that has a negatively charged molecule.

ACTH: Adrenocorticotropic hormone, a hormone secreted by the pituitary gland that stimulates the adrenal cortex.

Acuity: Sharpness of perception with respect to ability to resolve detail.

ADP: Adenosine diphosphate.

Aerosol: A system in which the dispersion medium is a gas and the dispersed phase is not large enough to settle out under the influence of gravity.

Aerosol particles: Solid particles from 10^{-12} to 10^{-1} μm in diameter dispersed in a gas.

ALA: δ-aminolevulinic acid, $COOH-CH_2-CH_2-\overset{\overset{\textstyle O}{\|}}{C}-CH_2-NH_2$, formed from succinyl coenzyme A and glycine (see Figure 4–3).

273

ALAD: δ-aminolevulinic acid dehydrase (syn. δ-aminolevulinic acid dehydratase, δ-aminolevulinic acid dehydrogenase): The enzyme found in cells that catalyzes formation of porphobilinogen from δ-aminolevulinic acid (see Figure 4–3).

ALAS: See δ-*aminolevulinic acid synthetase.*

Albuminuria: Presence in urine of albumin, a protein that is a normal constituent of blood.

Ambient air: The surrounding, mixed air; "ambient community air" refers to air in residential urban areas; "ambient urban air" refers to air in downtown areas with relatively heavy traffic.

δ-aminolevulinic acid synthetase: The enzyme that converts succinyl coenzyme A and glycine to A L A (see Figure 4–3).

Amyotrophic lateral sclerosis: A disease characterized by a hardening of the lateral columns of the spinal cord with muscular atrophy.

Anorexia: Loss of appetite.

Anoxia: Relative lack of oxygen; may be due to lack of blood carrying normal amounts of oxygen or to normal perfusion of blood carrying reduced amounts of oxygen.

Anterior pituitary (syn. anterior hypophysis): Part of the gland of internal secretion at the base of the brain, producing hormones that act on adrenal cortex, thyroid gland, gonads, and skeleton.

ASV: Anodic stripping voltammetry: An electrochemical method of analysis.

Ataxia: Failure of muscular coordination.

Atomization: Reduction to fine particles, usually in a spray.

BAL: 2,3-dimercapto-1-propanol (British anti-lewisite).

Balance experiments: Experiments on man or other animals that involve quantitative measurements of intake (via respiration and ingestion) and loss (via exhalation and excretion) of a specific element or substance. A positive balance means that more is taken in than is lost over a specified time.

Basophilic stippling: The characteristic appearance of some erythrocytes that contain cytoplasmic material that stains deeply with basic dyes.

Bender-Gestalt test: A performance test requiring reproduction of the configuration in line drawings.

Biosphere: The part of the earth's crust, waters, and atmosphere where living organisms can subsist.

Biota: The animal and plant life, collectively.

Biotransfer: The process by which living organisms, such as bacteria, can convert a chemical compound into another.

Blood–brain barrier: The barrier created by semipermeable cell walls and membranes to passage of some molecules from the blood to the cells of the central nervous system.

Body burden: The total amount of a specific substance (for example, lead) in an organism, including the amount stored and the amount absorbed.

CaEDTA: Edathamil calcium disodium, which is the calcium disodium salt of ethylenediaminetetraacetate, a chelating agent. CaEDTA is used in the study, diagnosis, and treatment of poisoning by various heavy metals, including lead.

CaEDTA mobilization test: A test in which a known quantity of CaEDTA is injected parenterally and the amount of lead excreted in urine during a known period beginning immediately thereafter is measured. This procedure is used both clinically and experimentally and is thought to provide an index of the mobile fraction of the total body lead burden.

Cerebellum: A large dorsally projecting part of the brain having the special function of muscle coordination and maintenance of equilibrium.

Cerebral anoxia: Relative lack of oxygen in the brain.

Chelate: A heterocyclic compound having a central metallic ion attached by covalent bonds to two or more nonmetallic atoms in the same molecule.

Chronic nephritis: Chronic inflammation of the kidneys.

Citraturia: The presence in the urine of citric acid. The term usually implies the presence of increased quantities of citric acid in the urine.

Colic: A paroxysmal pain in the abdomen, due to spasm, distention, or obstruction of any one of the hollow viscera.

Community exposure: Exposure of any community or group of persons to contaminant(s).

Complexing: In chemistry, the process of incorporation into other compounds, such as through hydration, oxygenation, halogenation, and chelation.

Contamination: Contact with an admixture of an unnatural agent, with the implication that the amount is measurable.

Conversion factors: For air, 1 $\mu g/m^3$ = approximately 8.5×10^{-4} ppm by weight; for water, 1 $\mu g/liter$ = 1 ppb; for soil, food, forage, etc., 1 $\mu g/g$ (dry, ashed, or wet weight) = 1 ppm, or 1 $\mu g/kg$ = 1 ppb.

Coordination site: Chemical configuration of a molecule where interaction between it and another molecule occurs.

COPRO (syn. CP): Coproporphyrin, the oxidized form of coproporphyrinogen. It is a by-product of intermediary heme biosynthesis found in tissue fluid and the excreta.

COPROGEN III: Coproporphyrinogen III, an intermediary metabolite in heme biosynthesis. It is a natural precursor of heme.

COPROGENASE: Coproporphyrinogenase, the enzyme that converts coproporphyrinogen III to protoporphyrin IX.

Coproporphyrinogen (syn. coprogen): A fully reduced colorless tetracarboxylic tetrapyrrole. Isomers I and III are found in biologic systems.

Corpus striatum: A subcortical mass of gray and white substance in each cerebral hemisphere, containing the caudate nucleus and the lentiform nucleus.

Cortical atrophy: Wasting away of the outer layer(s), e.g., of the brain or kidney.

Deionized water: Water that has been specially distilled or treated to remove inorganic ions and salts. Organic substances may be removed by special processes or prior distillation.

Demyelination: Destruction of the myelin, a fatlike substance forming a sheath around some nerve fibers.

Deposition: Removal of particles from the inhaled air.

Dithizone methods: Colorimetric methods of analysis for lead that involve the reaction of lead with dithizone (diphenylthiocarbazone) to form lead dithizonate, which is measured spectrophotometrically at 510 nm.

DNase: Deoxyribonucleic acidase, an enzyme.

dpm: Disintegrations per minute.

ECP: Erythrocyte coproporphyrin.

Edema: Abnormal accumulation of tissue fluid in the connective tissue or serous cavities.

EDTA: Ethylenediaminetetraacetic acid, used in the form of calcium–disodium salt as a chelating agent to complex with lead and other metals and remove them from the body by urinary excretion.

Effluent: The gaseous or liquid discharge of waste products, which may or may not contain environmental pollutants.

Electrostatic precipitator: A device for removing small particles of smoke, dust, oil, mist, etc., from air by passing the air first through an electrically charged screen, which gives a charge to the particles, and then between two charged plates, where the particles are attracted to one surface.

Elutriator: A machine for separating heavy and light mineral particles by washing and straining or decanting.

Emesis: Vomiting.

Encephalitis: Inflammation of the brain.

Endogenous lead: Lead that has already entered the body.

Endogenous urinary lead: Refers to the urinary excretion of lead that occurs normally in the absence of chelating agents.

Epithelioid cells: Cells resembling epithelium.

Erythroid hypoplasia: Decreased formation of erythroid elements of the blood (i.e., red blood cells).

Erythropoiesis: Formation of red blood cells.

Evoked-response technique: A technique widely used in electrophysiology whereby a stimulus (e.g., electric shock, light flash, click) is applied peripherally to the electrode used to detect the response.

Exposure level: The concentration of the contaminant to which the population in question is exposed.

Extensor muscles: The muscles under voluntary control that, when contracted, extend the limbs.

Fanconi syndrome: There are several Fanconi syndromes. As used in this document, the term refers to the triad of glycosuria, hyperaminoaciduria, and hypophosphatemia in the presence of hyperphosphaturia. This triad is associated with injury to proximal renal tubular cells.

FEC: Free erythrocyte coproporphyrin.

FEP: Free erythrocyte protoporphyrin.

Flicker-fusion: The fusion of intermittent flashes of light into a sensation of continuous brightness.

Fructosuria: The presence in the urine of fructose, a monosaccharide formed from the breakdown of more complex sugars and normally converted ultimately (during metabolism) to carbon dioxide and water.

Glycosuria: The presence in the urine of glucose, a monosaccharide formed from more complex sugars and normally retained in the body as a source of energy.

Gouty diathesis: Predisposition to gout.

G6PDH: Glucose-6-phosphate dehydrogenase, an enzyme important in the maintenance of adequate concentrations of reduced glutathione in red blood cells. Deficiency of this enzyme is inherited as a sex-linked trait.

GSH: Reduced glutathione.

Hematopoietic system: The system of cells in the bone marrow, spleen, and lymph nodes concerned with formation of the cellular elements of the blood.

Hemogram: A clinical term used to encompass several hematologic indices, including hematocrit, hemoglobin, and red blood cell count.

Hepatic porphyria: An inborn error of metabolism characterized by increased formation and accumulation of pyrroles in the liver.

Hepatocellular injury: Injury to the cells of the liver.

Histopathology: Abnormal structure of plant and animal cells at the microscopic level.

Hydrocephalus *"ex vacuo"*: Increased volume of cerebral spinal fluid within the cranial vault, associated with decreased volume of cortical tissue, as in severe cortical atrophy.

Hyperaminoaciduria: Presence in the urine of above-normal amounts of amino acids.

Hyperkinetic: Characterized by abnormally increased muscular movement.

Hyperkinetic–aggressive behavior disorder: A disorder characterized by overactivity, restlessness, distractibility, and short attention span.

Hyperphosphaturia: Above-normal amounts of phosphate compounds in the urine.

Hyperuricemia: Abnormal amounts of uric acid in the blood.

Hypochromic anemia: A condition characterized by a disproportionate reduction of red cell hemoglobin, compared with the volume of packed red cells.

Hypophosphatemia: Abnormally low amount of phosphate compounds in the blood.

Hypothalamus: The posterior portion of the forebrain that includes the nuclei of nerve cells that exert control over visceral activities, water balance, temperature, sleep, etc.

Illicitly distilled whiskey: Whiskey that is distilled and sold without payment of federal excise taxes.

Interstitial fibrosis: A progressive formation of fibrous tissue in the interstices in any structure; in the lungs, it reduces aeration of the blood.

Intranuclear inclusion bodies: Round, oval, or irregularly shaped bodies appearing in the nuclei of cells.

Iron deficiency: A deficiency of iron-containing foods in the diet such that not enough iron is available for incorporation into newly formed hemoglobin.

Knuckling: Involuntary flexing of the fetlock joint.

Laparotomy: Surgical incision through the abdominal wall.

Latency of response: The time between the application of a stimulus and the beginning of the response to that stimulus.

LDH: Lactic acid dehydrogenase.

Leached: Subjected to the action of percolating water or other liquid that removes the soluble parts.

Lead particles: Lead-containing particles.

Lead poisoning (syn. lead intoxication, plumbism, saturnism): A disease condition reflecting the adverse effect of the absorption of lead into the system.

Lead sesquioxide (syn. lead trioxide): Pb_2O_3.

Lead subacetate (syn. lead monosubacetate, monobasic lead acetate): $Pb(C_2H_3O_2)_2 \cdot 2Pb(OH)_2$.

Ligand: A molecule, ion, or atom that is attached to the central atom of a coordination compound, a chelate, or other complex.

Luting: A substance for packing a plumbing joint to make it impervious to gas or liquid.

Medical surveillance: Repeated medical examination, including physical examination and laboratory examination of blood and urine specimens, to discover any change from base-line ("normal") conditions.

Meningitis: Any disease producing inflammation of the meninges, membranes that envelop the brain and spinal cord.

Metabolites: End product of metabolic processes that transform one compound into another in living cells.

Metalloporphyrin: Any combination of a metal with porphyrin, e.g., iron and heme.

Metaphysis (plural, metaphyses): The wider part at the end of the shaft of a long bone, which during development contains the growth zone and consists of spongy bone.

Microcytic anemia: A condition in which the majority of the red cells are smaller than normal.

Microsome: One of the finer granular elements of protoplasm.

Mitochondria: Small granules or rod-shaped structures seen by differential staining in the cytoplasm of cells.

MMED (syn. MMD): Mass median equivalent diameter.

Mobile fraction of the body burden: The fraction of the total lead content of the body that can be removed by chelating agents.

Moonshine: Illicitly distilled whiskey (*q.v.*).

Motor skills: Skilled movements that depend on the integrity of the nervous system for control.

Myelopathy: Pathology of the muscle fiber.

Myocarditis: Inflammation of the heart muscle.

NASN: National Air Surveillance Networks.

Nerve conduction: Passage of a nerve impulse manifested by an electric impulse that travels along the nerve.

Nitrification: Oxidative process that converts ammonium salts to nitrites and nitrites to nitrates.

Nondestructive detectors: Instruments that can measure a variable without sampling or otherwise causing destruction of the material in which the variable occurs.

Normal blood lead: Range of 5–40 μg/100 g of whole blood.

Nutrient solution: A solution in which tissue cultures are grown that contains the necessary ingredients to nurture growth.

Obstipation: Extreme constipation.

Oliguria: Deficiency in the formation and excretion of urine.

Operant conditioning (syn. instrumental conditioning): The experimental procedure of presenting an animal with a reinforcing stimulus immediately after the occurrence of a specific response.

Organelle: A specific particle of organized living substance in most cells.

Organic brain damage: Structural impairment or change in the brain.

Paraplegia: Paralysis of both lower limbs due to spinal disease or injury.

Parental sequences: Sequential behaviors associated with rearing of the young of a species.

Parent material: The original rock from which the soil in question was made.

Paresis: Incomplete paralysis.

PBG: Porphobilinogen.

Pes cavus deformities: Exaggerated height of the longitudinal arch of the foot due to disturbed balance of the muscles.

pH: A symbol denoting the negative logarithm of the hydrogen ion concentration in gram-atoms per liter.

Phosphorylation: Introduction of the phosphoryl group into an organic compound.

Pica: Ingestion of nonfood items.

Pituitary–adrenal axis: The interrelation of the anterior pituitary and adrenal glands whereby the activity of one is stimulated or inhibited by a hormone of the other—e.g., regulation of ACTH secretion by the concentrations of adrenal corticoids in the blood.

Pituitary gonadotropic hormones: Hormones secreted in the anterior pituitary that control the gonads.

Pituitary–thyroid axis: The interrelated activities of the anterior pituitary and thyroid gland.

Plumbism: See *Lead poisoning.*

Pollution: Admixture of an agent with the implication that the effect is measurable.

Porphyria: A disturbance of porphyrin metabolism characterized by marked increase in formation and excretion of porphyrins or their precursors.

Porphyrin: Any of a group of iron- or magnesium-free pyrrole derivatives that occur universally in protoplasm and form the basis of the respiratory pigments of animals and plants.

Postictally: After a stroke or seizure, such as an acute epileptic attack.

Preganglionic transmission block: Blocking of nerve impulse transmission at the synapse before the nerve enters the ganglion.

Premature dementia: Premature organic brain deterioration.

Primary gout: A condition characterized by abnormal purine metabolism producing an excess of uric acid in the blood, chalky deposits (chiefly urates) in the joints, and attacks of acute arthritis.

Primary producers: Green plants that are able to fix carbon dioxide and give out oxygen.

Prodromal manifestations: Premonitory signs, indicating the approach of a disease or other morbid state.

PROTO: See *Protoporphyrin.*

PROTO 9: Protoporphyrin 9, an isomer of protoporphyrin.

Protoporphyrin: The most important natural porphyrin, $C_{34}H_{34}N_4O_4$, whose iron complex, united with protein, occurs as hemoglobin, myoglobin, catalase, and some respiratory pigments.

Pyrrole: A ring compound, consisting of four carbon atoms and one nitrogen atom with five hydrogen atoms, that is a component of chlorophyll, hemin, and many other important naturally occurring substances.

Reactive site: A chemical configuration on a molecule with which a bond is made by other specific molecules.

Renal insufficiency: A state in which the kidneys are unable to remove a sufficient proportion of the effete matter of the blood.

Rotameter: A device that measures the flow of a gas on the basis of the height in a calibrated cylinder to which it pushes a rotating bobble.

Sacral vertebrae: The five normally fused vertebrae at the posterior end of the spinal column that form the sacrum.

SC: Sickle cell–hemoglobin C disease, characterized by sickle cell anemia and the presence of C hemoglobin.

Schwann cell: One of the large nucleated masses of protoplasm lining the inner surface of the neurilemma, a membrane wrapping the nerve fiber.

Sequela: Any lesion or affection that follows or is caused by an attack of disease.

SH: Free sulfhydryl group consisting of sulfur and hydrogen atoms.

Sideroblasts: Early cells in the red blood cell series that contain granules of free iron as detected by the Prussian blue reaction.

Signs: Conditions that are evident to the examining physician but are not obvious to the patient, as are symptoms.

Spindle: The fine threads of achromatic material in the cell nucleus arranged in a spindle-shaped manner during mitosis.

SS: Sickle cell anemia, a hereditary, genetically determined hemolytic anemia accompanied by the presence of S hemoglobin.

Stanford-Binet intelligence test: A revised version of the Binet-Simon test for determining relative intellectual development; consists of a series of questions and tasks graded with reference to the ability of the "normal" child to deal with them at successive age levels.

Stoneware: A hard, opaque, vitrified ceramic ware.

Striatum: Corpus striatum.

Subclinical lead poisoning: Toxic effects of lead that do not produce clinically discernible signs.

Surface horizon: The earth's surface.

Synergistic effects: Joint effects of two or more agents, such as drugs, that, when taken together, increase each other's effectiveness.

Tared: Counterweighted before use in the sampling procedure to balance the weight of the filter alone.

TEL: Tetraethyl lead.

Thalassemia: A hereditary, genetically determined hemolytic anemia with familial and racial incidence; divided into a number of categories based on clinical severity and type(s) of hemoglobin contained in the red blood cells.

TML: Tetramethyl lead.

Translocation: The transfer of metabolites, nutritive material, or other substances from one part of a plant to another.

Tubular lesions: Lesions of the tubules of the kidney, causing impairment of its reabsorptive capacity.

UCP: Urinary coproporphyrin.

Upper horizon: The upper 6 in. of earth, immediately beneath the surface.

Urban atmosphere: The atmosphere over the center (downtown) of a city.

URO: Uroporphyrin, $C_{40}H_{38}O_{16}N_4$, a porphyrin occurring in the urine.

Vacutainers (trademark): Sealed ampules, maintained under a slight vacuum and containing an anticoagulant, into which blood samples may be drawn directly.

Vertigo: Dizziness.

References

1. Abernethy, R. G., M. J. Peterson, and F. H. Gibson. Spectrochemical Analyses of Coal Ash for Trace Elements. Bureau of Mines Report RI-7281. Washington, D.C.: U.S. Department of the Interior, 1969. 30 pp.
2. Acocella, G. Studio sulla chemioterapia dell'intossicazione sperimentale da piombo. Nota II. Effetti dell'acido nicotinico sulla coproporfirinuria da intossicazione saturnina nel ratto. Acta Vitaminol. (Milano) 20:195-202, 1966.
3. Allcroft, R. Lead as a nutritional hazard to farm livestock. IV. Distribution of lead in the tissues of bovines after ingestion of various lead compounds. J. Comp. Path. 60:190-208, 1950.
4. Allcroft, R. Lead poisoning in cattle and sheep. Vet. Rec. 63:583-590, 1951.
5. Allcroft, R., and K. L. Blaxter. Lead as a nutritional hazard to farm livestock. V. The toxicity of lead to cattle and sheep and an evaluation of the lead hazard under farm conditions. J. Comp. Path. 60:209-218, 1950.
6. Allen-Price, E. D. Uneven distribution of cancer in West Devon with particular reference to the divers water-supplies. Lancet 1:1235-1238, 1960.
7. Allison, A. C., and G. R. Patton. Chromosome damage in human diploid cells following activation of lysosomal enzymes. Nature 207:1170-1173, 1965.
8. Altshuller, L. F., D. B. Halak, B. H. Landing, and R. A. Kehoe. Deciduous teeth as an index of body burden of lead. J. Pediat. 60:224-229, 1962.
9. American Academy of Pediatrics. Subcommittee on Accidental Poisoning. Prevention, diagnosis, and treatment of lead poisoning in childhood. Pediatrics 44:291-298, 1969.

281

10. American Public Health Association. Committee on Chemical Procedures of the Occupational Health Section. Methods for Determining Lead in Air and in Biological Materials. New York: American Public Health Association, Inc., 1955. 69 pp.

11. Anderson, W. L., and P. L. Stewart. Relationships between inorganic ions and the distribution of pheasants in Illinois. J. Wild. Manage. 33:254–270, 1969.

12. Andrews, R., and J. R. Longcore. The killing efficiency of soft iron shot, pp. 337–345. Transactions of the Thirty-fourth North American Wildlife and Natural Resources Conferences, held in Washington, D.C., March 2–5, 1969. Washington, D.C.: Wildlife Management Institute, 1969.

13. Angevine, J. M., A. Kappas, R. L. DeGowin, and B. H. Spargo. Renal tubular nuclear inclusions of lead poisoning. A clinical and experimental study. Arch. Path. 73:486–494, 1962.

14. Angle, C. R., and M. S. McIntire. Lead poisoning during pregnancy. Amer. J. Dis. Child. 108:436–439, 1964.

15. Aring, C. D., and S. A. Trufant. Effects of heavy metals on the central nervous system, pp. 463–474. In H. H. Merritt and C. C. Hare, Eds. Metabolic and Toxic Diseases of the Nervous System. Proceedings of the Association for Research in Nervous and Mental Disease, Research Publications No. 32. Baltimore: The Williams & Wilkins Company, 1953.

16. Aronson, A. L., P. B. Hammond, and A. C. Strafuss. Studies with calcium ethylenediaminetetraacetate in calves; toxicity and use in bovine lead poisoning. Toxicol. Appl. Pharmacol. 12:337–349, 1968.

17. Association of Official Agricultural Chemists. Official Methods of Analysis. (10th ed.) Washington, D.C.: Association of Official Agricultural Chemists, 1965. 957 pp.

18. Atkins, P. R. Lead in a suburban environment. J. Air Pollut. Control Assoc. 19:591–594, 1969.

19. Aub, J. C., L. T. Fairhall, A. S. Minot, and P. Reznikoff. Lead Poisoning. Medicine Monographs. Vol. 7. Baltimore: The Williams & Wilkins Co., 1926. 265 pp.

20. Ault, W. U., R. G. Senechal, and W. E. Erlebach. Isotopic composition as a natural tracer of lead in the environment. Environ. Sci. Tech. 4:305–317, 1970.

21. Baader, E. W. L'aspect clinique de l'intoxication saturnine professionnelle. Maroc Med. 37:409–415, 1958.

22. Baernstein, H. D., and J. A. Grand. The relation of protein intake to lead poisoning in rats. J. Pharmacol. Exp. Ther. 74:18–24, 1942.

23. Baetjer, A. M. Effects of season and temperature on childhood plumbism. Ind. Med. Surg. 28:137–140, 1959.

24. Baetjer, A. M., and S. Horiguchi. Effects of environmental temperature and dehydration on lead poisoning in laboratory animals, pp. 795–797. In 14th International Congress on Occupational Health. Proceedings. Madrid, 16–21 Sept. 1963. Intern. Congr. Ser. No. 62. Amsterdam: Excerpta Medica Foundation, 1964.

25. Baetjer, A. M., S. N. D. Joardar, and W. A. McQuary. Effect of environmental temperature and humidity on lead poisoning in animals. Arch. Environ. Health 1:463–477, 1960.

26. Bagley, G. E., and L. N. Locke. The occurrence of lead in tissues of wild birds. Bull. Environ. Contam. Toxicol. 2:297–305, '1967.

27. Bagley, G. E., L. N. Locke, and G. T. Nightingale. Lead poisoning in Canada geese in Delaware. Avian Dis. 11:601–608, 1967.

28. Ball, G. V., and J. M. Morgan. Chronic lead ingestion and gout. South. Med. J. 61:21–24, 1968.

29. Ball, G. V., and L. B. Sorensen. Pathogenesis of hyperuricemia in saturnine gout. New Eng. J. Med. 280:1199–1202, 1969.

30. Barltrop, D. Lead poisoning in childhood. Postgrad. Med. J. 44:537–542, 1968.

31. Barltrop, D. The excretion of delta-aminolaevulinic acid by children. Acta Paediat. Scand. 56:265–268, 1967.

32. Barltrop, D. Transfer of lead to the human foetus, pp. 135–151. In D. Barltrop and W. L. Burland, Eds. Mineral Metabolism in Paediatrics. Philadelphia: F. A. Davis Co., 1969.

33. Barltrop, D., and N. J. P. Killala. Factors influencing exposure of children to lead. Arch. Dis. Child. 44:476–479, 1969.

34. Barltrop, D., and N. J. P. Killala. Faecal excretion of lead by children. Lancet 2:1017–1019, 1967.

35. Barry, P. S. I., and D. B. Mossman. Lead concentrations in human tissues. Brit. J. Ind. Med. 27:339–351, 1970.

36. Baumhardt, G. R. Absorption by and Growth of Corn (Zea mays L.) with Soil Applied Lead. Master's thesis, University of Illinois, 1970. 51 pp.

37. Beaver, D. L. The ultrastructure of the kidney in lead intoxication with particular reference to intranuclear inclusions. Amer. J. Path. 39:195–208, 1961.

38. Belknap, E. L. Clinical studies on lead absorption in the human. III. Blood pressure observations. J. Ind. Hyg. 18:380–390, 1936.

39. Bell, R. F., and J. C. Gilliland. Urinary lead-210 as index of mine radon exposure, pp. 411–423. In Radiological Health and Safety in Mining and Milling of Nuclear Materials. Vol. 2. Vienna: International Atomic Energy Agency, 1964.

40. Bell, W. B., W. R. Williams, and L. Cunningham. The toxic effects of lead administered intravenously. Lancet 2:793–800, 1925.

41. Benkö, A. Die gemeinsame Wirkung des Nikotinsäureamids und Cortigens auf die Porphyrinurie bei Bleivergiftung. Deutsch. Med. Wochenschr. 68:271–272, 1942.

42. Berk, P. D., D. P. Tschudy, L. A. Shepley, J. G. Waggoner, and N. I. Berlin. Hematologic and biochemical studies in a case of lead poisoning. Amer. J. Med. 48:137–144, 1970.

43. Bessis, M. C., and W. N. Jensen. Sideroblastic anaemia, mitochondria and erythroblastic iron. Brit. J. Haematol. 11:49–51, 1965.

44. Beutler, E. Glucose 6-phosphate dehydrogenase deficiency, pp. 1060–1089. In J. B. Stanbury, J. B. Wyngaarden, and D. S. Fredrickson, Eds. The Metabolic Basis of Inherited Disease. (2nd ed.) New York: McGraw-Hill, 1966.

45. Bischoff, F., L. C. Maxwell, R. D. Evans, and F. R. Nuzum. Studies on the toxicity of various lead compounds given intravenously. J. Pharmacol. Exp. Ther. 34:85–109, 1928.

46. Blair Bell, W., and J. Patterson. The effects of metallic ions on the growth of hyacinths. Ann. Appl. Biol. 13:157–159, 1926.

47. Blanchard, R. L. Relationship between polonium-210 and lead-210 in man and his environment, pp. 281–294. In B. Aberg and F. P. Hungate, Eds. Proceedings of the International Symposium on Radioecological Concentration Process. New York: Pergamon Press, 1966.

48. Blanksma, L. A., H. K. Sachs, E. F. Murray, and M. J. O'Connell. Failure of the urinary delta-aminolevulinic acid test to detect pediatric lead poisoning. Amer. J. Clin. Path. 53:956–962, 1970.

49. Blanksma, L. A., H. K. Sachs, E. F. Murray, and M. J. O'Connell. Incidence of high blood lead levels in Chicago children. Pediatrics 44:661–667, 1969.

50. Blaxter, K. L., and A. T. Cowie. Excretion of lead in the bile. Nature 157:588, 1946.

51. Bloomfield, J. J., and J. M. Dallavalle. The determination and control of industrial dust. Public Health Bulletin 217. Washington, D.C.: U.S. Treasury Department, 1935. 167 pp.

52. Bluhm, A. Hygienische Fürsorge für Arbeiterinnen und deren Kinder, pp. 83–106. In T. Weyl, Ed. Handbuch der Hygiene. Vol. 8. Jena: Verlag von Gustav Fischer, 1897.

53. Bolanowska, W. Distribution and excretion of triethyllead in rats. Brit. J. Ind. Med. 25:203–208, 1968.

54. Bolanowska, W., J. Piotrowski, and B. Trojanowska. Kinetics of distribution and excretion of lead (Pb-210) in rats. I. Distribution of a single intravenous dose in organism. Med. Pracy 18:29–41, 1967. (in Polish)

55. Bolanowska, W., J. Piotrowski, and B. Trojanowska. The kinetics of distribution and excretion of lead (Pb^{210}) in rats, pp. 420–422. In 14th International Congress on Occupational Health. Proceedings. Madrid, 16–21 Sept. 1963. Intern. Congr. Ser. No. 62. Amsterdam: Excerpta Medica Foundation, 1964.

56. Bond, E., and R. Kubin. Lead poisoning in dogs. Vet. Med. 44:118–123, 1949.

57. Bonsignore, D., P. Calissano, and C. Cartasegna. A simple method for determining delta-amino-levulinic-dehydratase in the blood. Med. Lav. 56:199–205, 1965. (in Italian)

58. Booker, D. V., A. C. Chamberlain, D. Newton, and A. N. B. Stott. Uptake of radioactive lead following inhalation and injection. Brit. J. Radiol. 42:457–466, 1969.

59. Bowen, H. J. Trace Elements in Biochemistry. New York: Academic Press Inc., 1966. 241 pp.

60. Boyland, E., C. E. Dukes, P. L. Grover, and B. C. V. Mitchley. The induction of renal tumours by feeding lead acetate to rats. Brit. J. Cancer 16:283–288, 1962.

61. Bradley, J. E., and R. J. Baumgartner. Subsequent mental development of children with lead encephalopathy, as related to type of treatment. J. Pediat. 53:311–315, 1958.

62. Bradley, J. E., A. E. Powell, W. Niermann, K. R. McGrady, and E. Kaplan. The incidence of abnormal blood levels of lead in a metropolitan pediatric clinic with observation on the value of coproporphyrinuria as screening test. J. Pediat. 49:1–6, 1956.

63. Bradley, W. R., and W. G. Fredrick. The toxicity of antimony; animal studies. Ind. Med. Ind. Hyg. 2 (Sect. 2):15–22, 1941.

64. Bradshaw, A. D., T. S. McNeilly, and R. P. G. Gregory. Industrialization, evolution and the development of heavy metal tolerance in plants, pp. 327–343. In G. T. Goodman, R. W. Edwards, and J. M. Lambert, Eds. Ecology and the Industrial Society. New York: John Wiley and Sons, 1965.

65. Brewer, R. F. Lead, pp. 213–217. In H. D. Chapman, Ed. Diagnostic Criteria for Plants and Soils. Berkeley: University of California, Division of Agricultural Sciences, 1966.

66. Britten, R. H., and L. R. Thompson. A Health Study of Ten Thousand Male Industrial Workers. Statistical Analysis of Surveys in Ten Industries. Public Health Bulletin 162. Washington, D.C.: U.S. Government Printing Office, 1926. 170 pp.

67. Brown, J. S. Ore leads and isotopes. Econ. Geol. 57:673–720, 1962.

68. Browning, E. Toxicity of Industrial Metals. (2nd ed.) New York: Appleton-Century-Crofts, 1969. 383 pp.

69. Buck, J. S., and D. M. Kumro. Toxicity of lead compounds. J. Pharm. 38:161–172, 1930.

70. Buck, W. B. Behavioral and Neurological Effects of Lead. Annual Progress Report 1. Contract CPA 22–69–NEG–107. College of Veterinary Medicine, Iowa State University, Ames, Iowa. July 15, 1970. 65 pp.

71. Buck, W. B. Lead and organic pesticide poisonings in cattle. J. Amer. Vet. Med. Assoc. 156:1468–1472, 1970.

72. Bullock, J. D., R. J. Wey, J. A. Zaia, I. Zarembok, and H. A. Schroeder. Effect of tetraethyllead on learning and memory in the rat. Arch. Environ. Health 13:21–22, 1966.

73. Burton, W. M., and N. G. Steward. Use of long-lived natural radioactivity as an atmospheric tracer. Nature 186:584–589, 1960.

74. Butler, E. J. Chronic neurological disease as a possible form of lead poisoning. J. Neurol. Neurosurg. Psychiat. 15:119–128, 1952.

75. Butt, E. M., R. E. Nusbaum, T. C. Gilmour, and S. L. Didio. Trace metal levels in human serum and blood. Arch. Environ. Health 8:52–57, 1964.

76. Butt, E. M., H. E. Pearson, and D. G. Simonsen. Production of meningoceles and cranioschisis in chick embryos with lead nitrate. Proc. Soc. Exp. Biol. Med. 79:247–249, 1952.

77. Byers, R. K. Lead poisoning. Review of the literature and report on 45 cases. Pediatrics 23:585–603, 1959.

78. Byers, R. K., and E. E. Lord. Late effects of lead poisoning on mental development. Amer. J. Dis. Child. 66:471–494, 1943.

79. Byers, R. K., C. A. Maloof, and M. Cushman. Urinary excretion of lead in children. Diagnostic application. Amer. J. Dis. Child. 87:548–558, 1954.

80. California Department of Public Health, Division of Environmental Sanitation and Division of Laboratories. Lead in the Environment and Its Effects on Humans. Berkeley: California Department of Public Health, 1967. 81 pp.

81. Calvery, H. O., E. P. Lang, and H. J. Morris. The chronic effects on dogs of feeding diets containing lead acetate, lead arsenate, and arsenic trioxide in varying concentrations. J. Pharm. Exp. Ther. 64:364–387, 1938.

82. Campbell, A. M. G., G. Herdan, W. F. T. Tatlow, and E. G. Whittle. Lead in relation to disseminated sclerosis. Brain 73:52–71, 1950.

83. Cannon, H. L., and J. M. Bowles. Contamination of vegetation by tetra-ethyl lead. Science 137:765–766, 1962.

84. Cantarow, A., and M. Trumper. Normal intake of lead, pp. 167–171. In Lead Poisoning. Baltimore: The Williams & Wilkins Co., 1944.

85. Carpenter, K. E. A study of the fauna of rivers polluted by lead mining in the Aberystwyth district of Cardiganshire. Ann. Appl. Biol. 11:1–23, 1924.

86. Carpenter, K. E. Further researches on the action of metallic salts on fishes. J. Exp. Zool. 56:407–422, 1930.

87. Carpenter, K. E. On the biological factors involved in the destruction of river-fisheries by pollution due to lead-mining. Ann. Appl. Biol. 12:1–13, 1925.

88. Carpenter, K. E. The lead mine as an active agent in river pollution. Ann. Appl. Biol. 13:395–401, 1926.

89. Carpenter, K. E. The lethal action of soluble metallic salts on fishes. Brit. J. Exp. Biol. 4:378–390, 1927.

90. Cassells, D. A. K., and E. C. Dodds. Tetra-ethyl lead poisoning. Brit. Med. J. 2:681–685, 1946.

91. Castellino, N., and S. Aloj. Intracellular distribution of lead in the liver and kidney of the rat. Brit. J. Ind. Med. 26:139–143, 1969.

92. Castellino, N., P. Lamanna, and G. Grieco. Biliary excretion of lead in the rat. Brit. J. Ind. Med. 23:237–239, 1966.

93. Catizone, O., and P. Gray. Experiments on chemical interference with the early morphogenesis of the chick. II. The effects of lead on the central nervous system. J. Exp. Zool. 87:71–83, 1941.

94. Catton, M. J., M. J. G. Harrison, P. M. Fullerton, and G. Kazantzis. Sub-clinical neuropathy in lead workers. Brit. Med. J. 2:80–82, 1970.

95. Chadwick, R. C., and A. C. Chamberlain. Field loss of radionuclides from grass. Atmos. Environ. 4:51–56, 1970.

96. Charlson, R. J., and J. M. Pierrard. Short communication. Visibility and lead. Atmos. Environ. 3:479–480, 1969.

97. Cheatham, J. S., and E. F. Chobot, Jr. The clinical diagnosis and treatment of lead encephalopathy. South. Med. J. 61:529–531, 1968.

98. Cheatum, E. L., and D. Benson. Effects of lead poisoning on reproduction of mallard drakes. J. Wild. Manage. 9:26–29, 1945.

99. Chiodi, H., and A. F. Cardeza. Hepatic lesions produced by lead in rats fed high fat diet. Arch. Path. 48:395–404, 1949.

100. Chiodi, H., and R. A. Sammartino. Nephrotoxic and renotropic effects of lead on white rats and its prevention by B.A.L. Nature 160:680–681, 1947.

101. Chisolm, J. J., Jr. Aminoaciduria as a manifestation of renal tubular injury in lead intoxication and a comparison with patterns of aminoaciduria seen in other diseases. J. Pediat. 60:1–17, 1962.

102. Chisolm, J. J., Jr. Chronic lead intoxication in children. Develop. Med. Child Neurol. 7:529–536, 1965.

103. Chisolm, J. J., Jr. Determination of δ-aminolevulinic acid in plasma. Anal. Biochem. 22:54–64, 1968.

104. Chisolm, J. J., Jr. Disturbances in the biosynthesis of heme in lead intoxication. J. Pediat. 64:174–187, 1964.
105. Chisolm, J. J., Jr. Lead poisoning (plumbism), pp. 313–319. In H. L. Barnett, Ed. Pediatrics. (14th ed.) New York: Appleton-Century-Crofts, 1968.
106. Chisolm, J. J., Jr. The use of chelating agents in the treatment of acute and chronic lead intoxication in childhood. J. Pediat. 73:1–38, 1968.
107. Chisolm, J. J., Jr. Treatment of lead poisoning. Mod. Treat. 4:710–728, 1967.
108. Chisolm, J. J., Jr., H. C. Harrison, W. R. Eberlein, and H. E. Harrison. Amino-aciduria, hypophosphatemia, and rickets in lead poisoning; study of a case. Amer. J. Dis. Child. 89:159–168, 1955.
109. Chisolm, J. J., Jr., and H. E. Harrison. Quantitative urinary coproporphyrin excretion and its relation to edathamil calcium disodium administration in children with acute lead intoxication. J. Clin. Invest. 35:1131–1138, 1956.
110. Chisolm, J. J., Jr., and H. E. Harrison. The exposure of children to lead. Pediatrics 18:943–957, 1956.
111. Chisolm, J. J., Jr., and E. Kaplan. Lead poisoning in childhood—comprehensive management and prevention. J. Pediat. 73:942–950, 1968.
112. Cholak, J. Further investigations of atmospheric concentration of lead. Arch. Environ. Health 8:314–324, 1964.
113. Cholak, J. The quantitative spectrographic determination of lead in urine. J. Amer. Chem. Soc. 57:104–107, 1935.
114. Cholak, J., and K. Bambach. Measurement of industrial lead exposure by analyses of blood and excreta of workmen. J. Ind. Hyg. 27:47–54, 1943.
115. Cholak, J., and R. V. Story. Spectrochemical determination of trace metals in biological material. J. Opt. Soc. Amer. 31:730–738, 1941.
116. Chow, T. J. Environmental pollution from industrial lead. In Y. Miyake, Ed. Proceedings of the International Symposium on Biogeochemistry and Hydrogeochemistry, held in Tokyo, Sept., 1970. (to be published)
117. Chow, T. J. Isotope analysis of seawater by mass spectrometry. J. Water Pollut. Control Fed. 40:399–411, 1968.
118. Chow, T. J. Lead accumulation in roadside soil and grass. Nature 225:295–296, 1970.
119. Chow, T. J., and J. L. Earl. Lead aerosols in the atmosphere: Increasing concentrations. Science 169:577–580, 1970.
120. Chow, T. J., J. L. Earl, and C. F. Bennett. Lead aerosols in marine atmosphere. Environ. Sci. Tech. 3:737–740, 1969.
121. Chow, T. J., and C. C. Patterson. The occurrence and significance of lead isotopes in pelagic sediments. Geochim. Cosmochim. Acta 26:263–308, 1962.
122. Christian, J. R., B. S. Celewycz, and S. L. Andelman. A three-year study of lead poisoning in Chicago. 1. Epidemiology. Amer. J. Public Health 54:1241–1251, 1964.
123. Clarke, E. G. C., and M. L. Clarke, Eds. Garner's Veterinary Toxicology. (3rd Ed.) Baltimore: The Williams & Wilkins Co., 1967. 477 pp.
124. Clarkson, T. W., and J. E. Kench. Uptake of lead by human erythrocytes in vitro. Biochem. J. 69:432–439, 1958.

125. Clarkson, T. W., and J. E. Kench. Urinary excretion of amino acids by men absorbing heavy metals. Biochem. J. 62:361–372, 1956.

126. Coburn, D. R., D. W. Metzler, and R. Treichler. A study of absorption and retention of lead in wild waterfowl in relation to clinical evidence of lead poisoning. J. Wild. Manage. 15:186–192, 1951.

127. Coes, L., Jr. Improving Water-Resistant Characteristics of Resins and Resinous Articles, and Resinous Products Resulting Therefrom. U.S. Patent 2,456,919. December 21, 1948.

128. Cogbill, E. C., and M. E. Hobbs. Transfer of metallic constituents of cigarettes to the main-stream smoke. Tobacco 144(19):24–29, 1957.

129. Cowdry, E. V., A. M. Lucas, and H. Fox. Distribution of nuclear inclusions in wild animals. Amer. J. Path. 11:237–253, 1935.

130. Cramér, K., and L. Dahlberg. Incidence of hypertension among lead workers. A follow-up study based on regular control over 20 years. Brit. J. Ind. Med. 23:101–104, 1966.

131. Cramér, K., and S. Selander. Studies in lead poisoning. Comparison between different laboratory tests. Brit. J. Ind. Med. 22:311–314, 1965.

132. Crandall, C. A., and C. J. Goodnight. The effects of sublethal concentrations of several toxicants to the common guppy Lebistes reticulatus. Trans. Amer. Microscop. Soc. 82:59–73, 1963.

133. Cremer, J. E. Toxicology and biochemistry of alkyl lead compounds. Occup. Health Rev. 17:14–19, 1965.

134. Dagg, J. H., A. Goldberg, A. Lochhead, and J. A. Smith. The relationship of lead poisoning to acute intermittent porphyria. Q. J. Med. 34:163–175, 1965.

135. Daines, R. H., H. Motto, and D. M. Chilko. Atmospheric lead: Its relationship to traffic volume and proximity to highways. Environ. Sci. Tech. 4:318–322, 1970.

136. Dalldorf, G., and R. R. Williams. Impairment of reproduction in rats by ingestion of lead. Science 102:668–670, 1945.

137. Danckwortt, P. W. Erhöhter Bleigehalt in niederen Organismen und in Haaren. Deutsch. Tieraerztl. Wochenschr. 50:28, 1942.

138. Danielson, L. Gasoline Containing Lead. Ecological Research Committee Bulletin 6. Stockholm: Swedish Natural Science Research Council, 1969. (Revised ed.)

139. Danilović, V. Chronic nephritis due to ingestion of lead-contaminated flour. Brit. Med. J. 1:27–28, 1958.

140. David, D. J., D. C. Wark, and M. Mandryk. Lead toxicity in tobacco resembles an early symptom of frenching. J. Aust. Inst. Agric. Sci. 21:182–185, 1955.

141. Davies, T. A. L., and S. G. Rainsford. Reporting blood–lead values. (Letter to the editor) Lancet 2:834–835, 1967.

142. Davis, R. K., A. W. Horton, E. E. Larson, and K. L. Stemmer. Inhalation of tetramethyllead and tetraethyllead. Arch. Environ. Health 6:473–479, 1963.

143. Dawson, A. B. The hemopoietic response in the catfish, Ameiurus nebulosus, to chronic lead poisoning. Biol. Bull. 68:335–346, 1935.

144. DeBarreiro, O. C. Effect of cysteine on 5-aminolaevulinate hydrolase from liver in two cases of experimental intoxication. Biochem. Pharmacol. 18:2267–2271, 1969.

145. de Bruin, A. Effect of lead exposure on the level of δ-aminolevulinic-dehydratase activity. Med. Lav. 59:411, 1968.

146. de Bruin, A., and H. Hoolboom. Early signs of lead-exposure. A comparative study of laboratory tests. Brit. J. Ind. Med. 24:203–212, 1967.

147. Dedolph, R., G. Ter Haar, R. Holtzman, and H. Lucas, Jr. Sources of lead in perennial ryegrass and radishes. Environ. Sci. Tech. 4:217–223, 1970.

148. Delves, H. T. A micro-sampling method for the rapid determination of lead in blood by atomic-absorption spectrophotometry. Analyst 95:431–438, 1970.

149. deTreville, R. T. P., H. W. Wheeler, and T. Sterling. Occupational exposure to organic lead compounds. The relative degree of hazard in occupational exposure to air-borne tetraethyllead and tetramethyllead. Arch. Environ. Health 5:532–536, 1962.

150. Dews, P. B. Drugs in psychology. A commentary on Travis Thompson and Charles R. Schuster's Behavioral Pharmacology. J. Exp. Anal. Behav. 13:395–406, 1970.

151. Diaz-Rivera, R. S., and R. C. Horn, Jr. Postmortem studies on hypertensive rats, chronically intoxicated with lead acetate. Proc. Soc. Exp. Biol. Med. 59:161–63, 1945.

152. Dilling, W. J. Influence of lead and the metallic ions of copper, zinc, thorium, beryllium and thallium on the germination of seeds. Ann. Appl. Biol. 13:160–167, 1926.

153. Dilling, W. J., C. W. Healey, and W. C. Smith. Experiments on the effects of lead on the growth of plaice (*Pleuronectes platessa*). Ann. Appl. Biol. 13:168–176, 1926.

154. Dingwall-Fordyce, I., and R. E. Lane. A follow-up study of lead workers. Brit. J. Ind. Med. 20:313–315, 1963.

155. Dodd, D. C., and E. L. J. Staples. Clinical lead poisoning in the dog. New Zealand Vet. J. 4:1–7, 1956.

156. Doe, B. R. Lead Isotopes, Minerals, Rocks and Inorganic Materials. Monograph Series of Theoretical and Experimental Studies No. 3. New York: Springer-Verlag, 1970. 39 pp.

157. Doudoroff, P., and M. Katz. Critical review of literature on the toxicity of industrial wastes and their components to fish. II. The metals, as salts. Sewage Ind. Wastes 25:802–839, 1953.

158. Dowdle, E. B., P. Mustard, and L. Eales. δ-Aminolaevulinic acid synthetase activity in normal and porphyric human livers. S. Afr. Med. J. 41:1093–1096, 1967.

159. Dreessen, W. C., T. I. Edwards, W. H. Reinhart, R. T. Page, S. H. Webster, D. W. Armstrong, and R. R. Sayers. The control of the lead hazard in the storage battery industry. Public Health Service Bulletin 262. Washington, D.C.: U.S. Government Printing Office, 1941.

160. Druyan, R., and B. Haeger-Aronsen. Aminoacetone excretion in porphyrias and in chronic lead intoxication. Scand. J. Clin. Lab. Invest. 16:498–502, 1964.

161. Duckering, G. E. The cause of lead poisoning in the tinning of metals. J. Hyg. 8:474–503, 1908.

162. Dukes, C. E. Clues to the causes of cancer of the kidney. Lancet 2:1157–1160, 1961.

163. Durfor, C., and E. Becker. Selected data on public supplies of the 100 largest cities in the United States, 1962. J. Amer. Water Works Assoc. 56:237–246, 1964.

164. Egan, D. A., and T. O'Cuill. Cumulative lead poisoning in horses in a mining area contaminated with galena. Vet. Rec. 86:736–737, 1970.

165. Egan, D. A., and T. O'Cuill. Opencast lead mining areas—A toxic hazard to grazing stock. Vet. Rec. 84:230, 1969.

166. Eisenbud, M., and M. E. Wrenn. Radioactivity Studies. Annual Report NYO–3086–10. Vol. 1. Sept. 1, 1970. Springfield, Va.: National Technical Information Service, 1970. 235 pp.

167. Ellis, M. M. Detection and measurement of stream pollution. U.S. Fish. Bull. 48:365–437, 1937. (Bulletin 22)

168. Emmerson, B. T. Chronic lead nephropathy: The diagnostic use of calcium EDTA and the association with gout. Australas. Ann. Med. 12:310–324, 1963.

169. Emmerson, B. T. The clinical differentiation of lead gout from primary gout. Arthritis Rheum. 11:623–634, 1968.

170. English, J. N., G. N. McDermott, and C. Henderson. Pollutional effects of outboard motor exhaust. Laboratory studies. J. Water Pollut. Control Fed. 35:923–931, 1963.

171. Enrione, R. E. Memorandum dated Oct. 20, 1970. Official File, Rm. B–47, C. P., APCO, Cincinnati, Ohio.

172. Ettinger, M. B. Lead in drinking water, pp. 21–27. In Symposium on Environmental Lead Contamination, sponsored by the U.S. Public Health Service, Dec. 13–15, 1965. Public Health Service Publication 1440. Washington, D.C.: U.S. Government Printing Office, 1966.

173. Everett, J. C., C. L. Day, and D. Reynolds. Comparative survey of lead at selected sites in the British Isles in relation to air pollution. Food Cosmet. Toxicol. 5:29–35, 1967.

174. Fairhall, L. T., and J. W. Miller. A study of the relative toxicity of the molecular components of lead arsenate. Public Health Rep. 56:1610–1625, 1941.

175. Fairhall, L. T., and J. W. Miller. The deposition and removal of lead in the soft tissues (liver, kidneys, and spleen). Public Health Rep. 56:1641–1650, 1941.

176. Falk, J. L. Drug effects on discriminative motor control. Physiol. Behav. 4:421–427, 1969.

177. Feldman, F., H. C. Lichtman, S. Oransky, E. S. Ana, and L. Reiser. Serum δ-aminolevulinic acid in plumbism. J. Pediat. 74:917–923, 1969.

178. Ferm, V. H., and S. J. Carpenter. Developmental malformations resulting from the administration of lead salts. Exp. Molec. Path. 7:208–213, 1967.

179. Ferster, C. B., and B. F. Skinner. Schedules of Reinforcement. New York: Appleton-Century-Crofts, 1957. 741 pp.

180. First, M. W. Process and system control, p. 298. In A. C. Stern, Ed. Air Pollution. Vol. 3. (2nd ed.) New York: Academic Press Inc., 1968.

181. Fleming, A. J. Industrial hygiene and medical control procedures. Manufacture and handling of organic lead compounds. Arch. Environ. Health 8:266–270, 1964.

182. Foreman, H. Toxic side effects of ethylenediaminetetraacetic acid. J. Chronic Dis. 16:319–323, 1963.

183. Foreman, H., H. L. Hardy, T. L. Shipman, and E. L. Belknap. Use of calcium ethylenediaminetetraacetate in cases of lead intoxication. A.M.A. Arch. Ind. Hyg. 7:148–151, 1953.

184. Fouts, P. J., and I. H. Page. Effect of chronic lead poisoning on arterial blood pressure in dogs. Amer. Heart J. 24:329–331, 1942.

185. Francis, C. W., G. Chesters, and W. H. Erhardt. ^{210}Polonium entry into plants. Environ. Sci. Tech. 2:690–695, 1968.

186. Francis, C. W., G. Chesters, and L. A. Haskin. Determinations of 210 Pb mean residence time in atmosphere. Environ. Sci. Tech. 4:586–589, 1970.

187. Franklin, B. Reprinted in Medical Affairs, pp. 26–27, Sept. 1965.

188. Freeman, R. Chronic lead poisoning in children: A review of 90 children diagnosed in Sydney, 1948–1967. 1. Epidemiological aspects. Med. J. Aust. 1:640–647, 1970.

189. Freeman, R. Reversible myocarditis due to chronic lead poisoning in childhood. Arch. Dis. Child. 40:389–393, 1965.

190. Fullerton, P. M. Chronic peripheral neuropathy produced by lead poisoning in guinea-pigs. J. Neuropath. Exp. Neurol. 25:214–236, 1966.

191. Fullerton, P. M. Toxic chemicals and peripheral neuropathy: Clinical and epidemiological features. Proc. Roy. Soc. Med. 62:201–204, 1969.

192. Gafafer, W. M., Ed. Occupational Diseases. A Guide to Their Recognition. Public Health Service Publication 1097. Washington, D.C.: U.S. Government Printing Office, 1964. 375 pp.

193. Galle, P., and L. Morel-Maroger. Les lésions rénales du saturnisme humain et expérimental. Nephron 2:273–286, 1965.

194. Gamble, J. F. A Study of Strontium, Barium, and Calcium Relationships in Soils and Vegetation. Final report NYO–10581 to the U.S. Atomic Energy Commission, Washington, D.C., 1963.

195. Gibson, K. D., A. Neuberger, and J. J. Scott. The purification and properties of δ-aminolaevulic acid dehydrase. Biochem. J. 61:618–629, 1955.

196. Gibson, S. L. M., J. C. Mackenzie, and A. Goldberg. The diagnosis of industrial lead poisoning. Brit. J. Ind. Med. 26:40–51, 1968.

197. Gillet, J. A. An outbreak of lead poisoning in the Canklow District of Rotherham. Lancet 1:1118–1121, 1955.

198. Goldberg. A., J. A. Smith, and A. C. Lochhead. Treatment of lead-poisoning with oral penicillamine. Brit. Med. J. 1:1270–1275, 1963.

199. Goldberg, E. D. Geochronology with lead-210, pp. 121–131. In Radioactive Dating: Proceedings of a Symposium, Athens, 19–23 November 1962, jointly sponsored by the IAEA and ICSU. Vienna: International Atomic Energy Agency, 1963.

200. Goldschmidt, V. M. The principles of distribution of chemical elements in minerals and rocks. J. Chem. Soc. 1937:655–673.

201. Goldsmith, J. R. Testimony presented before Air Resources Board, State of California. October 21, 1970.

202. Goldsmith, J. R., and A. C. Hexter. Respiratory exposure to lead: Epidemiological and experimental dose–response relationships. Science 158: 132–134, 1967.

203. Goldstein, A., L. Aronow, and S. M. Kalman. Principles of Drug Action, p. 312. New York: Hoeber, 1968.

204. Goldwater, L. J., and A. W. Hoover. An international study of "normal" levels of lead in blood and urine. Arch. Environ. Health 15:60–63, 1967.

205. Gontzea, I., P. Sutzesco, D. Cocora, and D. Lungu. Importance de l'apport de protéines sur la résistance de l'organisme a l'intoxication par le plomb. Arch. Sci. Physiol. (Paris) 18:211–224, 1964.

206. Goodwin, T. W., Ed. Biochemical Society Symposium 28: Porphyrins and Related Compounds. New York: Academic Press Inc., 1968. 162 pp.

207. Gordon, C. C. East Helena Reports for Director of Air Pollution Abatement. Dec. 16, 1968. 10 pp.

208. Goyer, R. A. The renal tubule in lead poisoning. I. Mitochondrial swelling and aminoaciduria. Lab. Invest. 19:71–77, 1968.

209. Goyer, R. A., and R. Krall. Ultrastructural transformation in mitochondria isolated from kidneys of normal and lead-intoxicated rats. J. Cell Biol. 41: 393–400, 1969.

210. Goyer, R. A., A. Krall, and J. P. Kimball. The renal tubule in lead poisoning. II. *In vitro* studies of mitochondrial structure and function. Lab Invest. 19:78–83, 1968.

211. Goyer, R. A., D. L. Leonard, J. F. Moore, B. Rhyne, and M. R. Krigman. Lead dosage and the role of the intranuclear inclusion body. Arch. Environ. Health 20:705–711, 1970.

212. Goyer, R. A., P. May, M. M. Cates, and M. R. Krigman. Lead and protein content of isolated intranuclear inclusion bodies from kidneys of lead-poisoned rats. Lab. Invest. 22:245–251, 1970.

213. Grabecki, J., T. Haduch, and H. Urbanowicz. Die einfachen Bestimmungsmethoden der δ-Aminolävulinsäure im Harn. Int. Arch. Gewerbepath. 23: 226–240, 1967.

214. Granick, S. Porphyrin biosynthesis in erythrocytes. I. Formation of δ-aminolevulinic acid in erythrocytes. J. Biol. Chem. 232:1101–1117, 1958.

215. Granick, S. The induction *in vitro* of the synthesis of δ-aminolevulinic acid synthetase in chemical porphyria: A response to certain drugs, sex hormones, and foreign chemicals. J. Biol. Chem. 241:1359–1375, 1966.

216. Granick, S., and D. Mauzerall. Porphyrin biosynthesis in erythrocytes. II. Enzymes converting δ-aminolevulinic acid to coproporphyrinogen. J. Biol. Chem. 232:1119–1140, 1958.

217. Green, R. G. The prevention of lead poisoning in waterfowl by the use of disintegrable lead shot, pp. 486–490. In Wildlife Restoration and Conservation: Proceedings of the North American Wildlife Conference Called by President Franklin D. Roosevelt, Washington, D.C., February 3–7, 1936. Washington, D.C.: U.S. Government Printing Office, 1936.

218. Greenburg, L., A. A. Schaye, and H. Shlionsky. A study of lead poisoning in a storage-battery plant. Public Health Rep. 44:1666–1698, 1929.

219. Griffith, J. Q., Jr., and M. A. Lindauer. Effect of chronic lead poisoning on arterial blood pressure in rats. Amer. Heart J. 28:295-297, 1944.

220. Griggs, R. C. Lead poisoning: Hematologic aspects, pp. 117-137. In C. V. Moore and E. B. Brown, Eds. Progress in Haematology. Vol. IV. New York: Grune & Stratton, Inc., 1964.

221. Griggs, R. C., I. Sunshine, V. A. Newill, B. W. Newton, S. Buchanan, and C. A. Rasch. Environmental factors in childhood lead poisoning. J.A.M.A. 187:703-707, 1964.

222. Gusev, M. I. Limits of allowable lead concentrations in the air of inhabited localities. In V. A. Ryazanov, Ed. Limits of Allowable Concentration of Atmospheric Pollutants. (Book 4, 1960.) Translated from the Russian. Washington, D.C.: U.S. Dept. Commerce, Office of Technical Services, Jan. 1961.

223. Habibi, K. Characterization of particulate lead in vehicle exhaust—experimental techniques. Environ. Sci. Tech. 4:239-248, 1970.

224. Habibi, K., E. S. Jacobs, W. G. Kunz, and D. L. Pastell. Characterization and control of gaseous and particulate exhaust emissions from vehicles. Paper presented at Air Pollution Control Association, West Coast Section, Fifth Technical Meeting, San Francisco, Calif., October 8-9, 1970. 33 pp.

225. Haeger-Aronsen, B. Evaluation of two methods for measuring δ-aminolaevulinic acid in urine. Scand. J. Clin. Lab. Invest. 25:19-23, 1970.

226. Haeger-Aronsen, B. Studies on urinary excretion of δ-aminolaevulic acid and other haem precursors in lead workers and lead-intoxicated rabbits. Scand. J. Clin. Lab. Invest. 12(Suppl. 47):1-128, 1960.

227. Hamilton, A. Lead poisoning in potteries, tile works, and porcelain enameled sanitary ware factories, pp. 56-58. U.S. Bureau of Labor Statistics, Bulletin 104, 1912.

228. Hamilton, A., and H. L. Hardy. Industrial Toxicology. (2nd ed.) New York: Hoeber, 1949. 574 pp.

229. Hamilton, E. I. Some problems concerning lead in the natural environment, pp. 355-358. In B. Aberg and F. P. Hungate, Eds. Radio-ecological Concentration Processes: Proceedings of an International Symposium held in Stockholm 25-29 April 1966. New York: Pergamon Press, 1966.

230. Hammer, D. I., J. F. Finklea, R. H. Hendricks, C. M. Shy, T. A. Minners, and W. B. Raggan. Trace metals in human hair as a simple epidemiologic monitor of environmental exposure. Amer. J. Epidemiol. 93:84-92, 1971.

231. Hammett, F. S. Studies in the biology of metals. III. The localization of lead within the cell of the growing root. Protoplasma 5:135-141, 1928.

232. Hammond, P. B., and A. L. Aronson. Lead poisoning in cattle and horses in the vicinity of a smelter. Ann. N.Y. Acad. Sci. 111:595-611, 1964.

233. Hammond, P. B., and A. L. Aronson. The mobilization and excretion of lead in cattle: A comparative study of various chelating agents. Ann. N.Y. Acad. Sci. 88:498-511, 1960.

234. Hammond, P. B., A. L. Aronson, and W. C. Olson. The mechanism of mobilization of lead by ethylenediaminetetraacetate. J. Pharmacol. Exp. Ther. 157:196-206, 1967.

235. Hammond, P. B., and D. K. Sorensen. Recent observations on the course and treatment of bovine lead poisoning. J. Amer. Vet. Med. Assoc. 130:23-25, 1957.

236. Hammond, P. B., H. N. Wright, and M. H. Roepke. A Method for the Detection of Lead in Bovine Blood and Liver. University of Minnesota Agricultural Experiment Station Technical Bulletin 221, Dec. 1956. 14 pp.

237. Hardy, H. L. Lead, pp. 73–83. In Symposium on Environmental Lead Contamination, Sponsored by the U.S. Public Health Service, Dec. 13–15, 1965. Public Health Service Publication 1440. Washington, D.C.: U.S. Government Printing Office, 1966.

238. Hardy, H. L. What is the status of knowledge of the toxic effect of lead on identifiable groups in the population? Clin. Pharmacol. Ther. 7:713–722, 1966.

239. Harley, J. H. Discussion. Sources of lead in perennial ryegrass and radishes. Environ. Sci. Tech. 4:225, 1970.

240. Harris, R. W., and W. R. Elsea. Ceramic glaze as a source of lead poisoning. J.A.M.A. 202:344–546, 1967.

241. Hart, F. L. A history of the adulteration of food before 1906. Food Drug Cosmet. Law J. 7:5–22, 1952.

242. Hasan, J., and S. Hernberg. Interactions of inorganic lead with human red blood cells. With special reference to membrane functions. A selective review supplemented by new observations. Work-Environment-Health 2:26–44, 1966.

243. Hasan, J., V. Vihko, and S. Hernberg. Deficient red cell membrane /Na$^+$ + K$^+$/-ATPase in lead poisoning. Arch. Environ. Health 14:313–318, 1967.

244. Hass, G. M., J. H. McDonald, R. Oyasu, H. A. Battifora, and J. T. Paloucek. Renal neoplasia induced by combinations of dietary lead subacetate and N-2-fluorenylacetamide, pp. 377–412. In J. S. King, Jr., Ed. Renal Neoplasia. Boston: Little, Brown and Company Inc., 1967.

245. Henderson, D. A. A follow-up of cases of plumbism in children. Australas. Ann. Med. 3:219–224, 1954.

246. Henderson, D. A., and J. A. Inglis. The lead content of bone in chronic Bright's disease. Australas. Ann. Med. 6:145–154, 1957.

247. Hernberg, S., J. Nikkanen, G. Mellin, and H. Lilius. δ-Aminolevulinic acid dehydrase as a measure of lead exposure. Arch. Environ. Health 21:140–145, 1970.

248. Hernberg, S., J. Nikkanen, S. Tola, S. Valkonen, and C.-H. Nordman. Erythrocyte ALA dehydratase as a test of lead exposure. Paper presented at International Conference on Chemical Pollution and Human Ecology, Prague, October 1970.

249. Hernberg, S., M. Nurminen, and J. Hasan. Nonrandom shortening of red cell survival times in men exposed to lead. Environ. Res. 1:247–261, 1967.

250. Heywood, H. Particle Size and Shape. Lecture delivered at Loughborough University of Technology, Loughborough, Leicestershire, England.

251. Hibbard, P. L. Accumulation of zinc on soil under long-persistent vegetation. Soil Sci. 50:53–55, 1940.

252. Hickman, J. R. Lead poisoning: Pottery glazes, an often-ignored hazard. Paper presented to the Canada Safety Council, Fredericton, N.B., Canada, May 26, 1970. 13 pp.

253. Hill, A. B. The environment and disease: Association or causation? Proc. Roy. Soc. Med. 58:295–300, 1965.

254. Hill, C. R. Lead-210 and polonium-210 in grass. Nature 187:211–212, 1960.

255. Hindle, E., and A. C. Stevenson. Hitherto undescribed intranuclear bodies in the wild rat and monkeys, compared with known virus bodies in other animals. Roy. Soc. Trop. Med. Hyg. Trans. 23:327, 1929–1930.

256. Hogan, A. W. Ice nuclei from direct reaction of iodine vapor with vapors from leaded gasoline. Science 158:800, 1967.

257. Holm, L. W., E. A. Rhode, J. D. Wheat, and G. Firch. Treatment of acute lead poisoning in calves with calcium disodium ethylenediaminetetraacetate. J. Amer. Vet. Med. Assoc. 123:528–533, 1953.

258. Holtzman, R. B. ^{226}Ra and the natural airborne nuclides ^{210}Pb and ^{210}Po in Arctic biota, pp. 1087–1096. In W. S. Snyder, H. H. Abee, L. K. Burton, R. Maushart, A. Benco, F. Duhamel, and B. M. Wheatley, Eds. Radiation Protection. Pt. 2. New York: Pergamon Press, Inc., 1968.

259. Homma, K. Experimental study for preparing metal fumes. Ind. Health 4:129–137, 1966.

260. Horiuchi, K., H. Noma, I. Asano, and K. Hashimoto. Studies on the industrial lead poisoning. An experimental study of lead intake in human being through the respiratory tract. Osaka City Med. J. 8:151–169, 1962.

261. Horiuchi, K., S. Horiguchi, and M. Suekane. Studies on the industrial lead poisoning. 1. Absorption, transportation, deposition and excretion of lead. 6. The lead contents in organ-tissues of the normal Japanese. Osaka City Med. J. 5:41–70, 1959.

262. Horiuchi, K., and I. Takada. Studies on the industrial lead poisoning. I. Absorption, transportation, deposition and excretion of lead. 1. Normal limits of lead in the blood, urine and feces among healthy Japanese urban habitants. Osaka City Med. J. 1:117–125, 1954.

263. Hsia, D. Y.-Y, and M. Page. Coproporphyrin studies in children. 1. Urinary coproporphyrin excretion in normal children. Proc. Soc. Exp. Biol. Med. 85:86–88, 1954.

264. Huber, G. No substitute yet for lead shot, p. A–24. The Evening Star, Washington, D.C., Dec. 1, 1970.

265. Huff, L. C. Abnormal copper, lead, and zinc content of soil near metalliferous veins. Econ. Geol. 47:517–542, 1952.

266. Hunt, W. F., Jr., C. Pinkerton, O. McNulty, and J. P. Creason. A study in trace element pollution of air in seventy-seven midwestern cities, pp. 56–68. In D. D. Hemphill, Ed. Trace Substances in Environmental Health. IV. Columbia: University of Missouri Press, 1971.

267. Hunter, B. F., and M. N. Rosen. Occurrence of lead poisoning in a wild pheasant (*Phasianus colchicus*). Calif. Fish Game 51:207, 1965.

268. Hursh, J. B., and T. T. Mercer. Measurement of ^{212}Pb loss rate from human lungs. J. Appl. Physiol. 28:268–274, 1970.

269. Hutchinson, R. R., R. E. Ulrich, and N. H. Azrin. Effects of age and related factors on the pain-aggression reaction. J. Comp. Physiol. Psychol. 69:365–369, 1965.

270. Imamura, Y. Studies on the industrial lead poisoning. 1. Absorption, transportation, deposition and excretion of lead. 3. An experimental study of lead intake in human being. Osaka City Med. J. 3:167–194, 1957.

271. Ingalls, T. H., E. A. Tiboni, and M. Werrin. Lead poisoning in Philadelphia, 1955–1960. Arch. Environ. Health 3:575–579, 1961.

272. Jacobs, M. B. The Analytical Toxicology of Industrial Inorganic Poisons, p. 170. New York: Interscience Publishers, 1967.

273. Jacobziner, H. Lead poisoning in childhood: Epidemiology, manifestations, and prevention. Clin. Pediat. 5:277–286, 1966.

274. James, L. F., V. A. Lazar, and W. Binns. Effects of sublethal doses of certain minerals on pregnant ewes and fetal development. Amer. J. Vet. Res. 27:132–135, 1966.

275. Jandl, J. H., J. K. Inman, R. L. Simmons, and D. W. Allen. Transfer of iron from serum iron-binding protein to human reticulocytes. J. Clin. Invest. 38:161–185, 1959.

276. Jenkins, C. D., and R. B. Mellins. Lead poisoning in children: A study of forty-six cases. Arch. Neurol. Psychiat. 77:70–78, 1957.

277. Jensen, W. N., G. D. Moreno, and M. C. Bessis. An electron microscopic description of basophilic stippling in red cells. Blood 25:933–943, 1965.

278. Johnstone, R. T. Clinical inorganic lead intoxication. Arch. Environ. Health 8:250–255, 1964.

279. Jones, J. R. E. Lead, zinc and copper: The "coagulation film anoxia" theory, pp. 53–65. In Fish and River Pollution. London: Butterworth & Co., 1964.

280. Jones, J. R. E. The metals as salts, pp. 66–82. In Fish and River Pollution. London: Butterworth & Co., 1964.

281. Jones, J. R. E. The relative toxicity of salts of lead, zinc and copper to the stickleback (Gasterosteus aculeatus L.) and the effect of calcium on the toxicity of lead and zinc salts. J. Exp. Biol. 15:394–407, 1938.

282. Jordan, J. S., and F. C. Bellrose. Lead poisoning in wild waterfowl. Illinois Natural Hist. Survey Biol. Notes 26:1–27, 1951.

283. Jowett, D. Populations of Agrostis spp. tolerant of heavy metals. Nature 182:816–817, 1958.

284. Jowett, D. Population studies on lead tolerant Agrostis tenuis. Evolution 18:70–80, 1964.

285. Joyce, C. R. B., H. Moore, and M. Weatherall. Effects of lead, mercury, and gold on potassium turnover of rabbit blood cells. Brit. J. Pharmacol. 9:463–470, 1954.

286. Jung, F. Zur Pathologie der roten Blutkörperchen. II. Mitteilung. Wirkungen einiger Metallsalze. Naunyn Schmiedebergs. Arch. Pharmakol. 204:139–156, 1947.

287. Kalabina, M. M., K. A. Mudretzova-Viss, A. S. Rasumov, and Z. I. Rogovskaja. Effect of the toxic substances of waste waters of non-ferrous metallurgy on microörganisms and biochemical process associated with self-purification of reservoirs. Gig. Sanit. 9:1–7, 1944. (in Russian)

288. Kaplan, E., and R. S. Shaull. Determination of lead in paint scrapings as an aid in the control of lead paint poisoning in young children. Amer. J. Public Health 51:65–69, 1961.

289. Kappas, A., C. S. Song, R. D. Levere, R. A. Sachson, and S. Granick. The induction of δ-aminolevulinic acid synthetase in vivo in chick embryo liver by natural steroids. Proc. Nat. Acad. Sci. U.S. 61:509–513, 1968.

290. Karnofsky, D. A., and L. P. Ridgway. Production of injury to the central nervous system of the chick embryo by lead salts. J. Pharmacol. Exp. Ther. 104:176–186, 1952.

291. Katz, A. I., and F. H. Epstein. The role of sodium–potassium-activated adenosine triphosphatase in the reabsorption of sodium by the kidney. J. Clin. Invest. 46:1999–2011, 1967.

292. Keaton, C. M. The influence of lead compounds on the growth of barley. Soil Sci. 43:401–411, 1937.

293. Keenan, R. G., D. H. Byers, B. E. Saltzman, and F. L. Hyslop. The "USPHS" method for determining lead in air and in biological materials. Amer. Ind. Hyg. Assoc. J. 24:481–491, 1963.

294. Kehoe, R. A. Experimental studies on the inhalation of lead by human subjects. Pure Appl. Chem. 3:129–144, 1961.

295. Kehoe, R. A. Lead absorption and lead poisoning. Med. Clin. N. Amer. 26:1261–1279, 1942.

296. Kehoe, R. A. Normal metabolism of lead. Arch. Environ. Health 8:232–243, 1964.

297. Kehoe, R. A. Responses of human subjects to lead compounds. Ind. Med. Surg. 28:156–159, 1959.

298. Kehoe, R. A. The metabolism of lead in man in health and disease. The Harben Lectures, 1960. J. Roy. Inst. Public Health Hyg. 24:1–81, 101–120, 129–143, 177–203, 1961.

299. Kehoe, R. A. Under what circumstances is ingestion of lead dangerous?, pp. 51–58. In Symposium on Environmental Lead Contamination, sponsored by the U.S. Public Health Service, Dec. 13–15, 1965. Public Health Service Publication 1440. Washington, D.C.: U.S. Government Printing Office, 1966.

300. Kehoe, R. A., J. Cholak, D. M. Hubbard, K. Bambach, and R. R. McNary. Experimental studies on lead absorption and excretion and their relation to the diagnosis and treatment of lead poisoning. J. Ind. Hyg. 25:71–79, 1943.

301. Kehoe, R. A., J. Cholak, D. M. Hubbard, K. Bambach, R. R. McNary, and R. V. Story. Experimental studies on the ingestion of lead compounds. J. Ind. Hyg. 22:381–400, 1940.

302. Kehoe, R. A., J. Cholak, and R. V. Story. A spectrochemical study of the normal ranges of concentration of certain trace metals in biological materials. J. Nutr. 19:579–592, 1940.

303. Kehoe, R. A., F. Thamann, and J. Cholak. An appraisal of the lead hazards associated with the distribution and use of gasoline containing tetramethyl lead. II. J. Ind. Hyg. Toxicol. 18:42–68, 1936.

304. Kehoe, R. A., F. Thamann, and J. Cholak. On the normal absorption and excretion of lead. I. Lead absorption and excretion in primitive life. J. Ind. Hyg. 15:257–272, 1933.

305. Kehoe, R. A., F. Thamann, and J. Cholak. On the normal absorption and excretion of lead. III. The sources of normal lead absorption. J. Ind. Hyg. 15:290–300, 1933.

306. Kelleher, R. T., and W. H. Morse. Determinants of the specificity of behavioral effects of drugs. Ergeb. Physiol. 60:1–56, 1968.

307. Keppler, J. F., M. E. Maxfield, W. D. Moss, G. Tietjen, and A. L. Linch. Interlaboratory evaluation of the reliability of blood lead analysis. Amer. Ind. Hyg. Assoc. J. 31:412–429, 1970.

308. Klein, M. Letter to the editor. New Eng. J. Med. 283:1292, 1970.

309. Klein, M., R. Namer, E. Harpur, and R. Corbin. Earthenware containers as a source of fatal lead poisoning. Case study and public-health considerations. New Eng. J. Med. 283:669, 1970.

310. Kleinkopf, M. D. Spectrographic determination of trace elements in lake waters of northern Maine. Bull. Geol. Soc. Amer. 71:1231–1241, 1960.

311. Kloke, A., and K. Riebartsch. Verunreinigung von Kulturpflanzen mit Blei aus Kraftfahrzeugabgasen. Naturwissenschaften 51:367–368, 1964.

312. Koeppe, D. E., and R. J. Miller. Lead effects on corn mitochondrial respiration. Science 167:1376–1377, 1970.

313. Konovalov, G. S., A. A. Ivanova, and T. K. Kolesnikova. Rare and trace elements in water and in suspended substance of the European U.S.S.R. rivers. Gidrokhim. Mater. 42:94–111, 1966. (in Russian)

314. Kopp, J. F., and R. C. Kroner. Trace Metals in Waters of the United States. A Five Year Summary of Trace Metals in Rivers and Lakes in the United States (Oct. 1, 1962–Sept. 30, 1967). Cincinnati: U.S. Department of the Interior, Federal Water Pollution Control Administration, Division of Pollution Surveillance, 1970.

315. Kostial, K., and V. B. Vouk. Lead ions and synaptic transmission in the superior cervical ganglion of the cat. Brit. J. Pharmacol. Chemother. 12:219–222, 1957.

316. Kradel, D. C., W. M. Adams, and S. B. Guss. Lead poisoning and eosinophilic meningoencephalitis in cattle. A case report. Vet. Med. 60:1045–1050, 1965.

317. Krafka, J., Jr. The effect of repeated leading on the blood picture in guinea pigs. J. Ind. Hyg. 17:13–17, 1935.

318. Kraut, H., and M. Weber. Ueber den Bleigehalt der Haare. Biochem. Z. 317:133–148, 1944.

319. Krigman, M. R., D. Crane, and R. A. Goyer. Lysosomal alterations in lead nephropathy. Fed. Proc. 27:410, 1968. (abstract)

320. Kumler, K., and T. P. Schreiber. Lead in blood—A rapid method for spectrochemical analysis. Amer. Ind. Hyg. Assoc. Q. 16:296–300, 1955.

321. Kurland, L. T., and D. Reed. Geographic and climatic aspects of multiple sclerosis. A review of current hypotheses. Amer. J. Public Health 54:588–597, 1964.

322. Lagerwerff, J. V. Heavy metal contamination of soils, pp. 343–364. In N. C. Brady, Ed. Agriculture and the Quality of Our Environment. Washington, D.C.: American Association for the Advancement of Science, 1967.

323. Lagerwerff, J. V., and A. W. Specht. Contamination of roadside soil and vegetation with cadmium, nickel, lead and zinc. Environ. Sci. Tech. 4:583–586, 1970.

324. Lampert, P. W., and S. S. Schochet, Jr. Demyelination and remyelination in lead neuropathy. Electron microscopic studies. J. Neuropath. Exp. Neurol. 27:527–545, 1968.

325. Landau, E., R. Smith, and D. A. Lynn. Carbon monoxide and lead—An environmental appraisal. J. Air Pollut. Control Assoc. 19:684–687, 1969.

326. Landsberg, H. H., L. L. Fischman, and J. L. Fisher. Resources in America's Future. Baltimore: Johns Hopkins Press, 1965. 465 pp.

327. Lane, R. E. Health control in inorganic lead industries. A follow-up of exposed workers. Arch. Environ. Health 8:243–250, 1964.

328. Lane, R. E. The care of the lead worker. Brit. J. Ind. Med. 6:125–143, 1949.

329. Lane, R. E. The clinical aspects of poisoning by inorganic lead compounds. Ann. Occup. Hyg. 8:31–34, 1965.

330. Lanza, A. J. Epidemiology of lead poisoning. J.A.M.A. 104:85–87, 1935.

331. Lascelles, J. Tetrapyrrole Biosynthesis and Its Regulation. New York: W. A. Benjamin, Inc., 1964. 132 pp.

332. Laug, E. P., and F. M. Kunze. Penetration of lead through skin. J. Ind. Hyg. Tox. 30:256–259, 1948.

333. Laug, E. P., and H. P. Morris. The effect of lead on rats fed diets containing lead arsenate and lead acetate. J. Pharmacol. Exp. Ther. 64:388–410, 1938.

334. Laurer, G. R., T. J. Kneip, R. E. Albert, and F. S. Kent. X-ray fluorescence: Detection of lead in wall paint. Science 172:466–468, 1971.

335. Laveskog, A. A method for determination of tetramethyl lead (TML) and tetraethyl lead (TEL) in air. Paper presented to the Second International Clean Air Congress of the International Union of Air Pollution Prevention Associations, Washington, D.C., Dec. 6–11, 1970.

336. Law, W. R., and E. R. Nelson. Gasoline-sniffing by an adult. Report of a case with the unusual complication of lead encephalopathy. J.A.M.A. 204: 1002–1004, 1968.

337. Lazrus, A. L., E. Lorange, and J. P. Lodge, Jr. Lead and other metal ions in United States precipitation. Environ. Sci. Tech. 4:55–58, 1970.

338. Leaf, A. The syndrome of osteomalacia, renal glycosuria, aminoaciduria, and increased phosphorus clearance (the Fanconi syndrome), pp. 1205–1220. In J. B. Stanbury, J. B. Wyngaarden, and D. S. Fredrickson, Eds. The Metabolic Basis of Inherited Disease. (2nd ed.) New York: McGraw-Hill, 1966.

339. Leake, J. P., and J. J. Bloomfield, pp. 31–38. In The Use of Tetraethyl Lead Gasoline and Its Relation to Public Health. Public Health Bulletin 163. Washington, D.C.: Department of the Treasury, 1926.

340. Lee, R. E., R. K. Patterson, and J. Wagman. Particle-size distribution of metal components in urban air. Environ. Sci. Tech. 2:288–290, 1968.

341. Legge, T. M. Thirty years' experience of industrial maladies. (Shaw lectures) J. Roy. Soc. Arts 77:1023–1039, 1929.

342. Legge, T. M., and K. W. Goadby. Lead Poisoning and Lead Absorption; the Symptoms, Pathology and Prevention, with Special Reference to the Industrial Origin, and an Account of the Principal Processes Involving Risk, p. 207. London: Edward Arnold, 1912.

343. Leh, H. O. Verunreinigungen von Kulturpflanzen mit Blei aus Kraftfahrzeugabgasen. Gesunde Pflanz. 18:21–24, 1966.

344. Lehnert, G. Chromosomal aberrations due to the effect of lead. Paper pre-

sented at conference on Chemical Pollution and Human Ecology held in Prague, October 12–17, 1970. 11 pp.

345. Lehnert, G., K. H. Schaller, A. Künner, and D. Szadkowski. Auswirkungen des Zigarettenrauchens auf den Blutbleispiegel. Int. Arch. Gewerbepath. Gewerbehyg. 23:358–363, 1967.

346. Leikin, S., and G. Eng. Erythrokinetic studies of the anemia of lead poisoning. Pediatrics 31:996–1002, 1963.

347. Levan, A. Cytological reactions induced by inorganic salt solutions. Nature 156:751–752, 1945.

348. Lewis, E. F., and J. C. Meikle. Notes on the use of calcium disodium versenate in heavy metal poisoning of livestock. Brit. Vet. J. 114:69–71, 1958.

349. Lewis, E. F., and J. C. Meikle. The treatment of acute lead poisoning in cattle with calcium versenate. Vet. Rec. 68:98–99, 1956.

350. Lewis, K. H. The diet as a source of lead pollution, pp. 17–20. In Symposium on Environmental Lead Contamination, sponsored by the U.S. Public Health Service, Dec. 13–15, 1965. Public Health Service Publication 1440. Washington, D.C.: U.S. Government Printing Office, 1966.

351. Lichtman, H. C., and F. Feldman. In vitro pyrrole and porphyrin synthesis in lead poisoning and iron deficiency. J. Clin. Invest. 41:830–839, 1963.

352. Liebig, G. F., Jr., A. P. Vanselow, and H. D. Chapman. Effects of aluminum on copper toxicity, as revealed by solution-culture and spectrographic studies of citrus. Soil Sci. 53:341–351, 1942.

353. Lightbody, H. D., and H. O. Calvery. Variations in the arginase concentrations in the livers of white rats caused by the administration of arsenic and lead. J. Pharm. 64:458–464, 1938.

354. Lilis, R., N. Gavrilescu, B. Nestorescu, C. Dumitriu, and A. Roventa. Nephropathy in chronic lead poisoning. Brit. J. Ind. Med. 25:196–202, 1968.

355. Linch, A. L., R. B. Davis, R. F. Stalzer, and W. F. Anzilotti. Studies of analytical methods for lead-in-air determination and use with an improved self-powered portable sampler. Amer. Ind. Hyg. Assoc. J. 25:81–93, 1964.

356. Linch, A. L., E. G. Wiest, and M. D. Carter. Evaluation of tetraalkyl lead exposure by personnel monitor surveys. Amer. Ind. Hyg. Assoc. J. 31:170–179, 1970.

357. Lin-Fu, J. S. Childhood lead poisoning . . . an eradicable disease. Children 17:2–9, 1970.

358. Lin-Fu, J. S. Lead Poisoning in Children. Social and Rehabilitation Service, U.S. Department of Health, Education, and Welfare, Children's Bureau Publication 452. Washington, D.C.: U.S. Government Printing Office, 1967. 25 pp.

359. Livingstone, D. A. Chemical composition of rivers and lakes, pp. G1–G64. Geological Survey Professional Paper 440–G. In M. Fleischer, Ed. Data of Geochemistry. (6th ed.) Washington, D.C.: U.S. Government Printing Office, 1963.

360. Locke, L. N., G. E. Bagley, and H. D. Irby. Acid-fast intranuclear inclusion bodies in the kidneys of mallards fed lead shot. Bull. Wild. Dis. Assoc. 2:127–131, 1966.

361. Locke, L. N., G. E. Bagley, and L. T. Young. The ineffectiveness of acid-

fast inclusions in diagnosis of lead poisoning in Canada geese. Bull. Wild. Dis. Assoc. 3:176, 1967.

362. Locke, L. N., H. D. Irby, and G. E. Bagley. Histopathology of mallards dosed with lead and selected suitable shot (*Anas platyrhynchos*). Bull. Wild. Dis. Assoc. 3:143–147, 1967.

363. London, I. M. The metabolism of the erythrocyte. Harvey Lect. 56:151–189, 1960–1961.

364. Lourie, R. S., E. M. Layman, and F. K. Millican. Why children eat things that are not food. Children 10:143–146, 1963.

365. Löwig, C. Ueber Methplumbäthyl. J. Prakt. Chem. 60:304–310, 1853.

366. Lucas, H. F., Jr., and J. E. Stanford. Excretion and Retention of Lead-210 in Rats, pp. 105–110. ANL-7360. Argonne National Laboratory. U.S. Atomic Energy Commission, July 1966.

367. Lund, C. The effect of chronic lead poisoning on reproductive capacity. Nord. Hyg. Tidskr. 18:12–20, 1936. (in Norwegian)

368. Lundgren, D. A. Atmospheric aerosol composition and concentration as a function of particle size and of time. J. Air Pollut. Control Assoc. 20:603–608, 1970.

369. MacLean, A. J., R. L. Halstead, and B. J. Finn. Extractability of added lead in soils and its concentration in plants. Can. J. Soil Sci. 49:327–334, 1969.

370. Makotchenko, V. M. The functional condition of suprarenal cortex in chronic poisoning with heavy metals (lead, mercury). Tr. Ukr. Nauch. Issled Inst. Eksp. Endokrinol. 20:162–170, 1965. (in Russian)

371. Mao, P., and J. J. Molnar. The fine structure and histochemistry of lead-induced renal tumors in rats. Amer. J. Path. 50:571–603, 1967.

372. Marten, G. C., and P. B. Hammond. Lead uptake by bromegrass from contaminated soils. Agron. J. 58:553–554, 1966.

373. Marver, H. S., D. P. Tschudy, M. G. Perlroth, A. Collins, and G. Hunter, Jr. The determination of aminoketones in biological fluids. Anal. Biochem. 14:53–60, 1966.

374. Matson, W. R. Trace Metals, Equilibrium, and Genetics of Trace Metal Complexes in Natural Media. M. A. Thesis, Massachusetts Institute of Technology, 1968. 272 pp.

375. Mauzerall, D., and S. Granick. Porphyrin biosynthesis in erythrocytes. III. Uroporphyrinogen and its decarboxylase. J. Biol. Chem. 232:1141–1162, 1958.

376. Mauzerall, D., and S. Granick. The occurrence and determination of δ-aminolevulinic acid and porphobilinogen in urine. J. Biol. Chem. 219:435–446, 1956.

377. Mayneord, W. V., R. C. Turner, and J. M. Radley. Alpha activity of certain botanical materials. Nature 187:208–211, 1960.

378. McAllister, R. G., Jr., A. M. Michelakis, and H. H. Sandstead. Plasma renin activity in chronic plumbism. Effect of treatment. Arch. Intern. Med. 127:919–923, 1971.

379. McCabe, L. J. Metal levels found in distribution samples. AWWA Seminar on Corrosion by Soft Water, Washington, D.C., 21 June 1970. 9 pp.

380. McCaldin, R. O. Estimation of sources of atmospheric lead and measured atmospheric lead levels, pp. 7–15. In Symposium on Environmental Lead

Contamination, sponsored by the U.S. Public Health Service, Dec. 13–15, 1965. Public Health Service Publication 1440. Washington, D.C.: U.S. Government Printing Office, 1966.

381. McClain, R. M., and B. A. Becker. Placental transport and teratogenicity of lead in rats and mice. Fed. Proc. 29:347, 1970. (abstract)

382. McCord, C. P. Lead and lead poisoning in early America. Benjamin Franklin and lead poisoning. Ind. Med. Surg. 22:393–399, 1953.

383. McCord, C. P. Lead and lead poisoning in early America—The lead pipe period. Ind. Med. Surg. 23:27–31, 1954.

384. McCulloch, E. C. Lead-arsenate poisoning of sheep and cattle. J. Amer. Vet. Med. 96:321–326, 1940.

385. McIntosh, I. G. Lead poisoning in animals. Vet. Rev. Annot. 2:57–60, 1956.

386. McMullen, T. B., R. B. Faoro, and G. B. Morgan. Profile of pollutant fractions in nonurban suspended particulate matter. J. Air Pollut. Control Assoc. 20:369–372, 1970.

387. Mehani, S. Lead retention by the lungs of lead-exposed workers. Ann. Occup. Hyg. 9:165–171, 1966.

388. Mellins, R. B., and C. D. Jenkins. Epidemiological and psychological study of lead poisoning in children. J.A.M.A. 158:15–20, 1955.

389. Menzel, R. G. Soil–plant relationships of radioactive elements. In Proceedings of the Hanford Symposium on Radiation and Terrestrial Ecosystems, Richland, Wash., 3–5 May, 1965. Health Physics 11:1325–1332, 1965.

390. Merrifield, D. B. Metal Stabilizers for Rubber. (Monsanto Chemical Company). U.S. Patent 2,954,356. September 27, 1960.

391. Millar, J. A., R. L. C. Cumming, V. Battistini, F. Carswell, and A. Goldberg. Lead and δ-aminolaevulinic acid dehydratase levels in mentally retarded children and in lead-poisoned suckling rats. Lancet 2:695, 1970.

392. Millican, F. K., E. M. Layman, R. S. Lourie, and L. Y. Takahashi. Study of an oral fixation: Pica. J. Amer. Acad. Child Psychiat. 7:79–107, 1968.

393. Mitchell, R. L., and J. W. S. Reith. The lead content of pasture herbage. J. Sci. Food Agric. 17:437–440, 1966.

394. Moeschlin, S. Lead, pp. 45–71. In Poisoning: Diagnosis and Treatment. (1st American ed., translated by J. Bickel from the 4th German ed.) New York: Grune & Stratton, Inc., 1965.

395. Molyneux, M. K. B. Use of single urine samples for the assessment of lead absorption. Brit. J. Ind. Med. 21:203–209, 1964.

396. Monaenkova, A. M. Functional state of the thyroid gland in chronic intoxication with some industrial poisons. Gig. Tr. Prof. Zabol. 1:44–48, 1957. (in Russian)

397. Moncrieff, A. A., O. P. Koumides, B. E. Clayton, A. D. Patrick, A. G. C. Renwick, and G. E. Roberts. Lead poisoning in children. Arch. Dis. Child. 39:1–13, 1964.

398. Monier-Williams, G. W. Trace Elements in Food. New York: John Wiley and Sons, Inc., 1950. 511 pp.

399. Moonshine: The Rotgut Racket. New York: Licensed Beverage Industries, Inc., 1969. 24 pp.

400. Morgan, G. B., G. Ozolins, and E. C. Tabor. Air pollution surveillance systems. Science 170:289–296, 1970.
401. Morgan, J. M. A simplified screening test for exposure to lead. South. Med. J. 60:435–438, 1967.
402. Morgan, J. M., M. W. Hartley, and R. E. Miller. Nephropathy in chronic lead poisoning. Arch. Intern. Med. 118:17–29, 1966.
403. Morris, H. P., E. P. Laug, H. J. Morris, and R. L. Grant. The growth and reproduction of rats fed diets containing lead acetate and arsenic trioxide and the lead and arsenic contents of newborn and suckling rats. J. Pharm. 64:420–445, 1938.
404. Morrison, P. X-ray shield. (To the United States of America, as represented by the Atomic Energy Commission) U.S. Patent 2,580,360. December 25, 1951.
405. Morrow, J. J., G. Urata, and A. Goldberg. The effect of lead and ferrous and ferric iron on δ-aminolaevulic acid synthetase. Clin. Sci. 37:533–538, 1969.
406. Motto, H. L., R. H. Daines, D. M. Chilko, and C. K. Motto. Lead in soils and plants: Its relationship to traffic volume and proximity to highways. Environ. Sci. Tech. 4:231–238, 1970.
407. Mueller, P. K. Discussion. (Characterization of particulate lead in vehicle exhaust—experimental techniques.) Environ. Sci. Tech. 4:248–251, 1970.
408. Mueller, P. K., and R. L. Stanley. Origin of Lead in Surface Vegetation. AIHL Report 87. Berkeley: State of California Department of Public Health, Air and Industrial Hygiene Laboratory, 1970. 15 pp.
409. Murashov, B. F. Functional state of the adrenal cortex in chronic poisoning with tetraethyl lead. Gig. Tr. Prof. Zabol. 10(8):46–47, 1966. (in Russian)
410. Muro, L. A., and R. A. Goyer. Chromosome damage in experimental lead poisoning. Arch. Path. 87:660–663, 1969.
411. Murozumi, M., T. J. Chow, and C. Patterson. Chemical concentrations of pollutant lead aerosols, terrestrial dusts, and sea salts in Greenland and Antarctic snow strata. Geochim. Cosmochim. Acta 33:1247–1294, 1969.
412. Murphy, G. P., J. C. Sharp, N. L. Lawson, R. B. Greer, and G. S. Johnston. The chronic functional and morphologic alterations caused by prolonged nephrotoxic states in the rat. Invest. Urol. 1:529–551, 1964.
413. Myerson, R. M., and J. H. Eisenhauer. Atrioventricular conduction defects in lead poisoning. Amer. J. Cardiol. 11:409–412, 1963.
414. Nakao, K., O. Wada, T. Kitamura, and K. Uono. Activity of amino-laevulinic acid synthetase in normal and porphyric human livers. Nature 210:838–839, 1966.
415. Nakao, K., O. Wada, and Y. Yano. Delta-aminolevulinic acid dehydratase activity in erythrocytes for the evaluation of lead poisoning. Clin. Chim. Acta 19:319–325, 1968.
416. Nandi, D. L., K. F. Baker-Cohen, and D. Shemin. δ-Aminolevulinic acid dehydratase of Rhodopseudomonas spheroides. J. Biol. Chem. 243:1224–1230, 1968.
417. Neal, P. A., W. C. Dreessen, T. I. Edwards, W. H. Reinhart, S. W. Webster, H. T. Castberg, and L. T. Fairhall. A study of the effect of lead arsenate

exposure on orchardists and consumers of sprayed fruit. Public Health Bulletin 267. Washington, D.C.: U.S. Government Printing Office, 1941.

418. Nelson, J. D., P. Dorn, L. E. Rogers, and P. Sartain. Fluorescence of erythrocytes in relation to erythrocyte protoporphyrin and to urinary lead excretion. Amer. J. Clin. Path. 50:297–301, 1968.

419. Nelson, K. W. Discussion. (Critical levels of lead in ambient air.) Presented at the Air Quality and Lead Symposium, Minneapolis, Minnesota, 1969. 2 pp.

420. Neumann, H. H. Pica—symptom or vestigial instinct? Pediatrics 46:441–444, 1970.

421. New directions in ion-selective electrodes. Chem. Eng. News 48(27):40–41, 1970.

422. Nix, J., and T. Goodwin. The simultaneous extraction of iron, manganese, copper, cobalt, nickel, chromium, lead, and zinc from natural water for determination by atomic absorption spectroscopy. Atomic Absorption Newsletter 9:119–122, 1970.

423. Novakova, S. Hygienic standards for combined presence of arsenic and lead in water. Hyg. Sanit. 34:96–101, Jan.–Mar. 1969.

424. Novick, R. P., and C. Roth. Plasmid-linked resistance to inorganic salts in *Staphylococcus aureus*. J. Bact. 95:1335–1342, 1968.

425. Nozaki, K. Method for studies on inhaled particles in human respiratory system and retention of lead fume. Ind. Health (Japan) 4:118–128, 1966.

426. Nusbaum, R. E., E. M. Butt, T. C. Gilmour, and S. L. DiDio. Relation of air pollutants to trace metals in bone. Arch. Environ. Health 10:227–232, 1965.

427. Nye, L. J. J. An investigation of the extraordinary incidence of chronic nephritis in young people in Queensland. Med. J. Aust. 2:145–159, 1929.

428. Oliver, T., Ed. Dangerous Trades, p. 296. London: John Murray, Albermarle Street, 1902.

429. Oswald, I. Sleep, dreaming and drugs. Proc. Roy. Soc. Med. 62:151–153, 1969.

430. Ott, W. R., and M. G. McLaren. Subsolidus studies in the system PbO–SiO$_2$. J. Amer. Ceram. Soc. 53:374–375, 1970.

431. Ottoboni, F., and E. Kahn. Study of Benicia area horse deaths. Interim report. California Dept. of Public Health, May 1, 1970. 12 pp.

432. Oyasu, R., H. A. Battifora, R. A. Clasen, J. H. McDonald, and G. M. Hass. Induction of cerebral gliomas in rats with dietary lead subacetate and 2-acetylaminofluorene. Cancer Res. 30:1248–1261, 1970.

433. Palmisano, P. A., R. C. Sneed, and G. Cassady. Untaxed whiskey and fetal lead exposure. J. Pediat. 75:869–871, 1969.

434. Pardoe, A. V., and M. Weatherall. Uptake and excretion of water in rats poisoned with lead. Brit. J. Pharm. 7:358–369, 1952.

435. Parungo, F. P., and J. O. Rhea. Lead measurement in urban air as it relates to weather modification. J. Appl. Meteorol. 9:468–475, 1970.

436. Passow, H., A. Rothstein, and T. W. Clarkson. The general pharmacology of the heavy metals. Pharmacol. Rev. 13:185–224, 1961.

437. Patterson, C. C. Contaminated and natural lead environments of man. Arch. Environ. Health 11:344–363, 1965.

438. Patterson, C. C., G. Tilton, and M. Inghram. Age of the earth. Science 121: 69–75, 1955.

439. Pecora, L., A. Silvestroni, and A. Brancaccio. Relations between the porphyrin metabolism and the nicotinic acid metabolism in saturnine poisoning. Panminerva Med. 8:284–288, 1966.

440. Pentschew, A. Morphology and morphogenesis of lead encephalopathy. Acta Neuropath. (Berlin) 5:133–160, 1965.

441. Pentschew, A., and F. Garro. Lead encephalo-myelopathy of the suckling rat and its implications on the porphyrinopathic nervous diseases. With special reference to the permeability disorders of the nervous system's capillaries. Acta Neuropath. (Berlin) 6:266–278, 1966.

442. Perlstein, M. A., and R. Attala. Neurologic sequelae of plumbism in children. Clin. Pediat. 5:292–298, 1966.

443. Pierrard, J. M., and R. A. Crane. The Effect of Gasoline Compositional Changes on Atmospheric Visibility and Soiling. (For presentation to the Air Pollution Control Association) Wilmington, Delaware: E. I. du Pont de Nemours & Company, Inc., Petroleum Laboratory, 1971. 14 pp.

444. Pines, A. G. Indexes of general reactivity in saturnine toxicity. Vrach. Delo 3:93–96, 1965. (in Russian)

445. Pinta, M. Detection and Determination of Trace Elements. (Translated from the French by M. Bivas.) Ann Arbor, Mich.: Humphrey Science Publishers, 1970. 31 pp.

446. Prendergast, W. D. The classification of the symptoms of lead poisoning. Brit. Med. J. 1:1164–1166, 1910.

447. Pringle, B. H., D. E. Hissong, E. L. Katz, and S. T. Mulawka. Trace metal accumulation by estuarine mollusks. J. Sanit. Eng. Div.; Proc. Amer. Soc. Civil Eng. 94:455–475, 1968.

448. Přerovská, I., and J. Teisinger. Excretion of lead and its biological activity several years after termination of exposure. Brit. J. Ind. Med. 27:352–355, 1970.

449. Radošević, Z., M. Šarić, T. Beritić, and J. Knežević. The kidney in lead poisoning. Brit. J. Ind. Med. 18:222–230, 1961.

450. Raule, A., and G. Morra. Prime ricerche sulla funzionalita' gonadotropica preipofisaria negli intossicati da piombo. Med. Lav. (Milano) 43:261–265, 1952.

451. Read, J. L., and J. P. Williams. Lead myositis: Report of a case. Amer. Heart J. 44:797–802, 1952.

452. Richet, G., C. Albahary, R. Ardaillou, C. Sultan, and A. Morel-Maroger. Le rein du saturnisme chronique. Rev. Fr. Etud. Clin. Biol. 9:188–196, 1964.

453. Richet, G., C. Albahary, L. Morel-Maroger, P. Guillaume, and P. Galle. Les altérations rénales dans 23 cas de saturnisme professionnel. Bull. Soc.•Med. Hop. Paris 117:441–466, 1966.

454. Robinson, E., and F. L. Ludwig. Particle size distribution of urban lead aerosols. J. Air Pollut. Control Assoc. 17:664–669, 1967.

455. Robinson, E., and F. Ludwig. Size Distributions of Atmospheric Lead Aerosols. Final Report PA–4788. Stanford Research Institute, Menlo Park, Calif., April 30, 1964. 36 pp.

456. Robinson, E., F. L. Ludwig, J. E. DeVries, and P. E. Hopkins. Variations of Atmospheric Lead Concentrations and Type with Particle Size. Final Report PA–4211. Stanford Research Institute, Menlo Park, Calif., Nov. 1, 1963. 93 pp.

457. Robinson, M. J., F. E. Karpinski, Jr., and H. Brieger. The concentration of lead in plasma, whole blood and erythrocytes of infants and children. Pediatrics 21:793–797, 1958.

458. Roe, F. J. C., E. Boyland, C. E. Dukes, and B. C. V. Mitchley. Failure of testosterone or xanthopterin to influence the induction of renal neoplasms by lead in rats. Brit. J. Cancer 19:860–866, 1965.

459. Rosen, M. N., and R. A. Bankowski. A diagnostic technic and treatment for lead poisoning in swans. Calif. Fish Game 46:81–90, 1960.

460. Rosenblum, W. I., and M. G. Johnson. Neuropathologic changes produced in suckling mice by adding lead to the maternal diet. Arch. Path. 86:640–648, 1968.

461. Rothstein, A. Cell membrane as site of action of heavy metals. Fed. Proc. 18:1026–1035, 1959.

462. Rubino, G. F., G. C. Coscia, G. Perrelli, and A. Parigi. Compartamento del glutatione, del test di stabilità del glutatione e dell'attività glucosio-6-fosfato-deidrogenasica nel saturnismo. Minerva Med. 54:930–932, 1963.

463. Rubino, G. F., E. Pagliardi, V. Prato, and E. Giangrandi. Erythrocyte copper and porphyrins in lead poisoning. Brit. J. Haematol. 4:103–107, 1958.

464. Ruhling, A., and G. Tyler. An ecological approach to the lead problem. Bot. Notiser. 121:321–342, 1968.

465. Sachs, H. K., L. A. Blanksma, E. F. Murray, and M. J. O'Connell. Ambulatory treatment of lead poisoning: Report of 1,155 cases. Pediatrics 46:389–396, 1970.

466. Sales Vazquez, M. Elvaler antitoxico del acido nicotinico. Rev. Clin. Esp. 10:40–43, 1943.

467. Salomon, K., and G. R. Cowgill. Porphyrinuria in lead poisoned dogs. Ind. Hyg. Toxicol. 30:114–118, 1948.

468. Sandstead, H. H. Effect of chronic lead intoxication on *in vivo* I-131 uptake by the rat thyroid. Proc. Soc. Exp. Biol. Med. 124:18–20, 1967.

469. Sandstead, H. H., A. M. Michelakis, and T. E. Temple. Lead intoxication. Its effect on the renin-aldosterone response to sodium deprivation. Arch. Environ. Health 20:356–363, 1970.

470. Sandstead, H. H., D. N. Orth, K. Abe, and J. Stiel. Lead intoxication: Effect on pituitary and adrenal function in man. Clin. Res. 18:76, 1970. (abstract)

471. Sandstead, H. H., E. G. Stant, and A. B. Brill. Lead intoxication and the thyroid. Arch. Intern. Med. 123:632–635, 1969.

472. Sano, S. Studies on the distribution of lead in animal tissues. Jap. J. Nation's Health 23:59–72, 1954. (English summary and tables)

473. Sano, S. The effect of mitochondria on porphyrin and heme biosynthesis in red blood cells. Acta Haematol. Jap. 21(Suppl. 2):337–351, 1958.

474. Sauer, R. M., B. C. Zook, and F. M. Garner. Demyelinating encephalo-

myelopathy associated with lead poisoning in nonhuman primates. Science 169:1091–1093, 1970.

475. Schaefer, V. J. Ice nuclei from automobile exhaust and iodine vapor. Science 154:1555–1557, 1966.

476. Schaefer, V. J. The inadvertent modification of the atmosphere by air pollution. Bull. Amer. Meteorol. Soc. 50:199–207, 1969.

477. Schepers, G. W. H. Tetraethyllead and tetramethyllead. Comparative experimental pathology. I. Lead absorption and pathology. Arch. Environ. Health 8:277–295, 1964.

478. Schmid, R. The porphyrias, pp. 813–870. In J. B. Stanbury, J. B. Wyngaarden, and D. S. Fredrickson, Eds. The Metabolic Basis of Inherited Disease. (2nd ed.) New York: McGraw-Hill, 1966.

479. Schmitt, N., G. Brown, E. L. Devlin, A. A. Larsen, E. D. McCausland, and J. M. Saville. Lead poisoning in horses. An environmental health hazard. Arch. Environ. Health 23:185–195, 1971.

480. Schroeder, H. A., J. J. Balassa, F. S. Gibson, and S. N. Valanju. Abnormal trace metals in man: Lead. J. Chron. Dis. 14:408–425, 1961.

481. Schroeder, H. A., J. J. Balassa, and W. H. Vinton, Jr. Chromium, lead, cadmium, nickel and titanium in mice: Effect on mortality, tumors and tissue levels. J. Nutr. 83:239–250, 1964.

482. Schroeder, H. A., and I. H. Tipton. The human body burden of lead. Arch. Environ. Health 17:965–978, 1968.

483. Schuck, E. A., and J. K. Locke. Relationship of automotive lead particulates to certain consumer crops. Environ. Sci. Tech. 4:324–332, 1970.

484. Schucker, G. W., E. H. Vail, E. B. Kelley, and E. Kaplan. Prevention of lead paint poisoning among Baltimore children: A hard-sell program. Public Health Rep. 80:969–974, 1965.

485. Schwartz, S., M. H. Berg, I. Bossenmaier, and H. Dinsmore. Determination of porphyrins in biological materials, pp. 221–294. In D. Glick, Ed. Methods of Biochemical Analysis. Vol. VIII. New York: Interscience Publishers, Inc., 1960.

486. Schwartz, S., L. Zieve, and C. J. Watson. An improved method for the determination of urinary coproporphyrin and an evaluation of factors influencing the analysis. J. Lab. Clin. Med. 37:843–859, 1951.

487. Selander, S. Treatment of lead poisoning. A comparison between the effects of sodium calciumedate and penicillamine administered orally and intravenously. Brit. J. Ind. Med. 24:272–282, 1967.

488. Selander, S., and K. Cramér. Determination of lead in blood by atomic absorption spectrophotometry. Brit. J. Ind. Med. 25:209–213, 1968.

489. Selander, S., and K. Cramér. Determination of lead in urine by atomic absorption spectrophotometry. Brit. J. Ind. Med. 25:139–143, 1968.

490. Selander, S., and K. Cramér. Interrelationships between lead in blood, lead in urine, and ALA in urine during lead work. Brit. J. Ind. Med. 27:28–39, 1970.

491. Selander, S., K. Cramér, and L. Hallberg. Studies in lead poisoning: Oral therapy with penicillamine: Relationship between lead in blood and other laboratory tests. Brit. J. Ind. Med. 23:282–291, 1966.

492. Selker, A. H. Effect of additives on resistance of PVC to gamma rays. Mod. Plast. 40(1):172, 244–245, 1962.

493. Shahidi, N. T., and M. L. Efron. Excretion of delta-aminolevulinic acid in the absence of demonstrable erythropoiesis. Proc. Soc. Exp. Biol. Med. 128:314–317, 1968.

494. Shalamberidze, O. P. Limit of allowable concentration of lead sulfide in atmospheric air, pp. 29–38. In V. A. Rjazanov, Ed. Maximum Permissible Concentrations of Atmospheric Pollutants. Book 5. Washington, D.C.: U.S. Public Health Service, 1962.

495. Shields, J. B., and H. H. Mitchell. The effect of calcium and phosphorus on the metabolism of lead. J. Nutr. 21:541–552, 1941.

496. Shiels, D. O. The elimination of lead in sweat. Australas. Ann. Med. 3:225–229, 1954.

497. Shupe, J. L., W. Binns, L. F. James, and R. F. Keeler. Lupine, a cause of crooked calf disease. J. Amer. Vet. Med. Assoc. 151:198–203, 1967.

498. Shupe, J. L., L. F. James, and W. Binns. Observations on crooked calf disease. J. Amer. Vet. Med. Assoc. 151:191–197, 1967.

499. Shy, C. M., D. I. Hammer, V. A. Newill, and W. C. Nelson. Health Hazards of Environmental Lead. In-House Technical Report, Community Research Branch, Bureau of Air Pollution Sciences, Environmental Protection Agency. (to be published)

500. Sibley, W. A., and J. M. Foley. Infection and immunization in multiple sclerosis. Ann. N.Y. Acad. Sci. 122:457–466, 1965.

501. Silver, W., and R. Rodriguez-Torres. Electrocardiographic studies in children with lead poisoning. Pediatrics 41:1124–1127, 1968.

502. Silverstein, E. Inhibition of certain mitochondrial oxidative enzymes by porphyrins and metalloporphyrins. Biochem. Pharmacol. 11:431–444, 1962.

503. Simpson, J. A., D. A. Seaton, and J. F. Adams. Response to treatment with chelating agents of anaemia, chronic encephalopathy, and myelopathy due to lead poisoning. J. Neurol. Neurosurg. Psychiat. 27:536–541, 1964.

504. Sir George Baker (1722–1809) discoverer of the pathogenesis of Devonshire colic. J.A.M.A. 204:541, 1968. (editorial)

505. Six, K. M., and R. A. Goyer. Enhancement of subclinical lead toxicity by low calcium diet. Fed. Proc. 29:568, 1970. (abstract)

506. Slingerland, D. W. The influence of various factors on the uptake of iodine by the thyroid. J. Clin. Endocrinol. 15:131–141, 1955.

507. Smith, H. D. Pediatric lead poisoning. Arch. Environ. Health 8:256–261, 1964.

508. Snyder, L. J. Determination of trace amounts of organic lead in air. Anal. Chem. 39:591–595, 1967.

509. Snyder, L. J., W. R. Barnes, and J. V. Tokos. Determination of lead in air. Rapid micromethod for field use. Anal. Chem. 20:772–776, 1948.

510. Snyder, L. J., and S. R. Henderson. A new field method for the determination of organolead compounds in air. Anal. Chem. 33:1175–1180, 1961.

511. Sobel, A. E., O. Gawron, and B. Kramer. Influence of vitamin D in experimental lead poisoning. Proc. Soc. Exp. Biol. Med. 38:433–435, 1938.

512. Sobel, A. E., I. B. Wexler, D. D. Petrovsky, and B. Kramer. Influence of

dietary calcium and phosphorus upon action of vitamin D in experimental lead poisoning. Proc. Soc. Exp. Biol. Med. 38:435–437, 1938.

513. Sobel, R. The psychiatric implications of accidental poisoning in childhood. Pediat. Clin. N. Amer. 17:653–685, 1970.

514. Specter, M. J., and V. F. Guinee. Epidemiology of lead poisoning in New York City–1970. Paper presented at the American Public Health Association's 98th annual meeting, Houston, Texas, Oct. 26, 1970. 23 pp.

515. Spector, W. S., Ed. Handbook of Biological Data, p. 267. Philadelphia: W. B. Saunders Company, 1956.

516. Spurný, K. R., J. P. Lodge, Jr., E. R. Frank, and D. C. Sheesley. Aerosol filtration by means of nuclepore filters. Structural and filtration properties. Environ. Sci. Tech. 3:453–464, 1969.

517. Sroczynski, J., G. Jonderko, and A. Wegiel. Effect of lead poisoning on the synthesis of ribonucleic acids in some rat organs. Pol. Med. J. 7:1148–1153, 1968.

518. Sroczynski, J., and B. Piekarski. Rabbit blood serum proteins in chronic lead poisoning. Postepy. Hig. Med. Dosw. 17:603–608, 1963. (in Polish)

519. Stadler, L. J. Mutations in barley induced by X-rays and radium. Science 68:186–187, 1928.

520. Stopps, G. J. Discussion. (Epidemiological bases for possible air quality criteria for lead.) J. Air Pollut. Control Assoc. 19:719–721, 1969.

521. Stopps, G. J., M. E. Maxfield, M. McLaughlin, and S. Pell. Lead research: Current medical developments. Trans. 31st Annual Meeting of the Industrial Hygiene Foundation of America, Inc. Trans. Bull. 40:73–91, 1966.

522. Swaine, D. J. The trace-element content of soils. Commonwealth Bur. Soil Sci. Tech. Comm. 48. York, England: Herald Printing Works, 1955. 157 pp.

523. Swaine, D. J., and R. L. Mitchell. Trace-element distribution in soil profiles. J. Soil Sci. 11:347–368, 1960.

524. Tanquerel des Planches, L. Lead Diseases: A Treatise. With Notes and Additions on the Use of Lead Pipe and Its Substitutes. (Translated from the French by S. L. Dana.) Lowell, Mass.: Daniel Bixby and Co., 1848. 441 pp.

525. Teisinger, J., F. Prevovska, V. Sedivec, J. Flek, and Z. Roth. Attempt on determination of biologically active lead in organism in experimental poisoning. Int. Arch. Gewerbepath. Gewerbehyg. 25:240–255, 1969.

526. Teisinger, J., and J. Srbova. The value of mobilization of lead by calcium ethylene-diamine-tetra-acetate in the diagnosis of lead poisoning. Brit. J. Ind. Med. 16:148–152, 1959.

527. Tenconi, L. T., and G. Acocella. Studio sulla chemioterapia dell'intossicazione sperimentale da piombo. Nota I. Effetti dell'avvelenamento da piombo sul metabolismo triptofano to acido nicotinico nel ratto. Acta Vitaminol. (Milano) 20:189–194, 1966.

528. Tepper, L. B. Renal function subsequent to childhood plumbism. Arch. Environ. Health 7:76–85, 1963.

529. Tepper, L. B. Seven-City Study of Air and Population Lead Levels. An Interim Report. Department of Environmental Health, College of Medicine, University of Cincinnati, 1971. 11 pp.

530. Tepper, L. B. Under what circumstances is direct contact with lead dangerous?, pp. 60–62. In Symposium on Environmental Lead Contamination,

sponsored by the U.S. Public Health Service, Dec. 13–15, 1965. Public Health Service Publication 1440. Washington, D.C.: U.S. Government Printing Office, 1966.

531. Ter Haar, G. L. Air as a source of lead in edible crops. Environ. Sci. Tech. 4:226–229, 1970.

532. Ter Haar, G. L., and M. A. Bayard. Composition of airborne lead particles. Nature 232:553–554, 1971.

533. Ter Haar, G. L., R. B. Holtzman, and H. F. Lucas, Jr. Lead and lead–210 in rainwater. Nature 216:353–355, 1967.

534. Thomas, A. Effects of certain metallic salts upon fishes. Trans. Amer. Fish. Soc. 44:120–124, 1915.

535. Thompson, T. I., and C. R. Schuster. Behavioral Pharmacology, pp. 1–7. Englewood Cliffs, N.J.: Prentice-Hall, Inc., 1968.

536. Thorsen, W. J. Estimation of cortical components in various wools. Textile Res. J. 28:185–197, 1958.

537. Thurston, D. L., J. N. Middelkamp, and E. Mason. The late effects of lead poisoning. J. Pediat. 47:413–423, 1955.

538. Tipton, I. H. The distribution of trace metals in the human body, pp. 27–42. In M. J. Seven and L. A. Johnson, Eds. Metal-binding in Medicine. Proceedings of a symposium sponsored by Hahnemann Medical College and Hospital, Philadelphia. Philadelphia: J. B. Lippincott Co., 1960.

539. Todd, J. R. A knackery survey of lead poisoning incidence in cattle in Northern Ireland. Vet. Rec. 74:116–118, 1962.

540. Todd, J. R. Notes on the use of calcium versenate in acute lead poisoning. Vet. Rec. 69:31–32, 1957.

541. Tomashefski, J. F., and R. I. Mitchell. Under what circumstances is inhalation of lead dangerous?, pp. 39–49. In Symposium on Environmental Lead Contamination, sponsored by the U.S. Public Health Service, Dec. 13–15, 1965. Washington, D.C.: U.S. Government Printing Office, 1966.

542. Tönz, O. Nierenveränderungen bei experimenteller chronischer Bleivergiftung (Ratten). Z. Gesamte. Exp. Med. 128:361–377, 1957.

543. Trainer, D. O., and R. A. Hunt. Lead poisoning of whistling swans in Wisconsin. Avian Dis. 9:252–264, 1965.

544. Tschudy, D. P., M. G. Perlroth, H. S. Marver, A. Collins, G. Hunter, Jr., and M. Rechcigl, Jr. Acute intermittent porphyria: The first "overproduction disease" localized to a specific enzyme. Proc. Nat. Acad. Sci. U.S. 53:841–847, 1965.

545. Tso, T. C., N. Harley, and L. T. Alexander. Source of lead–210 and polonium–210 in tobacco. Science 153:880–882, 1966.

546. Ulmer, D. D., and B. L. Vallee. Effects of lead on biochemical systems, pp. 7–27. In D. D. Hemphill, Ed. Trace Substances in Environmental Health. II. Columbia: University of Missouri Press, 1969.

547. U.S. Bureau of Mines. Minerals Yearbrook: Metals, Minerals and Fuels, Vol. 1–2. Washington, D.C.: U.S. Government Printing Office, 1969.

548. U.S. Bureau of the Census. Census of Agriculture, 1964. Statistics for the State and Counties, New York, Vol. 1, Part 7, p. 321. Washington, D.C.: U.S. Government Printing Office, 1966.

549. U.S. Bureau of the Census. Statistical Abstract of the United States, p. 682. (90th ed.) Washington, D.C.: U.S. Government Printing Office, 1969.

550. U.S. Congress. Public Law 91–695. 91st Congress. H.R. 19172, January 13, 1971. Lead-based Paint Poisoning Prevention Act. Washington, D.C.: U.S. Government Printing Office, 1971. 3 pp.

551. U.S. Department of Agriculture. Agricultural Statistics. Washington, D.C.: U.S. Government Printing Office, 1969. 631 pp.

552. U.S. Department of Health, Education, and Welfare, Public Health Service. Public Health Service Drinking Water Standards. Public Health Service Publication 956. (Revised) Washington, D.C.: U.S. Department of Health, Education, and Welfare, 1962. 61 pp.

553. U.S. Department of Health, Education, and Welfare, National Air Pollution Control Administration. Air Quality Data from the National Air Sampling Networks and Contributing State and Local Networks. 1966 Edition. NAPCA Publication APTD 68–9. Durham, N.C.: U.S. Department of Health, Education, and Welfare, 1968. 157 pp.

554. U.S. Department of Health, Education, and Welfare, Public Health Service, Division of Air Pollution. Survey of Lead in the Atmosphere of Three Urban Communities. Public Health Service Publication 999–AP–12. Cincinnati: Public Health Service, 1965. 94 pp.

555. U.S. Department of Health, Education, and Welfare, Public Health Service, Division of Air Pollution, Robert A. Taft Sanitary Engineering Center, Cincinnati. Air Pollution Measurements of the National Air Sampling Networks; Analyses of Suspended Particulates, 1957–1961. Public Health Service Publication 978. Washington, D.C.: U.S. Government Printing Office, 1962. 217 pp.

556. U.S. Department of Health, Education, and Welfare, Public Health Service, Division of Air Pollution. Air Quality Data of the National Air Sampling Networks, 1962. Cincinnati, Ohio: U.S. Department of Health, Education, and Welfare, 1964. 50 pp.

557. U.S. Department of Health, Education, and Welfare, Public Health Service, Division of Sanitary Engineering Services, Robert A. Taft Sanitary Engineering Center, Cincinnati. Air Pollution Measurements of the National Air Sampling Networks; Analyses of Suspended Particulates, 1953–1957. Public Health Service Publication 637. Washington, D. C.: U.S. Government Printing Office, 1958. 260 pp.

558. U.S. Department of Health, Education, and Welfare, Public Health Service, Environmental Health Service, National Air Pollution Control Administration. Air Quality Criteria for Particulate Matter. Public Health Service Environmental Health Service Publication AP–49. Washington, D.C.: U.S. Department of Health, Education, and Welfare, 1969. 211 pp.

559. U.S. Department of Health, Education, and Welfare, National Center for Air Pollution Control. Air Quality Data from the National Air Sampling Networks and Contributing State and Local Networks, 1964–1965. Cincinnati, Ohio: U.S. Department of Health, Education, and Welfare, 1966. 126 pp.

560. U.S. Department of Health, Education, and Welfare, Public Health Service, Division of Air Pollution, Robert A. Taft Sanitary Engineering Center, Cincinnati. Air Pollution Measurements of the National Air Sampling Networks; Analyses of Suspended Particulates, 1963. Washington, D.C.: U.S. Government Printing Office, 1965. 87 pp.

561. Urata, G., and S. Granick. Biosynthesis of α-aminoketones and the metabolism of aminoacetone. J. Biol. Chem. 238:811–820, 1963.

562. Van Esch, G. J., and R. Kroes. The induction of renal tumours by feeding basic lead acetate to mice and hamsters. Brit. J. Cancer 23:765–771, 1969.

563. Van Esch, G. J., H. Van Genderen, and H. H. Vink. The induction of renal tumours by feeding of basic lead acetate to rats. Brit. J. Cancer 16:289–297, 1962.

564. Vermande-Van Eck, G. J., and J. W. Meigs. Changes in the ovary of the Rhesus monkey after chronic lead intoxication. Fertil. Steril. 11:223–234, 1960.

565. Vigliani, E. C. Recenti studi sul saturnismo in Italia. Med. Lav. 41:105–123, 1950.

566. Voight, J. L., L. D. Edwards, and C. H. Johnson. Acute toxicity of arsenate of lead in animals. J. Amer. Pharm. Assoc. Sci. Ed. 37:122–123, 1948.

567. Waldron, H. A. The anaemia of lead poisoning: A review. Brit. J. Ind. Med. 23:83–100, 1966.

568. Warnick, S. L., and H. L. Bell. The acute toxicity of some heavy metals to different species of aquatic insects. J. Water Pollut. Control Fed. 41:280–284, 1969.

569. Warren, H. V. Trace elements and epidemiology. J. Coll. Gen. Pract. 6:517–531, 1963.

570. Warren, H. V., and R. E. Delavault. Lead in some food crops and trees. J. Sci. Food Agric. 13:96–98, 1962.

571. Water Quality Criteria. Report of the National Technical Advisory Committee to the Secretary of the Interior. Washington, D.C.: Federal Water Pollution Control Administration, 1968. 234 pp.

572. Watson, R. J., E. Decker, and H. C. Lichtman. Hematologic studies of children with lead poisoning. Pediatrics 21:40–46, 1958.

573. Waxman, H. S., and M. Rabinovitz. Control of reticulocyte polyribosome content and hemoglobin synthesis by heme. Biochim. Biophys. Acta 129:369–379, 1966.

574. Weir, P. A., and C. H. Hine. Effects of various metals on behavior of conditioned goldfish. Arch. Environ. Health 20:45–51, 1970.

575. Weiss, B., and V. G Laties. Behavioral pharmacology and toxicology. Ann. Rev. Pharmacol. 9:297–326, 1969.

576. Weller, C. V. The blastophthoric effect of chronic lead poisoning. J. Med. Res. 33:271–293, 1915.

577. Westerman, M. P., E. Pfitzer, L. D. Ellis, and W. N. Jensen. Concentrations of lead in bone in plumbism. New Eng. J. Med. 273:1246–1250, 1965.

578. Westfall, B. A. Coagulation film anoxia in fishes. Ecology 26:283–287, 1945.

579. Wetmore, A. Lead poisoning in waterfowl. U.S. Dept. Agric. Bull. 793:1–12, 1919.

580. Wetterberg. L. Acute porphyria and lead poisoning. Lancet 1:498, 1966.

581. Wiener, G. Varying psychological sequelae of lead ingestion in children. Public Health Rep. 85:19–24, 1970.

582. Wilkins, D. A. The measurement and genetic analysis of lead tolerance in *Festuca ovina*. Rep. Scottish Soc. Res. Pl. Breed. 1960:85–98.

583. Williams, H., E. Kaplan, C. E. Couchman, and R. R. Sayers. Lead poisoning in young children. Public Health Rep. 67:230–236, 1952.

584. Williams, H., W. H. Schulze, H. B. Rothchild, A. S. Brown, and F. R. Smith, Jr. Lead poisoning from the burning of battery casings. J.A.M.A. 100:1485–1489, 1933.

585. Williams, M. K., E. King, and J. Walford. An investigation of lead absorption in an electric accumulator factory with the use of personal samplers. Brit. J. Ind. Med. 26:202–216, 1969.

586. Wilson, D. O., and J. F. Cline. Removal of plutonium–239, tungsten–185, and lead–210 from soils. Nature 209:941–942, 1966.

587. Wilson, V. K., M. L. Thomson, and C. E. Dent. Amino-aciduria in lead poisoning. A case in childhood. Lancet 2:66–68, 1953.

588. Witschi, H. Desorption of some toxic heavy metals from human erythrocytes *in vitro*. Acta Haematol. (Basel) 34:101–115, 1965.

589. Wranne, L. Free erythrocyte copro- and protoporphyrin. A methodological and clinical study. Acta Paediat. 124(Suppl.):1–78, 1960.

590. Wright, J. R., R. Levick, and H. J. Atkinson. Trace element distribution in virgin profiles representing four great soil groups. Soil Sci. Soc. Amer. Proc. 19:340–344, 1955.

591. Xintaras, C., B. L. Johnson, C. E. Ulrich, and M. F. Sobecki. Application of the evoked response technique in air pollution toxicology. Toxicol. Appl. Pharmacol. 8:77–87, 1966.

592. Xintaras, C., M. F. Sobecki, and C. E. Ulrich. Sleep: Changes in rapid-eye-movement phase in chronic lead absorption. Toxicol. Appl. Pharmacol. 10:384, 1967.

593. Zaitseva, A. F. Hygienic determination of permissibly tolerable concentrations of lead in water-storage reservoirs. Gig. Sanit. 3:7–11, 1953. (in Russian)

594. Zawirska, B., and K. Medras. Tumoren und Störungen des Porphyrinstoffwechsels bei Ratten mit chronischer experimenteller Bleiintoxikation. I. Morphologische Studien. Zentralbl. Allg. Path. 111:1–12, 1968.

595. Zel'tser, M. E. The functional state of the thyroid gland in lead poisoning. Tr. Inst. Kraevoi. Patol. Akad. Nauk Kaz. SSR 10:116–120, 1962. (in Russian)

596. Ziegfeld, R. L. Importance and uses of lead. Arch. Environ. Health 8:202–212, 1964.

597. Zollinger, H. U. Durch chronische Bleivergiftung erzeugte Nierenadenome und -carcinome bei Ratten und ihre Beziehungen zu den entsprechenden Neubildungen des Menschen. Virchows Arch. Path. Anat. 323:694–710, 1953.

598. Zook, B. C. An animal model for human disease. Lead poisoning in nonhuman primates. Comp. Path. Bull. 3:3–4, 1971.

599. Zook, B. C., J. L. Carpenter, and E. B. Leeds. Lead poisoning in dogs. J. Amer. Vet. Med. Assoc. 155:1329–1342, 1969.

600. Zook, B. C., R. M. Sauer, and F. M. Garner. Lead poisoning in Australian fruit bats (*Pteropus poliocephalus*). J. Amer. Vet. Med. Assoc. 157:691–694, 1970.

Index

315

and weather modification, 203
control devices, effect of lead, 200
lead emissions, 200
particles in, 16
residence time in air, 27

Bacteria and lead biotransformation, 18
resistance to lead, 169
Bagley, G. E., 183, 184
Balance studies of lead in organisms,
50, 51, 52, 54, 61, 67. *See also*
Accumulation
Barltrop, D., 50, 75, 117, 162
Basophilic stippling in lead poisoning,
99, 103, 110, 132, 184
Battery casings, lead poisoning from,
79
Behavioral effects of lead. *See also*
Lead poisoning, mental effects;
Mental retardation
early exposure, 159–160
in experimental animals, 160–162,
184
lead poisoning in man, 85, 88, 95, 97,
157–160, 217
recommendation for study of, 217
Beverages. *See* Diet
Biliary secretion of lead, 55
Binding of lead
in blood, 103
in fresh water, 48
in soils, 34
Biochemical changes and behavioral
changes, 158
Biochemical defects and lead toxicity
in man, 155
Biochemical effects of lead, 164–167
Biologic availability of lead in body, 68
Biologic effects of lead, recommendations for study of, 219
Biologic materials, analysis for lead,
235–245
Biosphere, lead in, 25–31
Biotransformation of lead, 18, 28
recommendations for study of, 214
Birds, lead poisoning in, 182–184
Blindness. *See* Vision
Blood analysis for lead, 106, 242–244,
250–253

Blood–brain barrier and early lead
exposure, 162
Blood lead
and age, 133–136, 138
and airborne lead, correlation, 63,
216
and ALAD activity, correlation, 106,
107, 127
and anemia, 99, 112, 130
and CaEDTA mobilization test, 123
and exposure to lead alkyls, 195
and hematocrit values, 61
and lead absorption, 62, 65, 130
and symptoms, correlation, 91
and urinary ALA, correlation, 108–
109, 110, 111, 139
Blood lead concentration
and adverse effects, 127
in children, 109, 118, 127, 133,
135–138
in children with lead poisoning, 87,
92–94, 113, 118, 126
in encephalopathy, 88, 130
in man, 59–64, 74, 118
in mental retardation, 98
in nephropathy, 90
in occupational exposure, 73, 115
in zoo animals, 185
interpretation of, 118
Body lead burden, 53, 91, 94, 170
and leaded paint, 160
and remote exposure, 119
and renal insufficiency, 120
bone biopsies in, 119
distribution, 31, 59, 183
evaluation, 117–131
in low-level exposure, 159
recommendations for study of, 219
Body tissues and lead content, effect of
age, 67–68
Bone
deposition of lead in, 30, 59, 170,
199
deposition of metals in, and disease,
156
indirect effects of lead, 113
Bone biopsies as measure of body lead
burden, 119

614.71 N213lc1   AAK-1964
050101 000
Lead; airborne lead in perspec

0 0003 0149178 3
Lyndon State College